Overcoming Steroid Insensitivity in Respiratory Disease

Overcoming Steroid Insensitivity in Respiratory Disease

Edited by

Ian M. Adcock and Kian Fan Chung

National Heart and Lung Institute,
Imperial College London,
London, UK

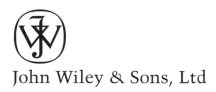

John Wiley & Sons, Ltd

Library of Congress Cataloging-in-Publication Data

Overcoming steroid insensitivity in respiratory disease / edited by Ian M.
Adcock and K. Fan Chung.
     p. ; cm.
  Includes bibliographical references and index.
  ISBN 978-0-470-05808-4 (alk. paper)
1. Respiratory organs–Diseases–Chemotherapy. 2. Steroid drugs. 3. Drug
resistance.   I. Adcock, Ian (Ian M.) II. Chung, K. Fan, 1951-
  [DNLM: 1. Respiratory Tract Diseases–drug therapy. 2. Adrenal Cortex
Hormones–therapeutic use. 3. Drug Resistance.
4. Glucocorticoids–therapeutic use. WF 145 O96 2008]
  RC735.C47O94 2008
  616.2'00461–dc22   2007033361

British Library Cataloguing in Publication Data

A catalogue record for this book is available from the British Library

ISBN   978-0-470-05808-4 (H/B)

Typeset in 10.5/13 pt Times by Thomson Digital
Printed and bound in Great Britain by Antony Rowe Ltd, Chippenham, Wiltshire.

Contents

List of Contributors

Ian M. Adcock   Airways Disease Section, National Heart and Lung Institute, Imperial College London, London, UK

David Adenuga   Department of Environmental Medicine, Division of Lung Biology and Disease, University of Rochester Medical Center, Rochester, NY, USA

Khusru Asadullah   Target Discovery, Bayer Schering Pharma AG, Muellerstrasse 178, Berlin, Germany

Pankaj Bhavsar   Airways Disease Section, National Heart and Lung Institute, Imperial College London, London, UK

John W. Bloom   Departments of Pharmacology and Medicine, Arizona Respiratory Center, University of Arizona College of Medicine, Tucson, AZ, USA

Gaetano Caramori   Centro di Ricerca su Asma e BPCO, Università di Ferrara, Ferrara, Italy

Evangelia Charmandari   Clarendon Wing, Leeds General Infirmary, Leeds, UK

George P. Chrousos   First Department of Pediatrics, Athens University Medical School, Aghia Sophia Children's Hospital, Athens, Greece

Kian Fan Chung   National Heart and Lung Institute, Imperial College London, London, UK

John A. Cidlowski   Laboratory of Signal Transduction, National Institute of Environmental Health Sciences, National Institutes of Health, Department of Health and Human Services, MD F307, Research Triangle Park, NC, USA

Wolf-Dietrich Döcke   Target Discovery, Bayer Schering Pharma AG, Berlin, Germany

Günther Hochhaus   College of Pharmacy, University of Florida, Gainsville, FL, USA

Kazuhiro Ito   Airways Disease Section, National Heart and Lung Institute, Imperial College London, London, UK

Iain Kilty   Allergy and Respiratory Therapeutic Area, Pfizer Global Research and Development, Sandwich, UK

Tomoshige Kino   Section on Pediatric Endocrinology, Reproductive Biology and Medicine Branch, National Institute of Child Health and Human Development, National Institutes of Health, Bethesda, MD, USA

Anna Miller-Larsson   Department of Medical Science, AstraZeneca R&D Lund, Sweden

Eric F. Morand   Centre for Inflammatory Diseases, Monash University, Monash Medical Centre, Melbourne, Victoria, Australia

Robert H. Oakley   Laboratory of Signal Transduction, National Institute of Environmental Health Sciences, National Institutes of Health, Department of Health and Human Services, MD F307, Research Triangle Park, NC, USA

Alberto Papi   Centro di Ricerca su Asma e BPCO, Università di Ferrara, Ferrara, Italy

Irfan Rahman   Department of Environmental Medicine, Lung Biology and Disease Program, University of Rochester Medical Center, Rochester, NY, USA

Heike Schäcke   Common Mechanism Research, Bayer Schering Pharma AG, Berlin, Germany

Olof Selroos   SEMECO AB, Selroos Medical Consulting, Lund, Sweden

Omar S. Usmani   National Heart and Lung Institute, Imperial College London, London, UK

Preface

The treatment of chronic inflammatory diseases was revolutionized by the discovery of the therapeutic utility of corticosteroids in the 1950s. Since this time they have been the mainstay of treatment for chronic inflammatory diseases. Their utility has been tempered, however, by the increasing risk of debilitating side effects with higher dose therapy. This is important because a reasonable proportion of patients with severe asthma do not respond well to high doses of inhaled or even oral corticosteroids. Thus 5% of asthmatics who do not respond to corticosteroid therapy account for >50% of the total healthcare costs for asthma. In addition, patients with chronic obstructive pulmonary disease also show little or no responsiveness to conventional corticosteroid therapy.

In the treatment of airways diseases side effects can be limited by targeted delivery to the airway and lung. Significant progress has been made through the use of increasingly selective molecules, and through a variety of lung-targeting strategies. Moreover, the recent developments in our understanding of the molecular and structural mechanisms of corticosteroid actions have suggested that it may be possible to develop a new corticosteroid, with intrinsically different pharmacology, that does not induce many of the pathways involved in the manifestation of side effects. A combination of these developments will enable the design of agents with an enhanced therapeutic index.

IAN M. ADCOCK
KIAN FAN CHUNG
Imperial College London

1

Molecular Mechanisms of Glucocorticoid Receptor Action

Pankaj Bhavsar and **Ian M. Adcock**

1.1   Introduction

Glucocorticoids are the most effective therapy for the treatment of many chronic inflammatory diseases such as asthma and inflammatory bowel disease (Ito et al., 2006a). In contrast to the situation in asthma, chronic obstructive pulmonary disease (COPD), a common and debilitating chronic inflammatory disease of the lung, is glucocorticoid insensitive (Barnes, 2000a, b; Culpitt et al., 2003).

Glucocorticoids act by binding to cytosolic glucocorticoid receptors (GRs), which upon binding become activated and rapidly translocate to the nucleus. Within the nucleus, GR either induces transcription of genes such as secretary leukocyte proteinase inhibitor (SLPI)(Abbinante-Nissen et al., 1995) and mitogen-activated kinase phosphatase-1(Lasa et al., 2002) by binding to specific DNA elements (glucocorticoid response element, GRE) at the promoter/enhancer of responsive genes, or reduces inflammatory gene transcription induced by nuclear factor-kappa B (NF-κB) or other pro-inflammatory transcription factors (Ito et al., 2006a). Binding of GR to p65-NF-κB is crucial for transrepression by glucocorticoids, however, it is not clear how the GR dissociates its ability to control inflammation by suppressing NF-κB from its ability to directly transactivate genes via binding to GRE (Ito et al., 2006b).

In the resting cell, chromatin is tightly compacted to prevent transcription factor accessibility. During activation of the cell this compact inaccessible chromatin is made available to DNA-binding proteins, thus allowing the induction of gene transcription (Lee and Workman, 2007; Li et al., 2007). There is compelling evidence that increased inflammatory gene transcription is associated with an increase in histone acetylation induced by transcriptional coactivators containing

Overcoming Steroid Insensitivity in Respiratory Disease   Edited by Ian M. Adcock and Kian Fan Chung
© 2008 John Wiley & Sons, Ltd.

histone acetyltransferase (HAT) activity, whereas hypoacetylation is correlated with reduced transcription or gene silencing (Lee and Workman, 2007; Li et al., 2007), which is controlled by histone deacetylases (HDACs). Investigation of the expression of key components of GR function in asthma and COPD may reveal the critical protein(s) required for glucocorticoid function in lung disease.

1.2   Glucocorticoid Receptor

Glucocorticoids exert their effects by freely diffusing across the plasma membrane of cells and binding to a ubiquitously expressed GR that is localized in the cytoplasm of target cells. Although unliganded GR is thought to remain in the cytoplasm, evidence using nuclear export inhibitors suggests that a rapid active cycling of GR between the nucleus and cytoplasm may occur (Hache et al., 1999; Kumar et al., 2004). Two GR isoforms (α and β) were originally described, with the nuclear GRβ having a dominant negative effect on GRα via the formation of GRα/GRβ heterodimers. Evidence is accumulating that this isoform may be important in certain disease states where GR nuclear translocation is deficient (Ito et al., 2006a; Zhou and Cidlowski, 2005). In addition, the use of different start sites has increased the number of potential isoforms present and differential expression may affect glucocorticoid function in an organ- or disease-specific manner (Lu and Cidlowski, 2005).

The crystal structure of the GR ligand binding domain (LBD) has been determined in a ternary complex with dexamethasone and a TIF2 coactivator peptide following point mutation of F602 (Bledsoe et al., 2002). The overall structure is similar to LBDs of other nuclear hormone receptors (NHRs) but contains a unique dimerization interface and a second charge clamp that may be important for cofactor selectivity. As with the results seen with the oestrogen antagonist raloxifene binding to oestrogen receptor, RU486 binding to the GR LBD results in a failure of helix 12 to correctly close over the binding cleft (Kauppi et al., 2003). This results in a conformation more able to recruit corepressors than the closed helix 12, which efficiently recruits coactivators (Garside et al., 2004; Kauppi et al., 2003) and has led to rational-based design of selective dissociated GR agonists (Barker et al., 2005). Modification of the dimerization interface by mutation of I628A resulted in reduced transactivation ability without affecting the ability to repress an NF-κB-driven reporter gene. The contrasting effects of this mutant suggest that the monomer and dimer forms of GR may regulate distinct signalling pathways confirming data obtained from the $dim(-/-)$ mouse (Karin, 1998).

1.3   Gene Induction by GR

Glucocorticoid binding to the cytoplasmic GR enables dissociation of chaperone proteins, including heat shock protein (hsp) 90, thereby allowing nuclear localization of

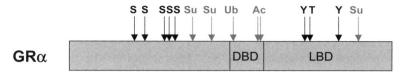

**Possible phosphorylation/
nitration sites**

Figure 1.1 Mechanism of gene activation by the glucocorticoid receptor (GR). Glucocorticoids can freely diffuse across the plasma membrane where they associate with the inactive cytosolic GR. Upon ligand binding the GR is activated and can translocate to the nucleus, where it binds to a glucocorticoid-response element (GRE) within the controlling region for glucocorticoid-responsive target genes. These GREs may be 5' or 3' to the start site for transcription. Once bound to DNA, GR recruits a complex containing basal transcription factors, coactivators (such as CBP and SRC-1), chromatin modifiers (such as SWI/SNF) and RNA polymerase II (RNAP II), which together induce histone modifications including acetylation (Ac) and chromatin remodelling and subsequent production of mRNAs encoding various genes including SLPI, MKP-1, CD163 and β2-adrenoceptor.

the activated GR–glucocorticoid complex utilizing selective importins (Chook and Blobel, 2001; Picard and Yamamoto, 1987; Savory et al., 1999). GR nuclear export is also tightly regulated; however, the role of the exportin-1 (CRM-1) pathway is currently unclear (Kumar et al., 2004; Picard and Yamamoto, 1987). Importantly, the nuclear localization signal (NLS)–importin-α interaction is often influenced directly by the phosphorylation status of the imported proteins (Chook and Blobel, 2001).

Within the nucleus GR dimerizes with another GR and binds to consensus DNA sites termed glucocorticoid response elements (GREs, GGTACAnnnTGTTCT) in the regulatory regions of glucocorticoid-responsive genes (Figure 1.1). This interaction allows GRs to recruit activated transcriptional coactivator proteins, including steroid receptor coactivator-1 (SRC-1) and cAMP response element binding protein (CBP), through LXXLL motifs (Smith and O'Malley, 2004). This produces a DNA-protein structure that allows enhanced gene transcription (Karin, 1998). Individual GR ligands can target GR to specific nuclear subdomains (Schaaf et al., 2005) and this, along with differences in the number of GREs, and the position of the GREs relative to the transcriptional start site (Wang et al., 2004), controls the magnitude and direction of the transcriptional response to glucocorticoids, dependent upon the particular ligand.

1.4   GR Transactivation and Histone Acetylation

Expression and repression of genes are associated with alterations in chromatin structure by enzymatic modification of core histones (Lee and Workman, 2007; Li et al., 2007).

Specific residues (lysines, arginines and serines) within the N-terminal tails of core histones are capable of being post-translationally modified by acetylation, methylation, ubiquitination or phosphorylation, all of which have been implicated in the regulation of gene expression (Lee and Workman, 2007; Li et al., 2007). The "histone code" refers to these modifications, which are set and maintained by histone-modifying enzymes and contribute to coactivator recruitment and subsequent increases in transcription (Jenuwein and Allis, 2001; Rice and Allis, 2001).

Transcriptional coactivators such as CBP, SRC-1, TIF2, GRIP-1 and p300/CBP associated factor (PCAF) have intrinsic HAT activity (Lee and Workman, 2007; Li et al., 2007), and increased GR-mediated gene transcription is associated with an increase in histone acetylation. In lung epithelial cells this occurs predominantly on histone H4 rather than H3, although it may be cell and/or gene specific (Ito et al., 2000; Li et al., 2003; Wu et al., 2005). In contrast, hypoacetylation induced by HDACs is correlated with reduced transcription or gene silencing (Lee and Workman, 2007; Li et al., 2007). Initially it was thought that acetylation neutralized positively charged lysine residues, thereby allowing reduced contacts with the negatively charged DNA. Subsequent data, however, have suggested that acetylation and other epigenetic tags on histones function as signalling marks enabling the recruitment of specific factors involved in gene transcription (Lee and Workman, 2007; Li et al., 2007). It is becoming clear that these two hypotheses are not mutually exclusive and interdependence can occur (Lee and Workman, 2007; Li et al., 2007). NHRs including GR do not necessarily recruit all these cofactors directly (Huang et al., 2003) as NHR-recruited cofactors can sequentially recruit other coactivators and chromatin remodelling complexes (Wu et al., 2005) that aid the formation of the transcription initiation complex and result in local chromatin remodelling (Lee and Workman, 2007; Li et al., 2007) (Figure 1.1).

A series of studies from Archer and others (Trotter and Archer, 2007) indicate that the ATP-dependent chromatin remodelling protein Brg1 is essential for GR-mediated transactivation at the MMTV promoter and a select number of endogenous promoters such as 11β-HSD and p21$^{CIP/WAF}$. Brg1 and associated factors are targeted to acetylated histone tails by bromodomains but they can also interact directly or indirectly with GR following GR ligand binding (Nie et al., 2000). More recently, it has become clear that Brg1 is also involved in GR-mediated transrepression and that the ultimate fate depends upon GR recruitment of cofactors (repressors or activators) at specific genes (Hebbar and Archer, 2007). In a similar manner perhaps STAMP (SRC-1- and TIF2-associated modulatory protein) can interact with TIF2 and SRC-1 to enhance both the transactivation and transrepression activities of GR (He and Simons, 2007).

In addition to the more classical modes of action, it is now clear that GR can bind to DNA as heterodimers with other transcription factors, such as members of the signal transducer and activator of transcription (STAT) family (Biola et al., 2000; Stocklin et al., 1996) and the ETS transcription factors (Mullick et al., 2001), leading to the recruitment of distinct coactivator (e.g. GRIP-1) or corepressor (e.g.

RIP140 or HDAC) complexes (Barnes et al., 2004; Garside et al., 2004; Stevens et al., 2003).

1.5 Post-translational Modifications of GR

GR is a phosphoprotein containing numerous potential phosphorylation sites, including those for extracellular signal-regulated kinase (ERK), p38 mitogen-activated protein kinase (MAPK), protein kinase C and protein kinase A. Altered GR phosphorylation status can affect GR-ligand binding (Irusen et al., 2002), hsp90 interactions (Hu et al., 1994), subcellular localization (Somers and DeFranco, 1992; Zuo et al., 1999), nuclear–cytoplasmic shuttling (Galigniana et al., 1999a; Hsu et al., 1992) and transactivation potential (Zuo et al., 1999), possibly through association with coactivator molecules (Somers and DeFranco, 1992) (Figure 1.2). The specific roles of these phosphorylation events are unclear (Zhou and Cidlowski, 2005) but phosphorylation of Ser-211 is a good marker of GR activation (Zhou and Cidlowski, 2005). MAPK activation or overexpression can also target other serine/threonine residues in GR, decreasing GR-mediated transactivation (Irusen et al., 2002; Szatmary et al., 2004) possibly via an effect on Ser-226 phosphorylation and increasing GR nuclear export (Itoh et al., 2002).

More recent evidence suggests that GR phosphorylation is also involved in receptor turnover and that phosphorylation can target the receptor for hormone-mediated

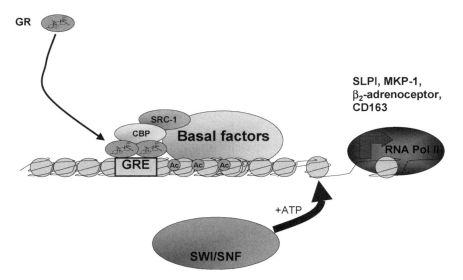

Figure 1.2 Post-translational modification of the glucocorticoid receptor (GR), particularly by phosphorylation and nitration, alters GR function and contributes to the potential for diverse function in distinct tissues. Other modifications such as ubiquitination (Ub), sumoylation (Su) and acetylation (Ac) are also shown.

proteasomal degradation (Wallace and Cidlowski, 2001). GR sumoylation appears to have the opposite effect of ubiquitination and results in increased GR activity (Le et al., 2002) possibly through changes in cofactor recruitment (Lin et al., 2003) (Figure 1.2). Interestingly, nitrosylation of GR at an hsp90 interaction site induced by the NO donor *S*-nitroso-DL-penicillamine has also been shown to prevent GR dissociation from the hsp90 complex and to reduced ligand binding (Galigniana et al., 1999b).

It has become clear that histones are not the only targets for histone acetylases and recent evidence has suggested that acetylation of transcription factors can modify their activity. For example, the p65 component of NF-κB can also be acetylated, thus modifying its transcriptional activity (Chen et al., 2001). Recent evidence suggests that GR is also acetylated (Figure 1.2) upon ligand binding and that deacetylation is critical for interaction with p65 at least at low (μM) dexamethasone concentrations (Ito et al., 2006b). Acetylation occurs within the GR nuclear retention signal (NRS) and may therefore possibly modify GR nuclear retention and GR-mediated transactivation and/or transrepression (Carrigan et al., 2007).

1.6   Repression of NF-κB-induced Inflammatory Gene Expression by GR–NF-κB

GR dimerization-deficient mice (Reichardt et al., 1998; Reichardt et al., 2001) indicate that the major anti-inflammatory effects of glucocorticoids are due mainly to an interaction between GR and transcription factors such as NF-κB, which mediate the expression of inflammatory genes (De Bosscher et al., 2006; Karin, 1998)(Figure 1.3). NF-κB is activated by numerous extracellular stimuli, including cytokines such as tumour necrosis factor-α (TNFα) and interleukin-1β (IL-1β), viruses and immune challenges (Baldwin, 2001). NF-κB is able not only to control induction of inflammatory genes in its own right but can enhance the activity of other cell- and signal-specific transcription factors (Barnes and Karin, 1997). Activation of NF-κB involves stimulation of a phosphorylation cascade resulting in phosphorylation and ubiquitination of a cytoplasmic inhibitor (IκBα) and release of NF-κB (generally a p65/p50 heterodimer) and its nuclear translocation (Ghosh and Karin, 2002). Subtle changes in p65 phosphorylation are also important in its activation (Sarkar et al., 2007); for example, inactive p65 is non-phosphorylated and is associated predominantly with HDAC1, whereas p65 is phosphorylated following IKK-2 stimulation and is able to bind to coactivator molecules such as p300/CBP (Zhong et al., 2002). NF-κB, as with GR, can induce histone acetylation and other histone modifications in a temporal manner (Ito et al., 2000; Lee et al., 2006) leading to recruitment of distinct coactivator and remodelling complexes and the induction of inflammatory gene expression. Adding to the complexity of NF-κB activation, p65 is also acetylated and its acetylation status by selective HDACs controls its association with, and loss of activity by, IκBα (Chen et al., 2001).

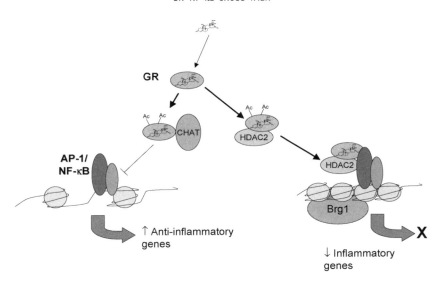

Figure 1.3   Deacetylation of the glucocorticoid receptor (GR) by histone deacetylase (HDAC)2 is essential for GR association with NF-κB. Upon ligand binding GR is acetylated at specific lysine residues within its hinge region, perhaps by chaperone acetylase (CHAT). Acetylated GR is able to translocate into the nucleus, bind to DNA and switch on anti-inflammatory genes. However, acetylated GR is unable to associate with activated NF-κB and must be deacetylated. Recruitment of HDAC2 by GR leads to deacetylation of GR, allows GR association with NF-κB and suppresses of inflammatory gene expression following alteration in the local histone acetylation status. This may require the involvement of remodelling factors such as Brg1.

NF-κB activated by distinct cellular stimuli can control the expression of different patterns of genes (Covert et al., 2005; Ogawa et al., 2005; Werner et al., 2005). Thus, lipopolysacchoride (LPS) and TNFα induced distinct gene profiles as a result of differences in the amplitude and duration of NF-κB activation, rate of IκBα decay and association with other factors such as IRF-3 (Covert et al., 2005; Nelson et al., 2004; Ogawa et al., 2005; Werner et al., 2005). Other signalling pathways such as the MAPKs may also affect the pattern and/or duration of NF-κB-mediated gene expression. Furthermore, it has also become clear that small changes in the consensus κB binding site and surrounding bases can have profound effects on the subsequent ability of activated NF-κB to activate gene expression (Luecke and Yamamoto, 2005).

1.7   GR–NF-κB Cross-talk

The precise mechanism for the ability of activated GR to repress NF-κB-induced gene transcription is still under debate and may alter depending upon GR expression levels (Simons, 2006) but it includes binding to, or recruiting, nuclear receptor corepressors (Ito et al., 2000; Nie et al., 2005; Rosenfeld and Glass, 2001), direct repression of coactivator complexes (Ito et al., 2000; Pascual et al., 2005), actions on histone phosphorylation status (Hasegawa et al., 2005) or effects on RNA polymerase II phosphorylation (Luecke and Yamamoto, 2005; Nissen and Yamamoto, 2000). We have previously reported that dexamethasone-induced NF-κB-mediated gene expression in epithelial cells is associated with changes in histone acetylation (Ito et al., 2000). Similar data have also been reported in primary airway smooth-muscle cells where fluticasone was able to attenuate TNFα-induced p65 association with the native CCL11 promoter and block TNFα-induced histone H4 acetylation (Nie et al., 2005).

Furthermore, these effects are context/gene dependent and repression often depends upon factors complexed with NF-κB. Thus, activated GR represses a large set of functionally related inflammatory genes stimulated by p65/IRF-3 complexes (Ogawa et al., 2005), perhaps by targeting the IRF-3–GRIP-1 interaction (Reily et al., 2006). In contrast, peroxisome proliforator -activated receptor gamma (PPARγ) and liver X receptors (LXRs) repress overlapping transcriptional targets in a p65/IRF-3-independent manner and cooperate with GR to suppress distinct subsets of pattern recognition receptor (PRR)-responsive genes (Ogawa et al., 2005). Designing drugs with the capacity to activate GR and other nuclear hormone receptors may, therefore, enhance the anti-inflammatory profile of glucocorticoids. Moreover, as the expression of many cofactors and nuclear receptors is tissue specific, there is the attractive possibility of designing tissue-specific ligands, although this approach will require a clearer understanding of the key tissues that are targeted by glucocorticoids.

Furthermore, GR–NF-κB interactions do not always result in gene repression. The context in which GRE and κB sites are found within a promoter of specific genes may drastically affect the final effect on gene expression (Hermoso et al., 2004; Sakai et al., 2004). For example, dexamethasone can enhance cytokine-inducible expression of TLR2 via a GR–p65 association on the promoter where the GRE overlaps with the κB site. This does not absolutely require the GRE and κB-RE to be in a close sequence alignment as similar effects of p65 and GR can be seen during the induction of stem cell factor (SCF) in human fibroblasts, despite the GRE and κB-RE being separated by ~1700 bp (Da Silva et al., 2004).

1.8 Role of HDAC2 in Glucocorticoid Function

We and others have reported that non-selective HDAC inhibitors are able to prevent GR repression of inflammatory genes (Ito et al., 2000; Jee et al., 2005; Marwick et al., 2004). Using siRNA we were able to show that HDAC2 was the only class I HDAC involved in GR-mediated gene repression (Ito et al., 2006b) and that this did not affect the ability of activated GR to undergo nuclear translocation or trans-activation (Ito et al., 2006b). GR is rapidly acetylated upon ligand binding at aa492-495 (KTKK) within the GR hinge region and only the deacetylated form of GR is able to associate with p65. Thus, recruitment of HDAC2 by acetylated GR leads to deacetylation of GR, interaction with the p65-NF-κB activated complex and subsequent suppression of inflammatory gene expression. This mechanism provides a molecular explanation for the ability of GR to distinguish between recruitment of coactivator and corepressor proteins as previously demonstrated for GRIP (Rogatsky et al., 2002) and the subsequent ability to transactivate or repress gene transcription (Ito et al., 2006b).

1.9   Overexpression of HDAC2 Restores Glucocorticoid Sensitivity in Alveolar Macrophages

HDAC2 expression and activity are decreased in smokers (Ito et al., 2001) and patients with COPD (Ito et al., 2005), who are known to be insensitive to the anti-inflammatory effects of glucocorticoids (Barnes, 2000a). In addition, there is a negative correlation between the repressive effect of dexamethasone on cytokine production and total HDAC activity in alveolar macrophages from smokers and non-smokers (Ito et al., 2001). In order to confirm a role for HDAC2 in glucocorticoid responsiveness in primary cells from these subjects, we overexpressed HDAC2 and examined cytokine repression by dexamethasone (Ito et al., 2006b). GR acetylation following dexamethasone treatment was increased in alveolar macrophages obtained from patients with COPD compared to normal subjects and these cells did not respond well to dexamethasone (Ito et al., 2006b). Overexpression of HDAC2, but not HDAC1, in primary macrophages from COPD patients restored dexamethasone efficacy towards suppressing LPS-induced GM-CSF release to levels seen in cells from healthy control subjects (Ito et al., 2006b). Furthermore, knockdown of HDAC2 in sputum macrophages from healthy non-smokers by RNAi reduced the inhibitory effect of dexamethasone (Ito et al., 2006b).

In support of this hypothesis, Bilodeau and colleagues (Bilodeau et al., 2006) have reported that GR-mediated repression of proopiomelanocortin (POMC) requires the ATPase-dependent chromatin remodelling enzyme Brg1 and the recruitment of HDAC2 to enable deacetylation of the POMC promoter. Bilodeau further hypothesized that loss of Brg1 and/or HDAC2 should induce glucocorticoid insensitivity and reports that 50% of glucocorticoid-resistant human and dog corticotroph adenomas, which are the hallmark of Cushing's disease, are deficient in the nuclear expression of either protein (Bilodeau et al., 2006).

Brg1-induced remodelling is essential for RNP2 initiation and re-initiation (Bilodeau et al., 2006), which involves changes in RNA polymerase II C-terminal domain (CTD) phosphorylation. Yamamoto and co-workers have shown previously that dexamethasone was able to reduce CTD serine 2 (Ser-2) phosphorylation induced by TNFα-induced NF-κB at the IL-8 promoter (Nissen and Yamamoto, 2000) via a reduction in the association of the Ser-2 CTD kinase, P-TEFb (Luecke and Yamamoto, 2005). Importantly, Bilodeau was able to show that a lack of HDAC2 leads to loss of Brg1 function resulting in RNP2 stalling on the promoter of responsive genes and a failure to remove the phospho tag from Ser-2 in the CTD (Bilodeau et al., 2006).

Taken together, these results indicate that HDAC2 is a key protein involved in the suppression of p65-mediated inflammatory gene expression. HDAC2 acts by deacetylating GR, thereby enabling p65 association and, in conjunction with Brg1, this results in subsequent attenuation of pro-inflammatory gene transcription. The importance of this mechanism in COPD and Cushing's disease, both glucocorticoid-insensitive diseases, is emphasized by: i) overexpression of HDAC2 restores glucocorticoid sensitivity in primary cells from COPD patients (Ito et al., 2006b), and ii) a lack of HDAC2 is associated with a lack of glucocorticoid responsiveness in adenocarcinomas from Cushing's patients (Bilodeau et al., 2006).

1.10 Acetylation of hsp90 and Regulation of GR Function

The actions of trichostatin A (TSA) on GR-mediated functions may not result from changes in GR acetylation. Chaperone proteins, including Hsp90 and p23 but not hsp70, also associate with GR at native GREs and modulate GR-mediated transactivation (Freeman and Yamamoto, 2002) and/or nuclear export (Kakar et al., 2006). The function of hsp90 is also regulated by its acetylation by chaperone acetyltransferase (CHAT) (Scroggins et al., 2007), a process that is specifically reversed by HDAC6 (Kovacs et al., 2005). Inactivation of HDAC6 by TSA or by selective knockdown using siRNA results in the accumulation of acetylated Hsp90, which is unable to interact stably with GR or with the critical co-chaperone p23 in A549 cells. This leads to defective GR ligand binding, nuclear translocation and transcriptional activation (Murphy et al., 2005).

1.11 Other Mechanisms of GR Action

Suppression of AP-1-induced gene transcription

The GR monomer can bind directly or indirectly with AP-1, which is also upregulated during inflammation (Demoly et al., 1995). Regulation of AP-1 activity has been thought to be similar to that of NF-κB. However, recent data has reported that a point mutation in the second zinc finger of the GR DNA binding domain (R488Q) results in a GR able to repress AP-1-mediated transcriptional responses but not those activated by NF-κB in three different cell lines, despite being able to physically associate with NF-κB (Bladh et al., 2005). In addition, this mutant had no effect on GRE-mediated events. The genes differentially regulated by this mutant were mainly involved in control of transcription and cell growth. The results indicate that different GR interaction surfaces or mechanisms are involved in the repression of NF-κB and AP-1, respectively (Bladh et al., 2005).

Other mechanisms for GR suppression of AP-1 and NF-κB have been proposed. The GR dimer can induce the expression of the NF-κB inhibitor IκB-α in certain cell types (Auphan et al., 1995; Heck et al., 1997). Similarly, induction of GILZ (glucocorticoid inducible leucine zipper) can prevent AP-1 DNA binding and activity in some cells (Mittelstadt and Ashwell, 2001).

Mutual suppression of MAPK activity

In addition, glucocorticoids may play a role in repressing the action of MAPKs, such as ERK and c-Jun N-terminal kinase (JNK) (Adcock, 2003). Caelles and colleagues have demonstrated that dexamethasone inhibits the phosphorylation and activation of JNK, resulting in a failure to phosphorylate c-Jun and Elk-1, reduced c-fos transcription and a marked reduction in AP-1 activity (Caelles et al., 1997). More recently, it has been shown that dexamethasone can rapidly induce the dual-specificity MAPK phosphatase-1 (MKP-1) and thereby attenuate p38-MAPK activation (Kassel et al., 2001; Lasa et al., 2001). Rogatsky and colleagues have, in turn, shown reciprocal inhibition of rat GR reporter gene activity by JNKs by direct phosphorylation of Ser-246, whereas ERK can inhibit GR action by an indirect effect, possibly through phosphorylation of a cofactor (Rogatsky et al., 1998). Furthermore, we and others have shown that p38-MAPK-mediated GR phosphorylation can attenuate GR function (Irusen et al., 2002; Szatmary et al., 2004).

In addition, p38-MAPK-mediated phosphorylation of Ser-10 of histone H3 is rapidly inhibited and redistributed away from sites of active gene transcription in a time- and concentration-dependent manner by dexamethasone in BEAS-2B cells (Hasegawa et al., 2005).

Regulation of mRNA stability

Glucocorticoids also appear to exert anti-inflammatory actions that do not depend on the receptor's ability to regulate transcription in the nucleus. Adenylate–uridylate-rich elements (AREs) are found within the 3′-UTR of many inflammatory genes and control the stability of mRNA (Fan et al., 2005; Meyer et al., 2004). These sequences are very heterogeneous and include both AUUUA pentamers and AT-rich stretches. Binding of mRNA to ARE-binding proteins results in the formation of messenger ribonucleoprotein (mRNP) complexes which control mRNA decay (Fan et al., 2005; Meyer et al., 2004). Several ARE-binding proteins have been reported and include tristetrapolin (TTP), which promotes mRNA decay, and HuR family members, which are associated with mRNA stability. Importantly, HuR binding to AREs is dependent upon p38 MAPK (Fan et al., 2005; Meyer et al., 2004). Dexamethasone has been reported to regulate the levels of HuR and TTP, thereby reducing the levels of inflammatory gene mRNAs such as COX-2 and CCL11 (Lu and Cidlowski, 2005; Shim and Karin, 2002) through a p38-MAPK-mediated pathway subsequent to induction of MKP-1 (Bergmann et al., 2004; Lasa et al., 2001). However, significant modulation of these genes often appears at 10 nM dexamethasone rather than the 1 nM concentrations associated with suppression of many inflammatory genes, although again these effects may be cell selective (Jalonen et al., 2005). Intriguingly, dexamethasone has recently been reported to decrease TTP expression in LPS-stimulated murine macrophages (Jalonen et al., 2005).

Non-genomic actions of glucocorticoids

Some very rapid effects of glucocorticoids, such as changes in bronchial blood flow, occur within minutes after inhaled corticosteroid dosing in asthmatics (Mendes et al., 2003) and this cannot be explained by the traditional genomic theory of steroid action. It has been proposed that these non-genomic actions are mediated by a distinct membrane receptor (Chen and Qiu, 1999; Norman and Mizwicki, 2004). Initially described in amphibians, these receptors have been described in mammalian cells and have distinctive hormone binding properties compared to the well-characterized cytoplasmic receptors and are probably linked to a number of intracellular signalling pathways acting through G-protein-coupled receptors and a number of kinase pathways (Evans et al., 2000; Norman and Mizwicki, 2004; Powell et al., 1999). In addition, the classical GR–hsp90 complex is associated with a number of kinases, phosphatases and acetylases (Adcock et al., 2002). These enzymes are released upon hormone binding and may also account for the rapid induction of tyrosine kinases seen in some cell types by glucocorticoids (Croxtall et al., 2000; Croxtall et al., 2002).

1.12   Conclusions

Overall, GR is able to selectively repress specific target genes by differing actions on promoter-specific components of NF-κB and AP-1 activation complexes and by effects on MAPKs. Explanations for the differences between the models may involve the concentration and timing of dexamethasone treatment of cells, GR expression levels and the precise inflammatory stimulus used (Simons, 2006). These pleiotropic effects of GR on suppressing inflammatory gene expression may underlie their effectiveness in most patients with airways disease but this also suggests that alteration of any of these pathways may result in a reduced ability of glucocorticoids to function effectively in patients with chronic inflammatory diseases of the lung. Understanding the molecular mechanisms of GR action may lead to the development of new anti-inflammatory drugs or enable clinicians to reverse the relative steroid insensitivity that is characteristic of severe asthma and COPD for example.

Acknowledgements

The literature in this area is extensive, and many important studies were omitted because of constraints on space, for which we apologize. We would like to thank other members of the Cell and Molecular Biology Group for their helpful discussions. Work in our group is supported by Asthma UK, The British Lung Foundation, The Clinical Research Committee (Brompton Hospital), The Medical Research Council (UK), The National Institutes of Health (USA), The Wellcome Trust, AstraZeneca, Boehringer Ingelheim, GlaxoSmithKline (UK), Mitsubishi Pharma (Japan), Novartis and Pfizer.

References

Abbinante-Nissen JM, Simpson LG, Leikauf GD. Corticosteroids increase secretory leukocyte protease inhibitor transcript levels in airway epithelial cells. *Am J Physiol* 1995; **268**: L601–L606.

Adcock IM. Glucocorticoids: new mechanisms and future agents. *Curr Allergy Asthma Rep* 2003; **3**: 249–257.

Adcock IM, Maneechotesuwan K, Usmani O. Molecular interactions between glucocorticoids and long-acting beta2-agonists. *J Allergy Clin Immunol* 2002; **110**: S261–S268.

Auphan N, Didonato JA, Rosette C, Helmberg A, Karin M. Immunosuppression by glucocorticoids: inhibition of NF-kappa B activity through induction of I kappa B synthesis [see comments]. *Science* 1995; **270**: 286–290.

Baldwin AS, Jr. Series introduction: the transcription factor NF-kappaB and human disease. *J Clin Invest* 2001; **107**: 3–6.

Barker M, Clackers M, Demaine DA, Humphreys D et al. Design and synthesis of new nonsteroidal glucocorticoid modulators through application of an "agreement docking" method. *J Med Chem* 2005; **48**: 4507–4510.

Barnes PJ. Inhaled corticosteroids are not beneficial in chronic obstructive pulmonary disease. *Am J Respir Crit Care Med* 2000a; **161**: 342–344.

Barnes PJ. Mechanisms in COPD: differences from asthma. *Chest* 2000b; **117**: 10S–14S.

Barnes PJ, Karin M. Nuclear factor-kappaB: a pivotal transcription factor in chronic inflammatory diseases. *N Engl J Med* 1997; **336**: 1066–1071.

Barnes PJ, Ito K, Adcock IM. Corticosteroid resistance in chronic obstructive pulmonary disease: inactivation of histone deacetylase. *Lancet* 2004; **363**: 731–733.

Bergmann MW, Staples KJ, Smith SJ, Barnes PJ, Newton R. Glucocorticoid inhibition of granulocyte macrophage-colony-stimulating factor from T cells is independent of control by nuclear factor-kappaB and conserved lymphokine element 0. *Am J Respir Cell Mol Biol* 2004; **30**: 555–563.

Bilodeau S, Vallette-Kasic S, Gauthier Y, Figarella-Branger D et al. Role of Brg1 and HDAC2 in GR trans-repression of the pituitary POMC gene and misexpression in Cushing disease. *Genes Dev* 2006; **20**: 2871–2886.

Biola A, Andreau K, David M, Sturm M et al. The glucocorticoid receptor and STAT6 physically and functionally interact in T-lymphocytes. *FEBS Lett* 2000; **487**: 229–233.

Bladh LG, Liden J, Hlman-Wright K, Reimers M et al. Identification of endogenous glucocorticoid repressed genes differentially regulated by a glucocorticoid receptor mutant able to separate between nuclear factor-kappaB and activator protein-1 repression. *Mol Pharmacol* 2005; **67**: 815–826.

Bledsoe RK, Montana VG, Stanley TB, Delves CJ et al. Crystal structure of the glucocorticoid receptor ligand binding domain reveals a novel mode of receptor dimerization and coactivator recognition. *Cell* 2002; **110**: 93–105.

Caelles C, Gonzalez-Sancho JM, Munoz A. Nuclear hormone receptor antagonism with AP-1 by inhibition of the JNK pathway. *Genes Dev* 1997; **11**: 3351–3364.

Carrigan A, Walther RF, Salem HA, Wu D et al. An active nuclear retention signal in the glucocorticoid receptor functions as a strong inducer of transcriptional activation. *J Biol Chem* 2007; **282**: 10963–10971.

Chen L, Fischle W, Verdin E, Greene WC. Duration of nuclear NF-kappaB action regulated by reversible acetylation. *Science* 2001; **293**: 1653–1657.

Chen YZ, Qiu J. Pleiotropic signaling pathways in rapid, nongenomic action of glucocorticoid. *Mol Cell Biol Res Commun* 1999; **2**: 145–149.

Chook YM, Blobel G. Karyopherins and nuclear import. *Curr Opin Struct Biol* 2001; **11**: 703–715.

Covert MW, Leung TH, Gaston JE, Baltimore D. Achieving stability of lipopolysaccharide-induced NF-kappaB activation. *Science* 2005; **309**: 1854–1857.

Croxtall JD, Choudhury Q, Flower RJ. Glucocorticoids act within minutes to inhibit recruitment of signalling factors to activated EGF receptors through a receptor-dependent, transcription-independent mechanism. *Br J Pharmacol* 2000; **130**: 289–298.

Croxtall JD, Van Hal PT, Choudhury Q, Gilroy DW, Flower RJ. Different glucocorticoids vary in their genomic and non-genomic mechanism of action in A549 cells. *Br J Pharmacol* 2002; **135**: 511–519.

Culpitt SV, Rogers DF, Shah P, De MC et al. Impaired inhibition by dexamethasone of cytokine release by alveolar macrophages from patients with chronic obstructive pulmonary disease. *Am J Respir Crit Care Med* 2003; **167**: 24–31.

Da Silva CA, Kassel O, Lebouquin R, Lacroix EJ, Frossard N. Paradoxical early glucocorticoid induction of stem cell factor (SCF) expression in inflammatory conditions. *Br J Pharmacol* 2004; **141**: 75–84.

De Bosscher K, Vanden BW, Haegeman G. Cross-talk between nuclear receptors and nuclear factor kappaB. *Oncogene* 2006; **25**: 6868–6886.

Demoly P, Chanez P, Pujol JL, Gauthier-Rouviere C et al. Fos immunoreactivity assessment on human normal and pathological bronchial biopsies. *Respir Med* 1995; **89**: 329–335.

Evans SJ, Murray TF, Moore FL. Partial purification and biochemical characterization of a membrane glucocorticoid receptor from an amphibian brain. *J Steroid Biochem Mol Biol* 2000; **72**: 209–221.

Fan J, Heller NM, Gorospe M, Atasoy U, Stellato C. The role of post-transcriptional regulation in chemokine gene expression in inflammation and allergy. *Eur Respir J* 2005; **26**: 933–947.

Freeman BC, Yamamoto KR. Disassembly of transcriptional regulatory complexes by molecular chaperones. *Science* 2002; **296**: 2232–2235.

Galigniana MD, Housley PR, DeFranco DB, Pratt WB. Inhibition of glucocorticoid receptor nucleocytoplasmic shuttling by okadaic acid requires intact cytoskeleton. *J Biol Chem* 1999a; **274**: 16222–16227.

Galigniana MD, Piwien-Pilipuk G, Assreuy J. Inhibition of glucocorticoid receptor binding by nitric oxide. *Mol Pharmacol* 1999b; **55**: 317–323.

Garside H, Stevens A, Farrow S, Normand C et al. Glucocorticoid ligands specify different interactions with NF-kappaB by allosteric effects on the glucocorticoid receptor DNA binding domain. *J Biol Chem* 2004; **279**: 50050–50059.

Ghosh S, Karin M. Missing pieces in the NF-kappaB puzzle. *Cell* 2002; **109**: S81–S96.

Hache RJ, Tse R, Reich T, Savory JG, Lefebvre YA. Nucleocytoplasmic trafficking of steroid-free glucocorticoid receptor. *J Biol Chem* 1999; **274**: 1432–1439.

Hasegawa Y, Tomita K, Watanabe M, Yamasaki A et al. Dexamethasone inhibits phosphorylation of histone H3 at serine 10. *Biochem Biophys Res Commun* 2005; **336**: 1049–1055.

He Y, Simons SS, Jr. STAMP, a novel predicted factor assisting TIF2 actions in glucocorticoid receptor-mediated induction and repression. *Mol Cell Biol* 2007; **27**: 1467–1485.

Hebbar PB, Archer TK. Chromatin-dependent cooperativity between site-specific transcription factors in vivo. *J Biol Chem* 2007; **282**: 8284–8291.

Heck S, Bender K, Kullmann M, Gottlicher M et al. I kappaB alpha-independent downregulation of NF-kappaB activity by glucocorticoid receptor. *EMBO J* 1997; **16**: 4698–4707.

Hermoso MA, Matsuguchi T, Smoak K, Cidlowski JA. Glucocorticoids and tumor necrosis factor alpha cooperatively regulate toll-like receptor 2 gene expression. *Mol Cell Biol* 2004; **24**: 4743–4756.

Hsu SC, Qi M, DeFranco DB. Cell cycle regulation of glucocorticoid receptor function. *EMBO J* 1992; **11**: 3457–3468.

Hu JM, Bodwell JE, Munck A. Cell cycle-dependent glucocorticoid receptor phosphorylation and activity. *Mol Endocrinol* 1994; **8**: 1709–1713.

Huang ZQ, Li J, Sachs LM, Cole PA, Wong J. A role for cofactor–cofactor and cofactor–histone interactions in targeting p300, SWI/SNF and Mediator for transcription. *EMBO J* 2003; **22**: 2146–2155.

Irusen E, Matthews JG, Takahashi A, Barnes PJ et al. p38 Mitogen-activated protein kinase-induced glucocorticoid receptor phosphorylation reduces its activity: role in steroid-insensitive asthma. *J Allergy Clin Immunol* 2002; **109**: 649–657.

Ito K, Barnes PJ, Adcock IM. Glucocorticoid receptor recruitment of histone deacetylase 2 inhibits interleukin-1beta-induced histone H4 acetylation on lysines 8 and 12. *Mol Cell Biol* 2000; **20**: 6891–6903.

Ito K, Chung KF, Adcock IM. Update on glucocorticoid action and resistance. *J Allergy Clin Immunol* 2006a; **117**: 522–543.

Ito K, Ito M, Elliott WM, Cosio B et al. Decreased histone deacetylase activity in chronic obstructive pulmonary disease. *N Engl J Med* 2005; **352**: 1967–1976.

Ito K, Lim S, Caramori G, Chung KF et al. Cigarette smoking reduces histone deacetylase 2 expression, enhances cytokine expression, and inhibits glucocorticoid actions in alveolar macrophages. *FASEB J* 2001; **15**: 1110–1112.

Ito K, Yamamura S, Essilfie-Quaye S, Cosio B et al. Histone deacetylase 2-mediated deacetylation of the glucocorticoid receptor enables NF-kappaB suppression. *J Exp Med* 2006b; **203**: 7–13.

Itoh M, Adachi M, Yasui H, Takekawa M et al. Nuclear export of glucocorticoid receptor is enhanced by c-Jun N-terminal kinase-mediated phosphorylation. *Mol Endocrinol* 2002; **16**: 2382–2392.

Jalonen U, Lahti A, Korhonen R, Kankaanranta H, Moilanen E. Inhibition of tristetraprolin expression by dexamethasone in activated macrophages. *Biochem Pharmacol* 2005; **69**: 733–740.

Jee YK, Gilmour J, Kelly A, Bowen H et al. Repression of interleukin-5 transcription by the glucocorticoid receptor targets GATA3 signaling and involves histone deacetylase recruitment. *J Biol Chem* 2005; **280**: 23243–23250.

Jenuwein T, Allis CD. Translating the histone code. *Science* 2001; **293**: 1074–1080.

Kakar M, Kanwal C, Davis JR, Li H, Lim CS. Geldanamycin, an inhibitor of Hsp90, blocks cytoplasmic retention of progesterone receptors and glucocorticoid receptors via their respective ligand binding domains. *AAPS J* 2006; **8**: E718–E728.

Karin M. New twists in gene regulation by glucocorticoid receptor: is DNA binding dispensable? *Cell* 1998; **93**: 487–490.

Kassel O, Sancono A, Kratzschmar J, Kreft B et al. Glucocorticoids inhibit MAP kinase via increased expression and decreased degradation of MKP-1. *EMBO J* 2001; **20**: 7108–7116.

Kauppi B, Jakob C, Farnegardh M, Yang J et al. The three-dimensional structures of antagonistic and agonistic forms of the glucocorticoid receptor ligand-binding domain: RU-486 induces a transconformation that leads to active antagonism. *J Biol Chem* 2003; **278**: 22748–22754.

Kovacs JJ, Cohen TJ, Yao TP. Chaperoning steroid hormone signaling via reversible acetylation. *Nucl Recept Signal* 2005; **3**: e004.

Kumar S, Chaturvedi NK, Nishi M, Kawata M, Tyagi RK. Shuttling components of nuclear import machinery involved in nuclear translocation of steroid receptors exit nucleus via exportin-1/CRM-1* independent pathway. *Biochim Biophys Acta* 2004; **1691**: 73–77.

Lasa M, Abraham SM, Boucheron C, Saklatvala J, Clark AR. Dexamethasone causes sustained expression of mitogen-activated protein kinase (MAPK) phosphatase 1 and phosphatase-mediated inhibition of MAPK p38. *Mol Cell Biol* 2002; **22**: 7802–7811.

Lasa M, Brook M, Saklatvala J, Clark AR. Dexamethasone destabilizes cyclooxygenase 2 mRNA by inhibiting mitogen-activated protein kinase p38. *Mol Cell Biol* 2001; **21**: 771–780.

Le DY, Mincheneau N, Le GP, Michel D. Potentiation of glucocorticoid receptor transcriptional activity by sumoylation. *Endocrinology* 2002; **143**: 3482–3489.

Lee KK, Workman JL. Histone acetyltransferase complexes: one size doesn't fit all. *Nat Rev Mol Cell Biol* 2007; **8**: 284–295.

Lee KY, Ito K, Hayashi R, Jazrawi EP et al. NF-{kappa}B and activator protein 1 response elements and the role of histone modifications in IL-1{beta}-induced TGF-{beta}1 gene transcription. *J Immunol* 2006; **176**: 603–615.

Li B, Carey M, Workman JL. The role of chromatin during transcription. *Cell* 2007; **128**: 707–719.

Li X, Wong J, Tsai SY, Tsai MJ, O'Malley BW. Progesterone and glucocorticoid receptors recruit distinct coactivator complexes and promote distinct patterns of local chromatin modification. *Mol Cell Biol* 2003; **23**: 3763–3773.

Lin DY, Lai MZ, Ann DK, Shih HM. Promyelocytic leukemia protein (PML) functions as a glucocorticoid receptor co-activator by sequestering Daxx to the PML oncogenic domains (PODs) to enhance its transactivation potential. *J Biol Chem* 2003; **278**: 15958–15965.

Lu NZ, Cidlowski JA. Translational regulatory mechanisms generate N-terminal glucocorticoid receptor isoforms with unique transcriptional target genes. *Mol Cell* 2005; **18**: 331–342.

Luecke HF, Yamamoto KR. The glucocorticoid receptor blocks P-TEFb recruitment by NFkappaB to effect promoter-specific transcriptional repression. *Genes Dev* 2005; **19**: 1116–1127.

Marwick JA, Kirkham PA, Stevenson CS, Danahay H et al. Cigarette smoke alters chromatin remodeling and induces proinflammatory genes in rat lungs. *Am J Respir Cell Mol Biol* 2004; **31**: 633–642.

Mendes ES, Pereira A, Danta I, Duncan RC, Wanner A. Comparative bronchial vasoconstrictive efficacy of inhaled glucocorticosteroids. *Eur Respir J* 2003; **21**: 989–993.

Meyer S, Temme C, Wahle E. Messenger RNA turnover in eukaryotes: pathways and enzymes. Crit. *Rev Biochem Mol Biol* 2004; **39**: 197–216.

Mittelstadt PR, Ashwell JD. Inhibition of AP-1 by the glucocorticoid-inducible protein GILZ. *J Biol Chem* 2001; **276**: 29603–29610.

Mullick J, Anandatheerthavarada HK, Amuthan G, Bhagwat SV et al. Physical interaction and functional synergy between glucocorticoid receptor and Ets2 proteins for transcription activation of the rat cytochrome P-450c27 promoter. *J Biol Chem* 2001; **276**: 18007–18017.

Murphy PJ, Morishima Y, Kovacs JJ, Yao TP, Pratt WB. Regulation of the dynamics of hsp90 action on the glucocorticoid receptor by acetylation/deacetylation of the chaperone. *J Biol Chem* 2005; **280**: 33792–33799.

Nelson DE, Ihekwaba AE, Elliott M, Johnson JR et al. Oscillations in NF-kappaB signaling control the dynamics of gene expression. *Science* 2004; **306**: 704–708.

Nie M, Knox AJ, Pang L. beta2-Adrenoceptor agonists, like glucocorticoids, repress eotaxin gene transcription by selective inhibition of histone H4 acetylation. *J Immunol* 2005; **175**: 478–486.

Nie Z, Xue Y, Yang D, Zhou S et al. A specificity and targeting subunit of a human SWI/SNF family-related chromatin-remodeling complex. *Mol Cell Biol* 2000; **20**: 8879–8888.

Nissen RM, Yamamoto KR. The glucocorticoid receptor inhibits NFkappaB by interfering with serine-2 phosphorylation of the RNA polymerase II carboxy-terminal domain. *Genes Dev* 2000; **14**: 2314–2329.

Norman AW, Mizwicki MT, Norman DP. Steroid-hormone rapid actions, membrane receptors and a conformational ensemble model. *Nat Rev Drug Discov* 2004; **3**: 27–41.

Ogawa S, Lozach J, Benner C, Pascual G et al. Molecular determinants of crosstalk between nuclear receptors and toll-like receptors. *Cell* 2005; **122**: 707–721.

Pascual G, Fong AL, Ogawa S, Gamliel A et al. A SUMOylation-dependent pathway mediates transrepression of inflammatory response genes by PPAR-gamma. *Nature* 2005; **437**: 759–763.

Picard D, Yamamoto KR. Two signals mediate hormone-dependent nuclear localization of the glucocorticoid receptor. *EMBO J* 1987; **6**: 3333–3340.

Powell CE, Watson CS, Gametchu B. Immunoaffinity isolation of native membrane glucocorticoid receptor from S-49++ lymphoma cells: biochemical characterization and interaction with Hsp 70 and Hsp 90. *Endocrinlogy* 1999; **10**: 271–280.

Reichardt HM, Kaestner KH, Tuckermann J, Kretz O et al. DNA binding of the glucocorticoid receptor is not essential for survival. *Cell* 1998; **93**: 531–541.

Reichardt HM, Tuckermann JP, Gottlicher M, Vujic M et al. Repression of inflammatory responses in the absence of DNA binding by the glucocorticoid receptor. *EMBO J* 2001; **20**: 7168–7173.

Reily MM, Pantoja C, Hu X, Chinenov Y, Rogatsky I. The GRIP1:IRF3 interaction as a target for glucocorticoid receptor-mediated immunosuppression. *EMBO J* 2006; **25**: 108–117.

Rice JC, Allis CD. Code of silence. *Nature* 2001; **414**: 258–261.

Rogatsky I, Logan SK, Garabedian MJ. Antagonism of glucocorticoid receptor transcriptional activation by the c-Jun N-terminal kinase. *Proc Natl Acad Sci USA* 1998; **95**: 2050–2055.

Rogatsky I, Luecke HF, Leitman DC, Yamamoto KR. Alternate surfaces of transcriptional coregulator GRIP1 function in different glucocorticoid receptor activation and repression contexts. *Proc Natl Acad Sci USA* 2002; **99**: 16701–16706.

Rosenfeld MG, Glass CK. Coregulator codes of transcriptional regulation by nuclear receptors. *J Biol Chem* 2001; **276**: 36865–36868.

Sakai A, Han J, Cato AC, Akira S, Li JD. Glucocorticoids synergize with IL-1beta to induce TLR2 expression via MAP kinase phosphatase-1-dependent dual inhibition of MAPK JNK and p38 in epithelial cells. *BMC Mol Biol* 2004; **5**: 2.

Sarkar SN, Elco CP, Peters KL, Chattopadhyay S, Sen GC. Two tyrosine residues of Toll-like receptor 3 trigger different steps of NF-kappaB activation. *J Biol Chem* 2007; **282**: 3423–3427.

Savory JG, Hsu B, Laquian IR, Giffin W et al. Discrimination between NL1- and NL2-mediated nuclear localization of the glucocorticoid receptor. *Mol Cell Biol* 1999; **19**: 1025–1037.

Schaaf MJ, Lewis-Tuffin LJ, Cidlowski JA. Ligand-selective targeting of the glucocorticoid receptor to nuclear subdomains is associated with decreased receptor mobility. *Mol Endocrinol* 2005; **19**: 1501–1515.

Scroggins BT, Robzyk K, Wang D, Marcu MG et al. An acetylation site in the middle domain of Hsp90 regulates chaperone function. *Mol Cell* 2007; **25**: 151–159.

Shim J, Karin M. The control of mRNA stability in response to extracellular stimuli. *Mol Cell* 2002; **14**: 323–331.

Simons SS, Jr. How much is enough? Modulation of dose-response curve for steroid receptor-regulated gene expression by changing concentrations of transcription factor. *Curr Top Med Chem* 2006; **6**: 271–285.

Smith CL, O'Malley BW. Coregulator function: a key to understanding tissue specificity of selective receptor modulators. *Endocr Rev* 2004; **25**: 45–71.

Somers JP, DeFranco DB. Effects of okadaic acid, a protein phosphatase inhibitor, on glucocorticoid receptor-mediated enhancement. *Mol Endocrinol* 1992; **6**: 26–34.

Stevens A, Garside H, Berry A, Waters C et al. Dissociation of steroid receptor coactivator 1 and nuclear receptor corepressor recruitment to the human glucocorticoid receptor by modification of the ligand-receptor interface: the role of tyrosine 735. *Mol Endocrinol* 2003; **17**: 845–859.

Stocklin E, Wissler M, Gouilleux F, Groner B. Functional interactions between Stat5 and the glucocorticoid receptor. *Nature* 1996; **383**: 726–728.

Szatmary Z, Garabedian MJ, Vilcek J. Inhibition of glucocorticoid receptor-mediated transcriptional activation by p38 mitogen-activated protein (MAP) kinase. *J Biol Chem* 2004; **279**: 43708–43715.

Trotter KW, Archer TK. Nuclear receptors and chromatin remodeling machinery. *Mol Cell Endocrinol* 2007; **265266**: 162–167.

Wallace AD, Cidlowski JA. Proteasome-mediated glucocorticoid receptor degradation restricts transcriptional signaling by glucocorticoids. *J Biol Chem* 2001; **276**: 42714–42721.

Wang JC, Derynck MK, Nonaka DF, Khodabakhsh DB et al. Chromatin immunoprecipitation (ChIP) scanning identifies primary glucocorticoid receptor target genes. *Proc Natl Acad Sci USA* 2004; **101**: 15603–15608.

Werner SL, Barken D, Hoffmann A. Stimulus specificity of gene expression programs determined by temporal control of IKK activity. *Science* 2005; **309**: 1857–1861.

Wu RC, Smith CL, O'Malley BW. Transcriptional regulation by steroid receptor coactivator phosphorylation. *Endocr Rev* 2005; **26**: 393–399.

Zhong H, May MJ, Jimi E, Ghosh S. The phosphorylation status of nuclear NF-kappa B determines its association with CBP/p300 or HDAC-1. *Mol Cell* 2002; **9**: 625–636.

Zhou J, Cidlowski JA. The human glucocorticoid receptor: one gene, multiple proteins and diverse responses. *Steroids* 2005; **70**: 407–417.

Zuo Z, Urban G, Scammell JG, Dean NM et al. Ser/Thr protein phosphatase type 5 (PP5) is a negative regulator of glucocorticoid receptor-mediated growth arrest. *Biochemistry* 1999; **38**: 8849–8857.

2

Side Effects of Topical and Oral Glucocorticoids

Heike Schäcke, Khusru Asadullah and Wolf-Dietrich Döcke

2.1   Introduction

For more than 50 years glucocorticoids (GCs) have been the most commonly used drugs in the treatment of acute and chronic inflammatory diseases. The therapeutic era of GCs started with the discovery that cortisol, a steroid hormone synthesized in adrenal cortex, was able to reduce the symptoms of Addison's disease (Mason et al., 1936). Ten years later it was shown that cortisol was effective in the treatment of rheumatoid arthritis (Hench et al., 1949). Since then the unparalleled progress of GCs has been enormous. They are successfully used in the treatment of most inflammatory disorders via distinct administration routes. In particular, rheumatoid, asthmatic, some dermatological conditions and organ transplantations can hardly be controlled without GCs (Schäcke et al., 2006).

In the 1950s and 1960s GCs of different strengths were used extensively and often without any critical supervision regarding possible undesired effects. As a consequence, strong side effects arose. Long-term systemic treatment with potent GCs can lead to several severe and also sometimes irreversible adverse effects. The strength of GCs, being active in many different cell types and tissues, is their problem. Nearly every organ or tissue of the body can be affected by GCs in an undesired fashion. One of the most frequently described side effects after long-term systemic GC treatment, which the patients are afraid of, is Cushing's syndrome. Cushing's syndrome is characterized by a moon face, central obesity, striae, proximal muscle weakness, insulin resistance and hypertension. However, as mentioned, many organs can be affected in different fashions by GCs. GC-induced osteoporosis, diabetes mellitus and hypertension are side effects that require additional treatments or hospitalization of

Overcoming Steroid Insensitivity in Respiratory Disease   Edited by Ian M. Adcock and Kian Fan Chung
© 2008 John Wiley & Sons, Ltd.

patients. Children who are treated over longer times with GCs often show a delayed or a reduced growth (Miner et al., 2005; Schäcke et al., 2006).

Introduction of local treatment options was a major step towards safer treatment opportunities. Targeted local administration of metabolically unstable GCs led to a significant reduction of systemic effects. These treatment options became of higher significance in dermatology, inflammatory bowel diseases, asthma and ophthalmology. Whereas in dermatology a huge number of differently formulated GCs are available, such as ointments, creams, milks, foams and others, for asthma treatment the drugs have to be formulated for inhalation (Hengge et al., 2006).

Especially for asthma therapy, inhaled GCs presented an enormous step forward to improve the benefit to risk ratio. They were a breakthrough in asthma management and resulted in improved symptom control and quality of life for many patients. Children present a huge group of asthma patients and therefore reducing side effects such as growth retardation is of major importance. For inhaled GC therapy the predominant potential side effects may be local, e.g. in the oropharyngeal cavity, or systemic due to absorption of inhaled GCs into the circulation through lung and gastrointestinal tract, respectively. For local side effects, the development of oral

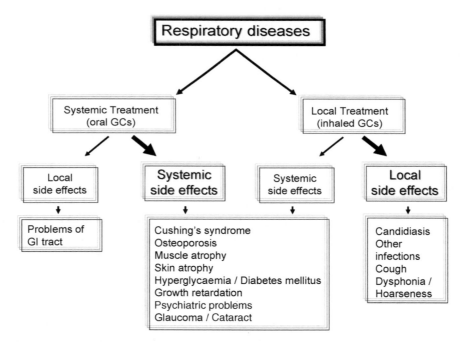

Figure 2.1   Both inhaled and oral glucocorticicoids (GCs) can lead to local and systemic side effects in subjects with respiratory disease. Local treatment with inhaled GCs is associated mainly with local side effects, including candidiasis, other infections, cough and dysphonia, with little systemic action. In contrast, oral corticosteroids result in some gastrointestinal (GI) tract problems but also have major systemic side effects, including Cushing's syndrome, osteoporosis, muscle and skin atrophy, diabetes mellitus, glaucoma and psychiatric problems.

Table 2.1 Factors that have an impact on the development of GC-induced adverse effects in the specific individual

	Characteristic
Drug	Strength
	Selectivity for the GR
	Pharmacokinetic properties
	Pharmacodynamic profile
Therapeutic regimen	Dose
	Duration
	Administration route
	Administration technique
Individual	Age[a]
	Sex[b]
	Predisposition[c]
	Concomitant diseases[d]
	Co-medications[e]

[a]Growth retardation – only children affected; glaucoma and cataract – preferentially in elderly patients (Allen et al., 2003).
[b]Skin atrophy – preferentially in women; osteoporosis – preferentially in post-menopausal women (Sambrook, 2002; Schoepe et al., 2006).
[c]Glaucoma and diabetes mellitus – family history, pre-treatment abnormalities (Allen et al., 2003).
[d]Glaucoma and cataract – increased risk in patients with diabetes mellitus (Allen et al., 2003).
[e]Drug-drug interaction with, for example, protease inhibitors in HIV patients or antibiotics (Bolland et al., 2004; Samaras et al., 2005).

candidiasis, dysphonia and/or cough have been described (Irwin and Richardson, 2006). However, dependent on dosage, type of inhaled GC and duration of therapy, systemic effects such as growth suppression, adrenal insufficiency, increased risk of fractures, cataract and / or glaucoma development, hyperglycaemia and psychological disorders might be induced. In particular, patients with severe asthma requiring high-dose inhaled GC therapy, patients additionally receiving intermittent oral therapy for disease exacerbation or patients getting GCs also by other routes (e.g. intranasal for allergic rhinitis or dermal for atopic dermatitis) are at increased risk of systemic side effects (Figure 2.1). Although the development of GC-induced adverse effects is undisputed, the individual risk depends on several factors outlined in Table 2.1.

In the following, the local side effects of inhaled GCs and systemic side effects of inhaled and oral GC therapy will be discussed.

2.2 Glucocorticoid-induced Side Effects

Local side effects of inhaled glucocorticoids

The most prominent local side effects after inhaled GC therapy are cough, dysphonia and hoarseness, and oral candidiasis.

Oral candidiasis (thrush) represents a fungal infection that is a common side effect in many adult patients receiving inhaled GCs. Diagnosis of this side effect is not easy and, therefore, reported incidences vary between 0 and 77% (Dubus et al., 2001). In a review by Irwin and Richardson (2006), differences in incidences for oral candidiasis between several drugs were discussed. In any case, development of this side effect is dose-dependent. The risk of inducing *Candida albicans* infection can be reduced by taking the drugs just prior to meals (Irwin and Richardson, 2006).

Oesophageal candidiasis, a second form of the infection, has also been reported as a dose-dependent undesired effect of inhalation therapy. A reduction of daily GC dose resolved the infection in some of the affected patients after 1 month (Kanda et al., 2003). Interestingly, oesophageal candidiasis seems to be more frequent in patients with diabetes (Kanda et al., 2003).

Induction of *dysphonia* and *hoarseness* seem to be direct effects of GCs after inhalation therapy. These undesired effects are observed in 5–50% of patients receiving inhaled GCs (National Asthma Education and Prevention Program, 1997). Dysphonia is associated with vocal stress and increasing dosages of inhaled GCs (Toogood et al., 1980).

Cough during inhaled GC therapy has been reported in 34% of adults, with no differences in incidence between two different GCs tested (Williamson et al., 1995). In children, cough seems to be the most prominent local effect of inhaled GCs (Irwin and Richardson, 2006).

In general, there is a high variability in local side effects reported for inhaled GC therapy dependent on drug, dose and device (Dubus et al., 2001). Much of this is also due to how side effects are defined and assessed.

Systemic side effects of inhaled and oral glucocorticoids

In principle, all inhaled GCs exhibit dose-dependent systemic adverse effects, although these are less frequent and less pronounced than those observed with a comparable dose of oral GCs. As systemic GCs, long-term local GC therapies can lead to the induction of systemic adverse effects, e.g. on adrenals, on bone and muscle, on skin, on eyes, and in children on growth (Allen, 2006; Allen et al., 2003; Irwin and Richardson, 2006; Lipworth, 1999).

Cushing's syndrome

Iatrogenic Cushing's syndrome, which is characterized by many adverse effects such as hypertension, disturbed glucose tolerance, osteoporosis and a cushingoid habitus (moon face, buffalo hump, central obesity), is not a common side effect of inhaled GC therapy. Nevertheless, case reports describe its occurrence in single patients (Chisholm and Chalkley, 1994). Moreover, the risk of developing Cushing's syndrome substantially increases when inhaled GCs are used in combination with drugs that interfere with their hepatic metabolism, e.g. antibiotics or protease inhibitors for treatment of HIV infection (Bolland et al., 2004; Samaras et al., 2005).

Cushing's syndrome is the consequence of an increased bioavailability of inhaled GCs, so the development of a cushingoid phenotype should trigger further diagnostics, e.g. for osteoporosis. Moreover, when reducing or withdrawing GCs, major attention has to be paid to possible risks, e.g. of established clinically relevant adrenal insufficiency (Hopkins and Leinung, 2005).

Adrenal insufficiency

The zona fasciculata cells of the adrenal cortex synthesize and secrete GCs in response to adrenocorticotrophic hormone (ACTH) as well as adrenergic stimuli. ACTH is generated in the corticotroph cells of the anterior pituitary by selective proteolytic processing of proopiomelanocortin (POMC). ACTH generation and secretion are predominantly controlled by the hypothalamic stimulatory factor corticotrophin-releasing hormone (CRH). GCs exert inhibitory feedback regulation on hypothalamic CRH secretion and ACTH generation and secretion in anterior pituitary via different mechanisms (Jacobson, 2005). Furthermore GC binding to extra-hypothalamic mineralocorticoid receptors contributes to the suppression of hypothalamic CRH secretion (Young et al., 1998). Moreover, whereas inhibitory effects of GCs on POMC mRNA expression in pituitary depend on DNA binding of the glucocorticoid receptor, the regulation of CRH expression and of ACTH secretion is DNA independent (Reichardt et al., 1998). Feedback inhibition occurs on distinct time domains, referred to as fast, delayed and slow feedback (Keller-Wood and Dallman, 1984). Slow feedback, reflecting chronic exposure to GCs, affects both basal and stimulated hypothalamic-pituitary activity. Prolonged exposure to high levels of GCs strongly inhibits ACTH secretion and causes apoptosis of adrenal cortex cells and loss of secretory capacity. Depending on the duration and level of GC exposure, the resulting adrenal insufficiency can take up to a year to reverse (Axelrod, 2003). Prolonged GC treatment is considered to be the main cause of adrenal insufficiency. Adrenal insufficiency becomes clinically relevant if exogenous GC therapy is withdrawn too rapidly (Bell, 1984) or in stressful situations (e.g. surgery) when higher GC levels might be required (Nicholson et al., 1998).

The suppressive effects of inhaled GCs on the hypothalamic-pituitary-adrenal (HPA) axis are markedly less than those of equivalent doses of oral GCs, and the corresponding risk of clinically relevant adrenal insufficiency due to inhaled GC therapy is rather low (Crowley, 2003; Irwin and Richardson, 2006; Storms & Theen, 1998). Nevertheless, both long-term effects of inhaled GCs on the HPA axis and even acute adrenal crisis due to withdrawal of inhaled GC treatment have been described. Moreover, observed effects of inhaled GC therapy on adrenal function might also be indicative of other systemic side effects.

Many studies describe effects of inhaled GCs on the HPA axis depending on the dosage and the drugs used. However, although biochemical evidence of adrenocortical insufficiency is demonstrated in some studies in a significant proportion of patients (up to 43% in high-dose inhaled therapy), clinical signs are rare (Chrousos and Harris, 1998; Chrousos et al., 2005; Crowley, 2003).

Remarkably, single patients seem to be very sensitive even to specific inhaled GCs. In a recent study in 13% of asthmatic children receiving inhaled GC therapy, a diminished response to a low-dose ACTH test and a decreased 24-h urinary free cortisol excretion were observed. Interestingly, half of the poor responders to the low-dose ACTH test showed a normal response to the standard-dose ACTH test (Ozbek et al., 2006). This indicates the necessity for refined diagnostics to assess the real incidence of HPA axis suppression. Among the tests used, the determination of the area under the cortisol concentration curve by measurement of 24-h sequential serum concentrations is considered to represent a definitive test of basal HPA axis function (Chrousos and Harris, 1998; Chrousos et al., 2005).

Clinical symptoms of adrenal insufficiency in patients receiving inhaled GC therapy are rare (Crowley, 2003). The clinical manifestations of adrenal insufficiency may include slow linear growth velocity, weight loss, anorexia, vomiting, diarrhoea, dizziness, orthostatic hypotension, hypoglycaemia, coma, convulsions, hyponatraemia and mild normocytic anaemia. Abrupt-onset adrenal failure in association with exogenous GC therapy has not been described (Oelkers, 1996).

Although acute adrenal insufficiency after discontinuation of moderate-dose therapy with inhaled GCs is rare, a series of case reports indicate that the frequency might be higher than expected (Macdessi et al., 2003; Patel et al., 2001). Moreover, most symptoms of adrenal insufficiency are not recognized by the patients themselves.

Periodic evaluation of adrenal function thus may be advisable whenever long-term high-dose inhaled GC therapy is necessary, or in patients who receive topical GCs by additional routes, e.g. for rhinitis or dermatitis (Allen, 2006). Moreover, any patient who reports suggestive symptoms of adrenal insufficiency or whose growth velocity is slow should have a dynamic test of HPA axis function performed (Crowley, 2003). Frequent short courses of oral glucocorticoids for acute asthma exacerbations, however, seem not to enhance the risk of adrenal insufficiency (Ducharme et al., 2003).

Growth retardation

Many parents of children who require long-term GC therapy, e.g. in the treatment of asthma or eczema, are especially afraid of growth suppression. This effect has been regularly described but it is debatable whether the final growth is really suppressed or just delayed. A review by Irwin and Richardson (2006) concludes that therapy with inhaled GCs is associated with a reduced short-term growth rate in children but that the overall effect is small and may not be sustained with long-term therapy. In a randomized, placebo-controlled study the effect of inhaled GCs on growth has been investigated in asthmatic and healthy children by determining the lower leg growth over time (Wolthers and Heuck, 2004). It was found that the mean lower leg growth rates were consistently lower in the asthma group than in the control group during the short-term periods of up to 12 weeks treatment. In contrast, lower leg growth rate changed very little up to 1 year following a 2–4 week treatment period. In another study that followed children treated with budesonide for 4 years, a height growth rate suppression of approximately 20% was found during the first year of treatment; thereafter, growth recovered in most children (Childhood Asthma Management Program Research Group, 2000).

Systemic GCs in comparison to inhaled GC therapy induce a much more prominent effect on the growth rate in children. Thus, it has been shown in patients with chronic lung diseases that systemic dexamethasone treatment affected the lower leg length significantly more than inhaled budesonide (Nicholl et al., 2002).

A final conclusion on the strength of effects on growth is not easily to make. In clinical studies either asthmatic children are compared to healthy probands or, in asthmatic patients, systemic versus inhaled GCs are compared. Thus, it is not possible to determine whether the disease itself also has an effect on growth. However, because of ethical reasons it is not possible to treat asthmatic children with a placebo. Mechanistically it is not completely clear how GCs affect growth but it has been shown that GCs negatively regulate the expression of growth hormone (Allen, 2004). Furthermore, the negative effects on bone (see below) also influence the growth rate.

All novel GCs, systemic as well as inhaled, should therefore be monitored with regard to their effects on lower leg growth during development. Lower leg growth seems to be an established parameter to get an idea of how the growth of children is affected by GCs.

Effects on bone

Osteoporosis is one of the undesired effects of GCs that patients are extremely afraid of. This fear is not baseless because GC therapy is the most common cause of osteoporosis in adults aged between 20 and 45 years (Alesci et al., 2005). Osteoporosis has been reported to occur in up to 50% of patients who receive systemic long-term GC therapy. However, even within the first months of treatment an increased risk of fractures has been seen in patients. Bone loss induced by GCs occurs most rapidly within the first 12 months after starting therapy. Thereafter it decelerates but continues during the whole treatment time. In young patients GC-induced bone loss can be reversible. This has been demonstrated by recovery in bone density following successful treatment of Cushing's syndrome (Pocock et al., 1987).

Under physiological conditions bones undergo a permanent remodelling process that balances bone resorption and bone formation. GCs directly affect bone metabolism by several mechanisms. Glucocorticoids can alter the regulation of bone cells (osteoblasts, osteoclasts, osteocytes), induce apoptosis in osteoblasts, affect the regulation of calcium flux and decrease gonadal steroid production (oestrogens and androgens).

The negative regulatory effect of GCs on bone formation is mainly due to inhibition of proliferation and possibly also differentiation of osteoblasts. Not only the reduced cell number but also a direct inhibitory effect of GCs on the synthesis of bone matrix proteins (such as osteocalcin, type I collagen, fibronectin and α1 integrin) are involved in a significantly decreased bone formation. It has been shown that GCs can inhibit synthesis of the anabolic growth factor (insulin growth factor [IGF]-1), the major bone matrix protein (BMP)-2, the osteoblastic transcription factor Cbfa1 and the osteoblast marker genes osteocalcin and osteopontin. They also exert a negative effect on osteocytes, which represent the first responders to changes in mechanical loading and microdamage of the bone. GCs inhibit formation as well as enhance apoptosis of both osteocytes and osteoblasts. GCs reduce bone mass not only due to a decrease in bone formation but also by an increased bone resorption. GC treatment increases the bone-resorbing activity of osteoclasts. They interfere with the receptor activator nuclear factor-κB ligand (RANKL)–osteoprotegerin (OPG) axis, which is part of osteoclastogenesis. RANKL expressed in osteoblasts binds to RANK on the surface of osteoclasts to induce osteoclast differentiation. OPG is also expressed by osteoblasts and functions as a decoy receptor of RANKL, avoiding the binding of RANKL to RANK and thus inhibiting osteoclast differentiation. GCs inhibit the expression of OPG and, in parallel, enhance the expression of RANKL, leading to a shift of the steady state to osteoclast differentiation (Miner et al., 2005; Sambrook, 2002).

In addition, long-term high-dose GC treatment can result in decreased intestinal calcium absorption, increased renal calcium excretion and increased serum parathyroid hormone levels (PTH). No changes in plasma 1,25-dihydroxyvitamin D are seen. As a consequence of these GC activities, a reduction in serum calcium level occurs that is available to form new bone (Miner et al., 2005).

Sex hormones are important to maintain the physiological bone metabolism. It has been shown that hypogonadism often is associated with the development of osteoporosis. Negative effects of GCs on sex hormones are mainly mediated via their inhibitory effects on the hypothalamic-pituitary-gonadal axis. They can inhibit the pituitary secretion of gonadotrophins. In parallel, GCs also have direct effects on target tissues of gonadal steroids (Miner et al., 2005). Glucocorticoid effects on muscle (see below) might also support the development of GC-induced osteoporosis.

To minimize the risk of fractures, patients undergoing long-term systemic GC treatment should be monitored carefully on a regular basis regarding their bone density. At best, prevention of GC-induced osteoporosis should start as soon as GC treatment begins. Wherever possible, unstable steroids delivered topically (e.g. inhaled, dermal) should be used for chronic GC treatment. Moreover, medical treatments of GC-induced osteoporosis to prevent and minimize bone loss and to increase bone mineral density should be used as long as GC therapy is required.

Effects on muscle

The loss of muscle mass and the development of muscle weakness are also consequences of long-term GC therapy. GC-induced myopathy and muscle atrophy can
increase the potential for falls and probably contribute to the high fracture rate
for patients. Frequencies of up to 50–60% have been described for myopathy and
muscle weakness in several patient populations (Batchelor et al., 1997; Lee et al.,
2005). In muscle biopsies from GC-treated patients, a selective atrophy of type IIa
muscle fibres associated with a relative increase of type IIb fibres and a decrease in
the number of type I fibres was found (Alesci et al., 2005).

Effects of GCs on muscle include an increased protein catabolism, inhibition of
glucose uptake into the muscle, inhibition of protein synthesis and an interference
with the fatty acid β-oxidation. There are hints from animal experiments that GC-
induced apoptosis of myocytes may also play a role in the development of myopathy
(Lee et al., 2005). Increased protein catabolism seems to be mediated at least in
part via a stimulation of the ubiquitin–proteasome-dependent protein breakdown
in skeletal muscle (Price et al., 2001). An increase in myostatin expression has
been shown to be associated with GC-induced muscle weakness (Ma et al., 2003)
and is suggested to play a key role in increased proteolytic activity in the muscle.
Dexamethasone treatment of myostatin knockout did not lead to an upregulation
of proteasome–ubibiquitin system components, and, in parallel, no muscle atrophy
has been found (Gilson et al., 2006). Glutamine synthetase, responsible for forming
glutamine, is also known to be upregulated by GCs. Glutamine efflux accounts for
25–30% of the total protein export from skeletal muscle during GC-induced myopathy (LaPier, 1997). Not only increased catabolic but also a decrease in anabolic
activities can be induced by GCs (Sjogren et al., 1999). GC treatment decreases the
expression of skeletal muscle IGF-1 (Gayan-Ramirez et al., 1999) which is involved
in the development of GC-induced muscle myopathy (Schakman et al., 2005).

Although a number of singular mechanisms are described in the context of GC-
induced muscle atrophy, the whole mechanism is not completely understood. In
comparison many more studies to investigate GC-induced osteoporosis have been
performed. However, myopathy and/or atrophy of the muscle seem to be associated with the development of GC-induced osteoporosis, and therefore this undesired
effect should be monitored in a similar manner to osteoporosis.

Hyperglycaemia/insulin resistance

High-dose and/or long-term oral GC treatment can result in the development of
hyperglycaemia and insulin resistance, which might end up in the manifestation or
exacerbation of diabetes mellitus. GC excess can induce both decreased beta-cell
insulin production and insulin resistance, which can lead to a reduced effectiveness
of insulin to suppress hepatic glucose production and increased glucose uptake in
muscle and fat tissue (Andrews and Walker, 1999). GC-related hyperglycaemia is

dose-dependent and can be induced even with low-dose GC treatment (Da Silva et al., 2006). Hyperglycaemia is usually rapidly reversed when GCs are stopped, but some patients will go on to develop persistent diabetes (Hricik et al., 1991).

Incidence of diabetes mellitus is about 30–40% in patients with hypercortisolism due to Cushing's syndrome (Biering et al., 2000). Diabetes is also a common complication in patients with organ transplants. In up to 40% of prednisone-treated renal transplant patients the development of a so-called post-transplant diabetes has been observed (Onwubgalili and Obineche, 1992). In heart and liver transplant patients the incidence is not as high as in renal transplant patients, with about 16% and 19%, respectively (Depczynski et al., 2000; Gonzales-Quintela et al., 1995).

Glucocorticoids decrease insulin receptor signalling molecules and reduce insulin-mediated increase in blood flow to muscles (Laakso et al., 1990), and, in parallel, they enhance glucose output by increasing the important enzymes of gluconeogenesis (Miner et al., 2005). Several enzymes that catabolize amino acids, such as tyrosine aminotransferase (TAT) or aspartate aminotransferase (AAT), have been shown to be induced by GCs. Promoters of both genes contain specific regulatory sequences for the glucocorticoid receptor (GR), so-called glucocorticoid response elements (GREs) (Beurton, 1999; Rigaud, 1991). Similar binding elements are found in genes of two enzymes that catalyse key steps of gluconeogenesis, glucose-6-phosphatase (G6Pase) and phosphoenolpyruvate carboxykinase (PEPCK) (Yoshiuchi, 1998). The GC-induced upregulation of gluconeogenic machinery leads to an increased glucose production followed by an increased glycogen storage in liver.

Immunological side effects

Due to their anti-inflammatory and immunomodulatory activity, GC therapy can lead to an enhanced risk of infection. On the other hand, inflammatory phenomena such as dermatitis and acne (see effects on skin) as well as an allergy to GC can result from inhaled GC therapy.

Systemic infection

Long-term oral GC therapy is associated with an enhanced risk of systemic and pulmonary infections (Stuck et al, 1989). Secondary infections may also occur in patients receiving short courses of systemic GCs for pulmonary disease exacerbations (Niewoehner, 2002). An association of inhaled GCs with pulmonary or systemic infections is discussed but has not been proven yet.

An enhanced risk of disseminated varicella infection, as is known for systemic GCs (Dowell and Bresee, 1993), has been indicated by case reports also for inhaled GC therapy and has raised the concerns of physicians (Choong et al., 1995; Irwin and

Richardson, 2006). However, no causal relationship has been shown (Welch, 1994), and varicella vaccination was not included in the recommendations for patients receiving inhaled GCs (National Asthma Education and Prevention Program, 1997). Reactivation of tuberculosis is also discussed as a side effect of inhaled GCs, and Shaikh (1992) reported 8 cases out of 548 asthmatics (1.46%) treated with inhaled beclomethasone seen over a 2-year period. Bahceciler et al. (2000), however, observed that inhaled GC therapy is safe in tuberculin-positive asthmatic children. Moreover, whereas GCs are used as adjuvant therapy in tuberculous meningitis and pericardial and pleural disease, an enhanced risk of tuberculosis reactivation is discussed but not proven for systemic GCs (Alzeer and FitzGerald, 1993; Jick et al., 2006).

Allergy to glucocorticoids

In the late 1950s the first case report of allergic contact dermatitis from hydrocortisone appeared (Burckhardt, 1959). The commonest GCs found to cause a reaction in patients who are patch-tested are non-halogenated steroids such as hydrocortisone and budesonide (Isaksson and Dooms-Gossens, 1997). Whereas contact dermatitis may be most frequent (English, 2000), mucocutaneous and respiratory reactions, and generalized eczematous reactions have been described (Cadinha et al., 2005; Kilpiö and Hannuksela, 2003; Poon and Fewings, 2001). Budesonide has been included in the European standard series as a marker for GC allergy. Cross-allergy between GCs is common (Ferguson et al., 2002). However, patients with GC allergy usually tolerate some other common GCs.

Glucocorticoid effects on skin

Skin atrophy

Skin atrophy represents the most frequent side effect of long-term topical GCs in the treatment of dermatoses. It also can be seen after short-term treatment of many acute and chronic conditions in children (Schou et al., 2003a, b). Clinical studies demonstrated that in patients receiving long-term inhaled GCs the risk of skin thinning and easy bruising was elevated (Irwin and Richardson, 2006).

Skin atrophy is characterized by a strongly increased transparency of skin, a cigarette-paper-like consistency accompanied by an increased fragility, bruising and a telangiectatic surface (Schoepe et al., 2006). The barrier function of the skin between the external milieu and the organism is disturbed leading to an increased transepidermal water loss. Histologically, a thinner epidermis, flattened dermal-epidermal junctions, reduced numbers of keratinocytes and fibroblasts, and reduced amounts of glycosaminoglycans are seen after GC treatment (Ahn et al., 2006; Schoepe et al., 2006).

Similarly as for many other side effects, several mechanisms are involved in the development of skin atrophy. First of all, GCs display negative effects on proliferation of keratinocytes and fibroblasts (Lange et al., 2000). As a consequence of the inhibition of keratinocyte proliferation, the epidermis becomes thinner leading to an increased permeability and water loss. Fibroblasts are the major synthesis places for many proteins of the extracellular matrix (ECM), so a reduced number of fibroblasts might contribute to the decrease in ECM proteins. Also, GCs directly inhibit the synthesis of collagens, some proteoglycans and other ECM proteins (Schoepe et al., 2006). Collagens represent a major component of the ECM, with 70% of the dry weight of the skin. Expression of type I and type III collagens has been shown to be inhibited by GCs on mRNA and protein levels. Prolyl hydroxylase, an enzyme important for the generation of collagen triple helices, is inhibited by GCs on the level of mRNA expression as well as on activity (Nuutinen et al., 2001; Oikarinen and Hannuksela, 1980).

Delayed wound healing

Delayed wound healing after systemic GC treatment is commonly observed and has been proven experimentally (Davidson, 1998; Grose et al., 2002, Schäcke et al., 2002). Wound healing is a complex process requiring tissue regeneration and is regulated by several cytokines and growth factors as well as by several constituents of the ECM (Beer et al., 2000; Martin, 1997; Singer and Clark, 1999).

In the beginning an inflammatory process is critical for an efficient wound healing, so the negative effects of GCs on wound healing might be (at least in part) a direct consequence of their anti-inflammatory activity (Anstead, 1998; Miner et al., 2005). In addition, the anti-proliferative effects of GCs on keratinocytes and dermal fibroblasts might contribute to the inhibition of wound healing (Hengge et al., 2006).

Other glucocorticoid side effects on skin

Inhaled GC therapy induces these side effects to a lesser extent than oral therapy. Several case reports describe acne (Monk et al., 1993) or perioral dermatitis (Held et al., 1997) induced by inhaled GC therapy. Furthermore, hirsutism has been observed sporadically in patients also showing other systemic side effects of inhaled GC therapy (Patel et al., 2001).

The undesired effects of systemic GCs on skin represent more than cosmetic problems only. The skin represents the barrier between the environment and the organism. If this barrier is disturbed, an increased risk of infections and a disturbance of water balance can be the consequences.

Glucocorticoid effects on the eye

GC treatment also can lead to the induction of adverse effects on eyes. Although adverse ocular effects seem to be rather rare, they can be severe and even irreversible. Many adverse ocular effects have been described, such as delayed wound healing, increased risk for infections and others. However, the most prominent adverse ophthalmic effects are cataracts and glaucoma (Allen et al., 2003).

Regarding inhaled GCs there are only limited data available on ocular effects. Although it is not clearly shown that long-term, high-dose inhaled GCs are involved in the induction of glaucoma and cataracts, clinical evidence is given at least in elderly patients and/or patients with a family history of glaucoma (Allen et al., 2003; Irwin and Richardson 2006).Especially for the induction of these adverse ocular effects, a correlation between dose, duration of treatment, administration route, the age of patients and the existence of concomitant diseases such as diabetes mellitus seems to be important.

Glaucoma

GCs can induce an increased intraocular pressure (IOP) that can lead to damage of the optic nerve and blindness as an end effect. Since the 1950s development of glaucoma is known as an undesired effect of the use of exogenous GCs. Glaucoma presents the second leading cause of blindness in the elderly in the USA whereas significant racial and ethnic differences regarding sensitivity exist (Allen et al., 2003).

In approximately 5% of the population the IOP starts to increase 2–4 weeks after starting GC therapy (Armaly, 1965). Ultimately, 18–36% of the population will respond to GC therapy with at least a moderate increase of IOP. The risk of GC responsiveness is dependent on age (>40 years), family history of glaucoma and the appearance of other systemic diseases such as diabetes mellitus. In patients with primary open-angle glaucoma the prevalence of GC responsiveness increases to 46–92% (Allen et al. 2003).

Long-term GC treatment leads to an accumulation of ECM proteins in the eye, resulting in an inhibited outflow of aqueous fluid through the Schlemm canal. Increased amounts of glycosaminoglycans, fibronectin, elastin, laminin, collagen types I and type IV and myocilin have been described as being involved in the increase of IOP. GCs increase the synthesis of these ECM proteins and in parallel they reduce proteolysis of these proteins by decreased synthesis of proteolytic enzymes. Additionally, a reduced phagocytic activity and a reorganization of cytoskeletal elements are induced by GCs.

Although older patients have a higher risk of developing an increase of IOP in response to exogenous GCs, induction of GC-induced glaucoma is a problem in children as well as adults. Often, inhaled GCs have to be supported by additional systemic GC treatments, dependent on disease activity. Therefore, it is not easy to describe the risk for an increased IOP in asthma therapy for both forms of therapy separately. By determining IOP on a regular basis, changes in IOP should be monitored carefully during long-term as well as short-term high-dose therapies.

Cataract

Development of posterior subcapsular cataract presents the second major adverse ocular effect in GC therapy (Allen at al., 2003). An increased risk for the development of cataracts has long been known for systemic GC treatment (Black et al., 1960). It is an adverse effect that typically requires long-term treatment and is developed only after months to years of GC therapy.

Cataract occurrence is related to age, with more than 50% of cataracts being developed in individuals older than 65. Secondary cataracts are developed in response to GC treatment or in patients suffering from diabetes mellitus (Allen et al., 2003).

Factors that participate in the development of GC-induced cataract include an increased glucose level, the inhibition of Na^+/K^+-ATPase, inhibition of RNA synthesis and, most importantly, a covalent binding of steroids to lens proteins forming the typical adducts of GC-induced cataracts (Kojima et al., 1995; Manabe et al., 1984).

In clinical studies, correlation of cataract occurrence with the current daily dose and duration of systemic therapy has been observed. This correlation could not be established for dose and duration of inhaled GC therapy. These results, however, did not exclude the possibility that inhaled GCs might also lead to cataracts, especially in older patients (Allen et al., 2003).

GC-induced psychotic and mood disorders

GCs can induce psychiatric syndromes, including depression, mania, psychosis and delirium, which are often subsumed as "steroid psychosis" representing an exogenous psychiatric disorder. However, steroid psychosis is not a specific clinical entity but consists of heterogeneous syndromes with likely different pathophysiological mechanisms. Moreover, GCs induce mood disorders in a higher frequency than psychoses. Dose-dependent changes and recurrent psychiatric syndromes are observed in clinical practice (Brown et al., 1999; Wada et al., 2001). In a recent study, a 1% prevalence of psychotic and mood disorders has been described for GC-treated patients (Wada et al., 2001).

Sporadic cases of neuropsychological and behavioural changes and even psychosis have also been reported for inhaled GC therapy in both adults and children. Symptoms disappear with termination of medication and recur when the inhalation of GCs is reinitiated at higher doses (Hederos, 2004). Short-term systemic treatment for acute asthma exacerbation may lead to acute behavioural effects (Kayani and Shannon, 2002). However, it has also been shown that poor disease control and poor adherence to inhaled steroids have the main impact on psychological morbidity in asthma patients (Cluley and Cochrane, 2001).

Whereas the mechanisms leading to GC-induced psychiatric syndromes are not clear and might be diverse, many lines of evidence, including animal experiments and clinical studies demonstrating HPA axis hyperactivity and therapeutic activity of CRH and GC antagonists in depression, indicate a general role of the stress mediator GCs for endogenous psychiatric disorders as well as for physiological control of behaviour (Holtzheimer and Nemeroff, 2006; Müller et al., 2004).

2.3 Summary

GCs have been used for more than 50 years very successfully in the treatment of acute and chronic inflammatory and autoimmune diseases. However, the success was also accompanied by the development of many adverse effects (Figure 2.1). The development and extent of adverse effects depend upon several factors that can be allocated to the drug, the therapy or the treated individual (see also Table 2.1). There are side effects that are present particularly in children (e.g. growth retardation), in elderly patients (e.g. osteoporosis, cataract and glaucoma, diabetes mellitus) or in women (e.g. more sensitive to develop skin atrophy, osteoporosis). Depending on the risk taken by an individual patient, monitoring of side effect induction should be initiated in parallel with the start of therapy.

The risk of developing systemic side effects is much higher for systemic GC therapy then for topical, including inhaled therapy. Nevertheless, for inhaled GC therapy, as for any other therapy, a risk/benefit decision has to be made by the physician and the patient. Risk of adverse effects should be minimized by using the lowest effective dose of a carefully selected inhaled GC, by using additive non-glucocorticoid anti-inflammatory therapies (e.g. long-acting β_2-agonists, theophyllines, leukotriene antagonists) instead of increasing GC dosage, and by minimizing systemic availability of the GC as well as local side effects through careful selection of the inhalation device as well as proper technique. For dose selection it has to be kept in mind that anti-inflammatory efficacy of current inhaled GCs might plateau at moderate doses whereas adverse effects do not, and that patients may show strong differences in sensitivity to specific GCs.

When assessing the patient's risk for adverse effects, additional GC treatments (e.g. nasal for rhinitis and dermal for atopic eczema) have to be taken into account.

Possible drug–drug interactions that hamper the systemic clearance of GCs have to be considered and should be avoided whenever possible. When long-term, high-dose inhaled GC therapy is required, periodic evaluations of adrenal function and bone density may be advisable. Any evidence of systemic side effects (e.g. growth retardation in children or the development of a cushingoid habitus) should be taken seriously and should lead to additional diagnostics. Whenever GCs are strongly reduced in dosage or withdrawn as well as in cases of severe stress (e.g. surgery), the potential risk for adrenal insufficiency has to be considered. Any symptom suspicious for adrenal insufficiency has to be followed up.

In conclusion, current inhaled GCs are highly effective and, when appropriately used, have a low risk of severe adverse effects. New drugs might further decrease the local and systemic side effects by better targeting drug activity to the lung (e.g. on-site activation) as well as by improving the pharmacological profile, resulting in a superior therapeutic index.

References

Ahn SK, Bak HN, Park BD et al. Effects of a multilamellar emulsion on glucocorticoid-induced epidermal atrophy and barrier impairment. *J Dermatol* 2006; **33**: 80–90.

Alesci S, De Martino MU, Ilias I et al. Glucocorticoid-induced osteoporosis: from basic mechanisms to clinical aspects. *Neuroimmunomodulation* 2005; **12**: 1–19.

Allen DB. Systemic effects of inhaled corticosteroids in children. *Curr Opin Pediatr* 2004; **16**: 440–444.

Allen DB. Effects of inhaled steroids on growth, bon metabolism, and adrenal function. *Adv Pediatr* 2006; **53**: 101–110.

Allen DB, Bielory L, Derendorf H et al. Inhaled corticosteroids: Past lessons and future issues. *J Allergy Clin Immunol* 2003; **112**: S1–40.

Alzeer AH, FitzGerald JM. Corticosteroids and tuberculosis: risks and use as adjunct therapy. *Tuber Lung Dis* 1993; **74**: 6–11.

Andrews RC, Walker BR. Glucocorticoids and insulin resistance: old hormones, new targets. *Clin Sci* 1999; **96**: 513–523.

Armaly MF. Statistical attributes of the steroid hypertensive response in clinically normal eye. I: The demonstration of three levels of response. *Invest Ophthalmol Vis Sci* 1965; **4**: 187–191.

Axelrod L. Perioperative management of patients treated with glucocorticoids. *Endocrinol Metab Clin North Am* 2003; **32**: 367–383.

Bahceciler NN, Nuhoglu Y, Nursoy MA et al. Inhaled corticosteroid therapy is safe in tuberculin-positive asthmatic children. *Pediatr Infect Dis J* 2000; **19**: 215–218.

Batchelor L, Nance J, Short B. An interdisciplinary team approach to implementing the ketogenic diet for the treatment of seizures. *Pediatr Nurs* 1997; **23**: 465–471.

Beer HD, Fässler R, Werner S. Glucocorticoid-regulated gene expression during cutaneous wound repair. *Vitam Horm* 2000; **59**: 217–223.

Bell NH. The glucocorticoid withdrawal syndrome. *Adv Exp Med Biol* 1984; **171**: 293–299.

Beurton F, Bandyopadhyay U, Dieumgard B et al. Delineation of insulin-responsive in rat cytosolic aspartate aminotransferase gene: binding sites for hepatocyte nuclear factor-3 and and nuclear factor I. *Biochem J* 1999; **343**: 687–695.

Biering H, Knappe G, Gerl H, Lochs H. Prevalence of diabetes in acromegali and Cushing's syndrome. *Acta Med Austr,* 2000; **27**: 27–31.

Black RL, Oglesby RB, von Sallmann L, Bunim JJ. Posterior subcapsular cataracts induced by corticosteroids in patients with rheumatoid arthritis. *JAMA* 1960; **1174**: 166–171.

Bolland MJ, Bagg W, Thomas MG et al. Cushing's syndrome due to interaction between inhaled corticosteroids and itraconazole. *Ann Pharmacother* 2004; **38**: 46–49.

Brown ES, Khan DA, Nejtek VA. The psychiatric side effects of corticosteroids Ann Allergy. *Asthma Immunol* 1999; **83**: 495–503.

Burckhardt W. [Contact eczema caused by hydrocortisone] *Hautarzt* 1959; **10**: 42–43.

Cadinha S, Malheiro D, Rodrigues J et al. Delayed hypersensitivity reactions to corticosteroids. *Allergol Immunopathol (Madr)* 2005; **33**: 329–332.

Childhood Asthma Management Program Research Group. Long-term effects of budesonide or nedocronial in children with asthma. *N Engl J Med* 2000; **343**: 1054–1063.

Chisholm D, Chalkley S. Cushing's syndrome from an inhaled glucocorticoid. *Med J Aust* 1994; **161**: 232.

Choong K, Zwaigenbaum L, Onyett H. Severe varicella after low dose inhaled corticosteroids *Pediatr Infect Dis J* 1995; **14**: 809–811.

Chrousos GP, Harris AG. Hypothalamic-pituitary-adrenal axis suppression and inhaled corticosteroid therapy. 1. General principles. *Neuroimmunomodulation* 1998; **5**: 277–287.

Chrousos GP, Ghaly L, Shedden A et al. Effects of mometasone furoate dry powder inhaler and beclomethasone dipropionate hydrofluoroalkane and chlorofluorocarbon on the hypothalamic-pituitary-adrenal axis in asthmatic subjects. *Chest* 2005; **128**: 70–77.

Cluley S, Cochrane GM. Psychological disorder in asthma is associated with poor control and poor adherence to inhaled steroids. *Respir Med* 2001; **95**: 37–39.

Crowley S. Inhaled glucocorticoids and adrenal function: an update. *Paediatr Respir Rev* 2003; **4**: 153–161.

Da Silva JAP, Jacobs JWG, Kirwan JR et al. Safety of low dose glucocorticoid treatment in rheumatoid arthritis: published evidence and prospective trial data. *Ann Rheum Dis* 2006; **65**: 285–293.

Davidson JM. Animal models for wound repair *Arch Dermatol Res 290 Suppl*: 1998, S1–11.

Depczynski B, Daly B, Campbell EV et al. Prediction the occurence of diabetes mellitus in recipients of heart transplants. *Diabet Med* 2000; **17**: 15–19.

Dowell SF and Bresee JS. Severe varicella associated with steroid use. *Pediatrics* 1993; **92**: 223–228.

Dubus JC, Marguet C, Deschildre A et al. Local side-effects of inhaled corticosteroids in asthmatic children: influence of drug, dose, age, and device. *Allergy* 2001; **56**: 944–948.

Ducharme FM, Chabot G, Polychronakos C et al. Safety profile of frequent short courses of oral glucocorticoids in acute pediatric asthma: impact on bone metabolism, bone density and adrenal function. *Pediatrics* 2003; **111**: 376–383.

English JS. Corticosteroid–induced contact dermatitis: a pragmatic approach. *Clin Exp Dermatol* 2000; **25**: 261–264.

Ferguson AD, Emerson RM, English JS. Cross-reactivity patterns to budesonide. *Contact Dermatitis* 2002; **47**: 337–340.

Gayan-Ramirez G, Vanderhoydonc F, Verhoeven G, Decramer M. Acute treatment with corticosteroids decreases IGF–1 and IGF–2 expression in the rat diaphragm and gastrocnemius. *Am J Respir Crit Care Med* 1999; **159**: 283–289.

Gilson H, Schakman O, Combaret L et al. Myostatin gene deletion prevents glucocorticoid–induced muscle atrophy. *Endocrinology* 2007; **148**: 452–460.

Gonzales-Quintela A, De la Mata M, Varo E et al. Incidence of new onset of diabetes mellitus in liver transplant recipients immunosuppressed with deflazacort. *TANSE* 1995; **6**: 107–115.

Grose R, Werner S, Kessler D et al. A role of endogenous glucocorticoids in wound repair. *EMBO Rep* 2002; **3**: 575–582.

Hederos CA. Neuropsychologic changes and inhaled corticosteroids. *J Allergy Clin Immunol* 2004; **114**: 451–452.

Held E, Ottevanger V, Petersen CS, Weismann K. [Perioral dermatitis in children under steroid inhalation therapy] *Ugeskr Laeger* 1997; **159**: 7002–7003.

Hench PS, Kendall EC, Slocumb CH, Polley HF. Effects of hormone of adrenal cortex (17-hydroy-11-dehydrocorticosterone, Compound E) and of pituitary adrenocorticotropic hormone on rheumatoid arthritis: preliminary report. *Proc Staff Meet, Mayo Clin* 1949; **24**: 181–197.

Hengge UR, Ruzicka T, Schwartz RA, Cork MJ. Adverse effects of topical glucocorticosteroids. *J Am Acad Dermatol* 2006; **54**: 1–15.

Holtzheimer PE 3rd, Nemeroff CB. Emerging treatments for depression. *Expert Opin Pharmacother* 2006; **7**: 2323–2339.

Hopkins RL, Leinung MC. Exogenous Cushing's syndrome and glucocorticoid withdrawal. *Endocrinol Metab Clin North Am* 2005; **34**: 371–384, ix.

Hricik DE, Bartucci MR, Moir EJ et al. Influence of corticosteroid withdrawal on posttransplant diabetes mellitus in cyclosporine–treated renal transplant recipients. *Transplant Proc 23* 1991; **2**: 1007–1008.

Irwin RS, Richardson ND. Side effects with inhaled corticosteroids: the physicians perception. *Chest* 2006; **130**: 41S–53S.

Isaksson M, Dooms-Goossens AN. Contact allergens – what's new? Corticosteroids. *Clin Dermatol* 1997; **15**: 527–553.

Jacobson L. Hypothalamic-pituitary-adrenocortical axis regulation. *Endocrinol Metab Clin North Am* 2005; **34**: 271–292.

Jick SS, Lieberman ES, Rahman MU, Choi HK. Glucocorticoid use other associated factors and the risk of tuberculosis. *Arthritis Rheum* 2006; **55**: 19–26.

Kanda N, Yasuba H, Takahashi T et al. Prevalence of esophageal candidiasis among patients treated with inhaled fluticasone propionate. *Am J Gastroenterol* 2003; **98**: 2146–2148.

Kayani S, Shannon DC. Adverse behavioral effects of treatment for acute exacerbation of asthma in children: a comparison of two doses of oral steroids. *Chest* 2002; **122**: 624–628.

Keller-Wood ME, Dallman MF. Corticosteroid inhibition of ACTH secretion. *Endocr Rev* 1984; **5**: 1–24.

Kilpio K, Hannuksela M. Corticosteroid allergy in asthma. *Allergy* 2003; **58**: 1131–1135.

Kojima M, Shui YB, Sasaki K. Topographic distribution of prednisolone in the lens after organ culture. *Ophthalmol Res* 1995; **27**: 25–33.

Laakso M, Edelman SV, Brechtel G, Baron AD. Decreased effect of insulin to stimulate skeletal muscle blood flow in obese man. A novel mechanism for insulin resistance. *J Clin Invest* 1990; **85**: 1844–1852.

Lange K, Kleuser N, Gysler A et al. Cutaneous inflammation and proliferation in vitro: differential effects and mode of action of topical glucocorticoids. *Skin Pharmacol Appl Skin Physiol* 2000; **13**: 93–103.

Lapier TK. 9C-induced muscle atrophy. The role of exercise in treatment and prevention. *J Cardiopulm Rehabil* 1997; **17**: 76–84.

Lee MC, Wee GG, Kim JH. Apoptosis of skeletal muscle on steroid-induced myopathy in rats. *J Nutr* 2005; **135**: 1806S–1808S.

Lipworth BJ. Systemic adverse effects of inhaled corticosteroid therapy: A systematic review and meta-analysis. *Arch Intern Med* 1999; **159**: 941–955.

Ma K, Mallidis C, Bhansin S et al. Glucocorticod–induced skeletal muscle atrophy is associated with upregulation of myostatin gene expression. *Am J Physiol Endocrinol Metab* 2003; **285**: E363–371.

Macdessi JS, Randell TL, Donaghue KC et al. Adrenal crises in children treated with high–dose inhaled corticosteroids for asthma. *Med J Aust* 2003; **178**: 214–216.

Manabe S, Bucala R, Cerami A. Nonenzymatic addition of GCs to lens proteins in steroid–induced cataracts. *J Clin Invest* 1984; **74**: 1803–1810.

Martin P. Wound healing – aiming for perfect skin regeneration. *Science* 1997; **276**: 75–81.

Mason HC, Myers CS and Kendall EC. The chemistry of crystalline substances isolated from the suprarenal gland. *J Biol Chem* 1936; **114**: 613–631.

Miner J, Hong MH, Negro-Vilar. A New and improved glucocorticoid receptor ligands. *Expert Opin Invest Drugs* 2005; **14**: 1527–1545.

Monk B, Cunliffe WJ, Layton AM, Rhodes DJ. Acne induced by inhaled corticosteroids. *Clin Exp Dermatol* 1993; **18**: 148–150.

Müller MB, Uhr M, Holsboer F, Keck ME. Hypothalamic-pituitary-adrenocortical system and mood disorders: highlights from mutant mice. *Neuroendocrinology* 2004; **79**: 1–12.

National Asthma Education and Prevention *Program. Expert Panel Report 2: Guidelines for the Diagnosis and Management of Asthma*, publication No 97–4051. Bethesda MD: National Institutes of Health, 1997.

Nicholl RM, Greenough A, King M et al. Growth effects of systemic versus inhaled steroids in chronic lung diseases. *Arch Dis Child Fetal Neonatal Ed* 2002; **87**: F59–F61.

Nicholson G, Burrin JM, Hall GM. Peri-operative steroid supplementation. *Anaesthesia* 1998; **53**: 1091–1104.

Niewoehner DE. The role of systemic corticosteroids in acute exacerbation of chronic obstructive pulmonary disease. *Am J Respir Med* 2002; **1**: 243–248.

Nuutinen P, Autio P, Hurskainen T, Oikarinen A. Glucocorticoid action on skin collagen. overview on clinical significance and consequences. *J Eur Acad Dermatol Venerol* 2001; **15**: 361–362.

Oelkers W. Adrenal insufficiency. *N Engl J Med* 1996; **335**: 1206–1212.

Oikarinen A, Hannuksela M. Effect of hydrocortisone-17-butyrat hydrocortisone and clobetasol-17-propionate on prolyl hydroxylase activity in human skin. *Arch Derm Res* 1980; **267**: 79–82.

Onwubalili JK, Obineche EN. High incidence of post-transplant diabetes mellitus in a single-centre study. *Nephrol Dial Transplant* 1992; **7**: 346–349.

Ozbek OY, Turktas I, Bakirtas A, Bideci A. Evaluation of hypothalamic-pituitary-adrenal axis suppression by low-dose (0.5 μg) and standard-dose (250 μg) adrenocorticotropic hormone (ACTH) tests in asthmatic children treated with inhaled corticosteroid. *J Pediatr Endocrinol Metab* 2006; **19**: 1015–1023.

Patel L, Wales JK, Kibirige MS et al. Symptomatic adrenal insufficiency during inhaled corticosteroid treatment. *Arch Dis Child* 2001; **85**: 330–334.

Pocock NA, Eisman JA, Dunstan CR et al. Recovery from steroid–induced osteoporosis. *Ann Intern Med* 1987; **107**: 319–323.

Poon E, Fewings JM. Generalized eczematous reaction to budesonide in a nasal spray with cross-reactivity to triamcinolone. *Australas J Dermatol* 2001; **42**: 36–37.

Price JM, Du JD, Bailey JL, Griffin MR. Molecular mechanisms regulating protein turnover in muscle. *Am J Kidney Dis* 2001; **37**: S112–S114.

Reichardt HM, Kaestner KH, Tuckermann J et al. DNA binding of the glucocorticoid receptor is not essential for survival. *Cell* 1998; **93**: 531–541.

Rigaud G, Roux J, Pictet R, Grange T. In vivo footprinting of rat TAT gene: dynamic interplay between GC receptor and a liver-specific factor. *Cell* 1991; **67**: 977–986.

Samaras K, Pett S, Gowers A et al. Iatrogenic Cushing's syndrome with osteoporosis and secondary adrenal failure in human immunodeficiency virus-infected patients receiving inhaled corticosteroids and ritonavir-boosted protease inhibitors: six cases. *J Clin Endocrinol Metab* 2005; **90**: 4394–4398.

Sambrook PN. Glucocorticoid osteoporosis. *Curr Pharm Design* 2002; **8**: 1877–1883.

Schäcke H, Döcke WD, Asadullah K. Mechanisms involved in the side effects of glucocorticoids. *Pharmacol Ther* 2002; **96**: 23–43.

Schäcke H, Rehwinkel H, Asadullah K, Cato AC. Insight into the molecular mechanisms of glucocorticoid receptor action promotes identification of novel ligands with an improved therapeutic index. *Exp Dermatol* 2006; **15**: 565–573.

Schoepe S, Schäcke H, May E, Asadullah K. Glucocorticoid therapy-induced skin atrophy. *Exp Dermatol* 2006; **15**: 406–420.

Schou AJ, Heuck C, Wolthers OD. Differential effects of short-term prednisolone treatment on peripheral and abdominal subcutaneous thickness in children assessed by ultrasound. *Steroids* 2003; **68**: 525–531.

Schou AJ, Heuck C, Wolthers OD. Ultrasound of skin in prednisolone-induced short-term growth suppression. *J Pediatr Endocrinol & Metab* 2003b; **16**: 973–980.

Shaikh WA. Pulmonary tuberculosis in patients treated with inhaled beclomethasone. *Allergy* 1992; **47**: 327–330.

Shakman O, Gilson H, de Conink V et al. Insulin-like growth factor-I gene transfer by electropoation prevents skeletal muscle atrophy in glucocorticoid-treated rats. *Endocrinology* 2005; **146**: 1789–1797.

Singer AJ, Clark RA. Cutaneous wound healing. *N Engl J Med* 1999; **341**: 738–746.

Sjogren K, Liu JL, Blad K et al. Liver-derived insulin-like growth factor I IGF-I is the principal source of IGF-I in blood but is not required for postnatal body growth in mice. *Proc Natl Acad Sci USA* 1999; **96**: 7088–7092.

Storms WW, Theen C. Clinical adverse effects of inhaled corticosteroids: results of a questionnaire survey of asthma specialists. *Ann Allergy Asthma Immunol* 1998; **80**: 391–394.

Stuck AE, Minder CE, Frey FJ. Risk of infectious complications in patients taking glucocorticosteroids. *Rev Infect Dis* 1989; **11**: 954–963.

Toogood JH, Jenning B, Greenway RW, Chuang L. Candidiasis and dysphonia complicating beclomethasone treatment of asthma. *J Allergy Clin Immunol* 1980; **65**: 146–153.

Wada K, Yamada N, Sato T et al. Corticosteroid-induced psychotic and mood disorders: diagnosis defined by DSM-IV and clinical pictures. *Psychosomatics* 2001; **42**: 461–466.

Welch MJ. Inhaled steroids and severe viral infections. *J Asthma* 1994; **31**: 43–50.

Williamson IJ, Matusiewicz SP, Brown PH et al. Frequency of voice problems and cough in patients using pressurized aerosol inhaled steroid preparations. *Eur Respir J* 1995; **8**: 590–592.

Wolthers OD, Heuck C. Assessment of relation between short and intermediate term growth in children with asthma treated with inhaled glucocorticoids. *Allergy* 2004; **59**: 1193–1197.

Yoshiuchi I, Shingu R, Nakajima H et al. Mutation / polymorphism scanning of glucose-6-phosphatase gene promoter in noninsulin-dependent diabetes mellitus patients. *J Clin Metab* 1998; **83**: 1016–1019.

Young EA, Lopez JF, Murphy-Weinberg V et al. The role of mineralocorticoid receptors in hypothalamic-pituitary-adrenal axis regulation in humans. *J Clin Endocrinol Metab* 1998; **83**: 3339–3345.

3
Glucocorticoid Receptor Subtypes and Steroid Sensitivity

Robert H. Oakley and **John A. Cidlowski**

3.1 Introduction

Glucocorticoids are endogenous hormones released by the adrenal cortex in a circadian manner and in response to stressful stimuli. These hormones are essential for life and play critical roles in many diverse physiological processes, including lung and central nervous system development, protein, lipid and carbohydrate metabolism, skeletal growth, immune system function and apoptosis (Barnes, 1998; Sapolsky et al., 2000). The ability of glucocorticoids to inhibit inflammation and suppress the immune system has made them one of the most widely prescribed therapeutic agents in the world over the last half-century (Rhen and Cidlowski, 2005). Exogenous glucocorticoids are used to treat inflammatory diseases such as asthma, rheumatoid arthritis and ulcerative colitis. They are used also to prevent transplant rejection and are important chemotherapeutic agents for treating certain leukaemias, lymphomas and myelomas. The ability of both natural and synthetic glucocorticoids to elicit specific cellular effects is dependent on the presence of the glucocorticoid receptor (GR). The GR belongs to the nuclear receptor superfamily of intracellular proteins that function as ligand-dependent transcription factors (Evans, 1988). Upon binding glucocorticoids, GRs enhance or repress expression of target genes leading to specific changes in cellular function.

Cellular responsiveness to glucocorticoids is remarkably diverse in both health and disease (Lamberts et al., 1996). Sensitivity to glucocorticoids varies among individuals and among tissues of the same individual (Bronnegard, 1996). Changes in glucocorticoid responsiveness are even observed in the same tissue during development and in the same cell during the cell cycle (Gorovits et al., 1994; Hsu and

Overcoming Steroid Insensitivity in Respiratory Disease Edited by Ian M. Adcock and Kian Fan Chung
© 2008 John Wiley & Sons, Ltd.

DeFranco, 1995). In the treatment of disease, the beneficial effects of glucocorticoids are often limited by the development of resistance in the diseased tissue. Tissue-specific glucocorticoid resistance has been reported in patients with rheumatoid arthritis, asthma, Crohn's disease, ulcerative colitis and osteoarthritis (Kino et al., 2003). Understanding the molecular basis for these alterations in glucocorticoid responsiveness in both physiological and pathophysiological conditions is necessary for better patient care and is a major focus of current research.

As the principal mediator of glucocorticoid action, the GR is the primary target for regulatory events that alter target cell sensitivity to hormone. Regulation can be achieved in two primary ways: altering the level of receptor expression and/or altering the ability of the receptor to function as a transcription factor (Oakley and Cidlowski, 1993, 2001). The GR is derived from a single gene and the prevailing assumption over the last several decades has been that a single receptor isoform is responsible for the myriad effects of glucocorticoids. Recent studies, however, have challenged this simple one-gene–one-receptor paradigm by revealing the presence of an astonishing array of GR isoforms that arise from alternative processing of the GR gene (Chrousos and Kino, 2005; Lu and Cidlowski, 2005, 2006). The combination of alternative splicing and alternative translation initiation generates multiple receptor subtypes with distinct expression, function and gene regulatory profiles. Consequently, glucocorticoid responsiveness will ultimately be determined by the composition of these isoforms in a particular cell type or tissue. In the following chapter, we review the origin and nature of these GR subtypes and discuss their potential role in the regulation of glucocorticoid signalling.

3.2 Overview of Classic GR Function

Like other members of the steroid/thyroid/retinoic acid receptor superfamily of transcription factors, the GR is a modular protein consisting of three major domains: an amino-terminal transactivation domain (NTD), a central DNA binding domain (DBD) and a carboxyl-terminal ligand binding domain (LBD) (Figure 3.1A) (Kumar and Thompson, 2005; Oakley and Cidlowski, 2001). The sequence separating the DBD and LBD is referred to as the hinge region. Each domain contains additional sequences and/or subdomains with important roles in GR function. The NTD contains the ligand-independent transcriptional activation function-1 (AF-1) that plays a major role in gene activation by associating with the basal transcription machinery and vari-ous coregulators. The DBD contains two zinc finger regions critical for recognition of target DNA sequences and for receptor homodimerization. The LBD contains sites for binding hormone and interacting with chaperone proteins such as heat shock protein 90 (hsp90). The LBD also contains the ligand-dependent transcriptional activation function-2 (AF-2) that modulates transcription via interactions with coactivators and corepressors. Two nuclear localization signals have also been mapped in the protein, one spanning the DBD/hinge region junction and the other residing in the LBD.

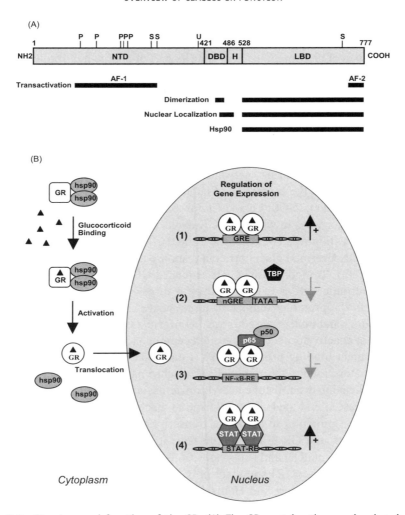

Figure 3.1 Structure and function of the GR. (A) The GR contains three major domains: the amino-terminal transactivation domain (NTD), the DNA binding domain (DBD) and the ligand binding domain (LBD). Regions important for transactivation (AF-1 and AF-2), dimerization, nuclear localization and hsp90 binding are also indicated. The human receptor can be post-translationally modified by: phosphorylation (P) on Ser-119, Ser-141, Ser-203, Ser-211 and Ser-226; sumoylation (S) on Lys-277, Lys-293 and Lys-703; and ubiquitination (U) on Lys-417. Numbers are for the human glucocorticoid receptor. H, hinge region. (B) Signal transduction pathway for glucocorticoids. In the absence of glucocorticoids (▲), the GR resides in the cytoplasm of cells in a complex with chaperone proteins such as hsp90. Upon binding the hormone, the receptor undergoes a change in conformation (activation), dissociates from accessory proteins and translocates into nucleus. The receptor dimerizes and regulates gene expression in four basic ways: (1) by binding directly to a glucocorticoid response element (GRE) and enhancing the transcription of target genes, (2) by binding directly to a negative GRE (nGRE) and repressing transcription of target genes, (3) by associating with a transcription factor such as nuclear factor-κB (NF-κB) and impairing its activity on responsive genes, and (4) by associating with a transcription factor such as signal transducer and activator of transcription (STAT)5 and enhancing its activity on responsive genes

Consistent with the widespread actions of glucocorticoids, the GR is expressed in almost every cell of the body. In the absence of hormone, the receptor is retained in the cytoplasm of cells in an inactive state as part of a large multiprotein complex that includes the chaperone protein hsp90 (Figure 3.1B) (Pratt, 1993; Pratt and Toft, 1997). The association with hsp90 appears to maintain the receptor in a conformation that favours high-affinity hormone binding. Glucocorticoids are lipophilic in nature and passively diffuse across the plasma membrane into the cell. Binding of hormone induces a conformational change in the receptor, resulting in the dissociation of hsp90 and exposure of the nuclear localization signals (Figure 3.1B). This transcriptionally competent or "activated" form of GR then translocates into the nucleus where it alters the expression of hundreds to thousands of genes (Cidlowski et al., 1990; Htun et al., 1996; Lu and Cidlowski, 2006).

One of the major ways in which the GR elicits these genomic effects is by direct binding to DNA (Figure 3.1B, schemes 1 and 2). The receptor recognizes specific sequences of DNA termed glucocorticoid response elements (GREs) (Beato, 1989; Freedman, 1992). The consensus GRE sequence GGTACAnnnTGTTCT consists of two palindromic half-sites separated by a three-base-pair spacer and is most often found in the promoter regions of target genes. The receptor binds the GRE as a homodimer and undergoes additional conformational changes resulting in the recruitment of coactivators such as steroid receptor coactivator-1 (SRC-1) and cAMP response element binding protein (CBP) (Lonard and O'Malley, 2005). Many of these coactivators induce the remodelling of chromatin structure and unwinding of DNA by their intrinsic histone acetyltransferase and methyltransferase activity. RNA polymerase II and the basal transcription machinery are then recruited to the newly accessible promoter to stimulate transcription of the linked gene. In some promoter contexts, the GR binds a more heterogeneous response element termed a "negative" GRE (nGRE) and suppresses transcription. In contrast to the positive GRE described above, nGREs contain only one conserved half-site and bind GR with lower affinity (Dostert and Heinzel, 2004). The mechanism underlying the repression involves GR interfering with the binding or activity of other positive-acting transcription factors.

The activated GR can also regulate gene expression, apart from DNA binding, by physically associating with other transcription factors and modulating their activity on responsive genes (Figure 3.1B, schemes 3 and 4) (Necela and Cidlowski, 2004; Smoak and Cidlowski, 2004). For example, the GR interacts with the *c*-jun and *c*-fos components of activator protein-1 (AP-1) and represses AP-1 responsive genes. Similarly, the receptor inhibits the transcriptional activity of nuclear factor-κB (NF-κB) by associating with the p65 subunit. How the interaction with GR disrupts the ability of AP-1 and NF-κB to regulate gene expression is controversial. The receptor may prevent these transcription factors from binding their cognate response elements. Alternatively, the GR may tether to the DNA-bound proteins and interfere with chromatin remodelling and/or recruitment of basal transcription machinery. Since both NF-κB and AP-1 are key mediators of the inflammatory response, the ability of GR to interact with these proteins and antagonize their activity appears to be the major mechanism underlying the anti-inflammatory and immunosuppressive actions of glucocorticoids. In contrast to the inhibitory effects of GR on AP-1 and NF-κB, the physical association of the receptor with members of the signal transduction and activator of transcription (STAT) family can lead to enhanced transcription of STAT-regulated genes (Necela and Cidlowski, 2004; Smoak and Cidlowski, 2004).

The GR protein is a substrate for several types of post-translational modifications that regulate glucocorticoid responsiveness by modulating the levels and/or transcriptional activity of the receptor (Figure 3.1A). For example, the GR is a phosphoprotein that becomes hyperphosphorylated after binding glucocorticoids (Bodwell et al., 1991). Five different serine residues have been identified as sites of phosphorylation in the human GR NTD. Phosphorylation enhances the transcriptional activity of GR in a promoter-specific fashion and regulates both the basal and glucocorticoid-induced turnover of the receptor (Wang et al., 2002; Webster et al., 1997). The GR is also post-translationally modified by attachment of the small ubiquitin-related modifier-1 (SUMO-1) at three consensus sites. Sumoylation of the receptor is facilitated by hormone and regulates the stability of the receptor protein and the ability of GR to transactivate certain reporter genes (Holmstrom et al., 2003; Le Drean et al., 2002; Tian et al., 2002). Finally, ubiquitination of the GR at a lysine residue near the NTD/DBD juncture limits glucocorticoid responsiveness by targeting the activated receptor to proteasomes for degradation (Wallace and Cidlowski, 2001).

3.3   GR Subtypes Arising from Alternative Splicing

To date, only one GR gene has been identified in every species examined. The human GR gene was first cloned in 1985 and subsequently mapped to chromosome 5q31-32 (Francke and Foellmer, 1989; Hollenberg et al., 1985; Theriault et al., 1989). The gene is comprised of nine exons (Figure 3.2) (Encio and Detera-Wadleigh, 1991; Oakley et al., 1996). Exon 1 and the proximal part of exon 2 contain a 5′ untranslated region, exon 2 encodes the NTD, exons 3 and 4 encode the two zinc fingers of the DBD and exons 5–9 encode the hinge region and LBD. Exon 9 also contains a large 3′ untranslated region. Alternative splicing has been shown to occur at both the 5′ and 3′ ends of the GR primary transcript. Three different exon 1 sequences (1A, 1B and 1C), each under the control of a distinct promoter, can be spliced into the same acceptor site in exon 2 (Breslin et al., 2001). Although these exon 1 variants encode the same GR protein, the unique 5′ untranslated region alone or in combination with the specific promoter may regulate GR expression in a cell-type specific manner. At the 3′ end of the human GR primary transcript, alternative splicing in exon 9 generates two different GR protein isoforms termed GRα and GRβ (Encio and Detera-Wadleigh, 1991; Hollenberg et al., 1985; Oakley et al., 1996). GRα, the

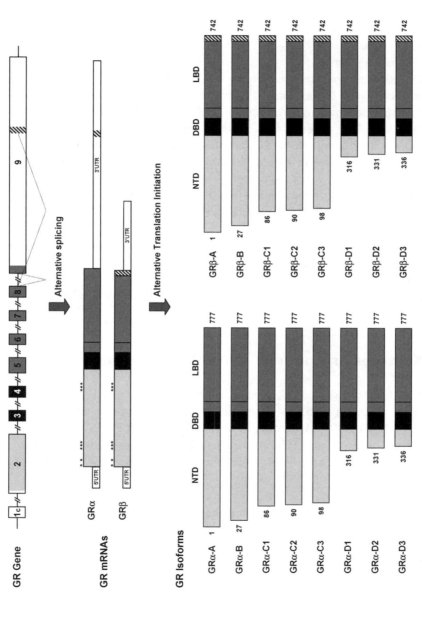

Figure 3.2 Multiple GR isoforms are generated by alternative processing of the GR gene. The human GR gene is comprised of nine exons. Alternative splicing in exon 9 of the primary transcript generates GRα and GRβ mRNAs, which encode the GRα and GRβ proteins that differ only at the carboxyl-terminal end of the ligand binding domain (LBD). Alternative translation initiation of the GRα and GRβ mRNA molecules generates additional protein isoforms that differ only at the amino-terminal end of the amino-terminal transactivation domain (NTD). The positions of the eight AUG start codons within the GR mRNA are indicated with an asterisk (*). Numbers denote the first and last residues for the human GR isoforms. Only exon 1C is shown for the GR gene

classic GR protein, results from the end of exon 8 being joined to the beginning of exon 9, whereas GRβ results from the end of exon 8 being joined to downstream sequences in exon 9 (Figure 3.2). Consequently, the two GR subtypes are identical through amino acid 727 (corresponding to the end of exon 8) but then diverge with each isoform having a unique carboxyl-terminus. GRα contains an additional 50 amino acids that encode helices 11 and 12 of the LBD and play a crucial role in both hormone binding and transactivation of gene expression (Bledsoe et al., 2002; Zhang et al., 1996). In contrast, GRβ contains an additional, non-homologous 15 amino acids. When compared to GRα, the unique GRβ sequence is predicted to be largely disordered and is missing helix 12 altogether (Yudt and Cidlowski, 2003).

As a consequence of its altered carboxyl-terminus, GRβ functions quite differently from GRα (Lewis-Tuffin and Cidlowski, 2006; Lu and Cidlowski, 2004). GRβ does not bind glucocorticoids, resides predominantly in the nucleus of cells and does not directly activate or repress glucocorticoid-responsive reporter genes. However, when coexpressed with GRα, the splice variant inhibits the transcriptional activity of GRα on target genes. This dominant negative activity of GRβ has been observed in many systems on genes both positively and negatively regulated by glucocorticoids (Bamberger et al., 1995; Fruchter et al., 2005; Hauk et al., 2002; Oakley et al., 1996, 1999). GRβ retains the ability to specifically bind GREs, and has been shown to physically associate with GRα in a heterodimer (Oakley et al., 1999). Thus, the mechanism underlying GRβ antagonism of GRα may involve competition for GRE binding and/or the formation of transcriptionally deficient GRα/GRβ heterodimers. Additionally, GRβ interacts with various transcription factors such as the p160 coactivator glucocorticoid receptor interacting protein-1 (GRIP-1), suggesting that competition with GRα for needed coactivators may also be involved in the suppression (Charmandari et al., 2005). Recent work has demonstrated that the unique GRβ carboxyl-terminus, particularly amino acids Lys-733 and Pro-734, is necessary for the dominant negative activity by localizing the GRβ in the nucleus (Yudt et al., 2003).

The ability of GRβ to antagonize GRα suggests that the ratio of these two isoforms may play a major role in regulating cellular sensitivity to glucocorticoids. The GRβ mRNA has been shown by reverse transcription-polymerase chain reaction (RT-PCR) to be expressed in almost all tissues and cell lines, though at levels significantly less than GRα (Bamberger et al., 1995; Oakley et al., 1996; Pujols et al., 2002). The GRβ protein has also been detected in various tissues using GRβ-specific antibodies made against its unique 15-amino-acid carboxyl-terminus (de Castro et al., 1996; Oakley et al., 1997). Consistent with the mRNA studies, the GRβ protein appears to be expressed at lower levels than GRα. The relative ratio of GRα and GRβ found in tissues, however, may not reflect the actual ratio in individual cells. Immunocytochemistry performed on human tissue sections has revealed that GRβ levels vary considerably among different cell types (Oakley et al., 1997). GRβ was most abundant in certain epithelial cells, including those lining the terminal bronchiole of the lung, those forming the outer layer of Hassall's corpuscles in the thymus and those lining the bile duct in the liver. Studies have also shown high levels of GRβ expression in neutrophils (Strickland et al., 2001). In addition, the relative ratio of GRα and GRβ determined at a single stage, time point or condition may not reflect the ratio in response to certain signalling events or in diseased tissue. Treatment of a variety of cell types with pro-inflammatory cytokines selectively increases the expression of GRβ and confers glucocorticoid resistance (Orii et al., 2002; Strickland et al., 2001; Tliba et al., 2006; Webster et al., 2001). A preferential induction in GRβ and resulting glucocorticoid insensitivity also occurs in peripheral blood monocytes exposed to microbial superantigens (Hauk et al., 2000). Finally, the potential importance of GRβ in disease is underscored by its enhanced expression in glucocorticoid-resistant forms of asthma, rheumatoid arthritis, ulcerative colitis, nasal polyposis and chronic lymphocytic leukaemia (Chikanza, 2002; Hamid et al., 1999; Hamilos et al., 2001; Honda et al., 2000; Leung et al., 1997; Shahidi et al., 1999; Sousa et al., 2000).

Changes in the efficiency of the GRβ alternative splicing event is one mechanism by which GRβ could be selectively increased over GRα. Although our understanding of the factors involved in GR splicing is in its infancy, recent work has identified the alternative splicing factor serine–arginine-rich protein p30c (SRp30c) as necessary for the specific generation of GRβ transcripts over GRα transcripts in neutrophils (Xu et al., 2003). Moreover, expression of the splicing protein was induced by the same agent (interleukin-8) that stimulated a selective increase in GRβ in these cells (Xu et al., 2003). An important goal of future studies will be to evaluate the activity of this enzyme in pathological conditions of glucocorticoid resistance.

New functions are emerging for GRβ that suggest that this receptor isoform may play an even greater physiological role than previously thought. The canonical view that GRβ does not bind glucocorticoids and is transcriptionally inactive apart from its dominant negative activity on GRα has been challenged by recent work from our laboratory (Lewis-Tuffin et al., 2007). We found that GRβ binds the anti-glucocorticoid RU486 with a K_d of approximately 100 nM, and as a result of this interaction GRβ molecules residing in the cytoplasm of cells translocate into the nucleus. We also investigated the transcriptional activity of GRβ by performing microarray analysis in cells stably expressing GRβ in the absence of GRα. In contrast to earlier studies using transfected reporter gene constructs, this approach allows the transcriptional activity of GRβ to be evaluated on endogenous genes in their chromatin context. To our surprise, GRβ by itself regulated a large set of unique genes and administration of RU486 antagonized this activity. These results demonstrate that GRβ can function directly as a ligand-independent regulator of gene expression, and they suggest that GRβ may contribute to glucocorticoid resistance by genomic effects distinct from its inhibition of GRα. Furthermore, they raise the possibility that some of the side effects reported for the abortifacient RU486 may be due to alterations in GRβ-mediated gene regulation.

Several additional GR subtypes have also been identified that result from alternative splicing at sites more centrally located in the receptor primary transcript. Use of an alternative splice donor site in the intron between exons 3 and 4 generates an isoform termed GRγ which contains an insertion of three nucleotides that encode an arginine residue between the two zinc fingers of the DBD (Ray et al., 1996). The GRγ variant has a widespread tissue distribution but possesses less than 50% of the transcriptional activity of GRα. The mRNA for this isoform has been detected in various pathologies displaying glucocorticoid resistance, including small-cell lung carcinoma cells, corticotroph adenomas and haematological cells isolated from patients with acute lymphoblastic leukaemia (Beger et al., 2003; Ray et al., 1996; Rivers et al., 1999). Two GR splice variants with altered LBDs have been identified in human multiple myeloma cells and both have been associated with glucocorticoid-resistant phenotypes (Krett et al., 1995; Moalli et al., 1993). GR-A is missing exons 5, 6 and 7 (which encode the amino-terminal half of the LBD) due to alternative splicing linking the end of exon 4 to the beginning of exon 8. GR-P is missing exons 8 and 9 (which encode the carboxyl-terminal half of the LBD) and possesses a unique carboxyl-terminus due to a splicing failure resulting in the retention of intronic sequences after exon 7. The GR-P mRNA has been found at high levels in certain myeloma and other GR-resistant haematological malignancies (de Lange et al., 2001). Interestingly, *in vitro* studies have demonstrated that GR-P enhances the transcriptional activity of GRα on reporter genes (de Lange et al., 2001).

3.4 GR Subtypes arising from Alternative Translation Initiation

Alternative translation initiation is another important mechanism by which a single gene can give rise to diverse protein isoforms with distinct physiological functions. Our laboratory has recently discovered that the GRα mRNA undergoes alternative translation initiation to generate eight receptor subtypes with progressively shorter amino-terminal domains (Figure 3.2) (Lu and Cidlowski, 2005). All eight AUG start codons are located in exon 2 and are 100% conserved in human, monkey, rat and mouse. The names of the translational isoforms and positions of the initiator methionine are as follows: GRα-A (Met-1), GRα-B (Met-27), GRα-C1 (Met-86), GRα-C2 (Met-90), GRα-C3 (Met-98), GRα-D1 (Met-316), GRα-D2 (Met-331) and GRα-D3 (Met-336). Notably, the GRβ mRNA also contains the identical start codons and would be expected to generate a similar complement of subtypes (Figure 3.2). GRα-A is the classic full-length 777-amino-acid protein. It is generated from the first initiator AUG codon, which lies within a weak KOZAK translation initiation consensus sequence (Yudt and Cidlowski, 2001). Production of the shorter isoforms from internal AUG codons involves both ribosomal leaky scanning and ribosomal shunting. Interestingly, immunoblots performed on tissue and cell extracts with GR antibodies had previously revealed a heterogeneous population of proteins smaller in size than the full-length 94-kDa receptor. These immunoreactive species, however, were assumed to be receptor degradation products and were ignored for many years. Only when the internal AUG start codons were mutated and the presence of the lower molecular weight proteins was eliminated did the appreciation for trans-lation re-initiation in GR biology emerge (Lu and Cidlowski, 2005; Yudt and Cidlowski, 2001).

The GRα subtypes have been evaluated for functional differences (Lu and Cidlowski, 2005). All eight isoforms bind glucocorticoids with similar high affinity, as would be expected since they each retain an intact LBD. Additionally, each iso-form is found in the nucleus of cells following glucocorticoid treatment. Surprisingly, however, the subcellular distribution of the isoforms differed in the absence of hor-mone. In contrast to the cytoplasmic location of GRα-A, GRα-B, GRα-C1, GRα-C2 and GRα-C3, the three D isoforms were found in the nucleus of cells. This result suggests that sequences in the NTD play a previously unappreciated role in nuclear localization, nuclear export and/or cytoplasmic retention. Alternatively, the severe amino-terminal truncation may simply alter the conformation of the D isoforms such that one or both of the NLS are exposed even in the unoccupied receptor.

The ability of the GRα translational isoforms to function as ligand-dependent transcription factors was evaluated initially on several different glucocorticoid-responsive reporter genes (Lu and Cidlowski, 2005). All eight isoforms induced expression of the reporter genes with similar potencies following glucocorticoid treatment. However, the extent of transactivation differed among the isoforms. The weakest activity was observed for the three D isoforms as their maximal activa-tion was only 50% of the full-length GRα-A. The D isoforms are missing all five sites of phosphorylation and the entire AF-1 transactivation domain, and would be expected to have a compromised ability to communicate with the basal tran-scription machinery for stimulation of gene expression. Surprisingly, the GRα-C3 subtype exhibited the greatest amount of transcriptional activity that was approxi-mately twice that measured for GRα-A. The remaining isoforms GRα-B, GRα-C1 and CRα-C2 possessed intermediate levels of reporter gene activity that were similar to GRα-A. The reason for the enhanced activity of GRα-C3 is not clear. It differs from GRα-C1 and GRα-C2 subtypes by the absence of only 12 and 8 amino acids, respectively, but possesses a markedly stronger transactivation profile in this in vitro system. Perhaps the conformation adopted by the GRα-C3 amino-terminal domain or the sequence itself interacts more favourably with a coactiva-tor or less favorably with a corepressor. Other reports have also implicated a role for the extreme amino-terminus in modulating the transcriptional activity of GRα (Dahlman-Wright et al., 1994; Yudt and Cidlowski, 2001).

The transcriptional activity of the GRα isoforms was further explored by evaluat-ing their capacity to regulate endogenous genes in their chromatin context (Lu and Cidlowski, 2005). Microarray analyses performed on U2OS cells stably expressing wild-type GRα, GRα-A, GRα-B, GRα-C3 or GRα-D3 revealed that approximately 200 genes were commonly regulated by all receptor isoforms. For instance, each GRα subtype induced expression of the regulator of G protein signalling 2 (RGS2) gene and repressed expression of the immediate early response 3 gene. In addition to this common set of genes, each GRα subtype also regulated a unique set of approximately 200–400 genes when compared to wild-type GRα. Consequently, of the 20 186 genes measured in this experimental system, over 2000 were regulated by at least one of the GRα isoforms.

Expression of the eight GRα isoforms has been investigated in a variety of human cell lines and in both rat and mouse tissues (Lu and Cidlowski, 2005). These studies demonstrated that the subtypes have a widespread tissue distribution but their levels vary significantly both between and within tissues. For example, the GRα-C isoforms were expressed at higher levels in the pancreas than in the lung, and the GRα-D subtypes were most abundant in spleen. Within the same tissue, GRα-B was found to be more abundant than GRα-A in liver, pancreas, stomach and thymus but not in the other tissues examined. Variations in the expression of the GRα subtypes are predicted to have two important ramifications (Figure 3.3). First, differences in the cellular composition of GRα isoforms would account for cell-type-specific glucocorticoid responses because, as discussed above, each isoform regulates a unique set of genes. Second, variations in GRα subtype expression would account for alterations in cellular sensitivity to glucocorticoids. In support of the latter claim, we have found that cells expressing different combinations of two GRα subtypes exhibit a transcriptional response reflecting the composite action of both isoforms (Lu and Cidlowski, 2005). Addition of GRα-C3 into cells expressing GRα-A led to enhanced glucocorticoid responsiveness whereas addition of GRα-D3 did not. Clearly, the potential role for the GRα subtypes in regulating both the type and magnitude of glucocorticoid signalling makes it especially important for future studies to investigate the expression of these isoforms in disease and to elucidate the factors that promote the selective expression of one GRα isoform over another.

3.5 Conclusions

The traditional view that glucocorticoids exert their effects on cells through one receptor isoform has dramatically changed in recent years with the finding of additional GR subtypes arising from alternative processing of the single GR gene. Alternative splicing and alternative translation initiation generate a diverse set of GR isoforms with unique expression, function and gene regulatory profiles. We propose that glucocorticoid signalling is mediated by as many as eight GRα subtypes and eight GRβ subtypes. The potential for these isoforms to undergo post-translational modifications and to function as monomers, homodimers and heterodimers provides cells with a wealth of possibilities for controlling a wide range of cellular functions with fine-tuned precision. In addition, alterations in the relative levels of these isoforms may underlie diseased states characterized by hyposensitivity or hypersensitivity to glucocorticoids. Development of synthetic

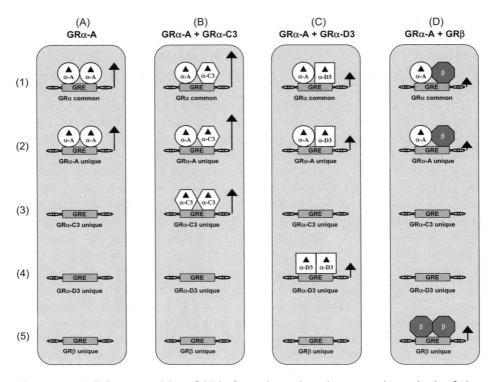

Figure 3.3   Cellular composition of GR isoforms determines the type and magnitude of glucocorticoid response. The Cartoon depicts glucocorticoid regulation of the same five genes in cells expressing predominantly GRα-A (A), GRα-A and GRα-C3 (B), GRα-A and GRα-D3 (C) or GRα-A and GRβ (D). Cell-type-specific responses can be achieved by GR isoform-specific regulation of unique genes. For example, a subset of genes regulated in cell B will differ from those regulated in cell C due to the presence of GRα-C3 (cf. gene 3 in B and C). Similarly, a subset of genes regulated in cell C will differ from those regulated in cell B due to the presence of GRα-D3 (cf. gene 4 in B and C). Gradations in the magnitude of the glucocorticoid response can be achieved on both common and unique genes by cross-talk among the GR subtypes via heterodimerization (pictured), competition for GRE binding and/or competition for cofactors. For example, the presence of the more transcriptionally competent GRα-C3 isoform confers a greater capacity for transactivation of responsive genes than do the less competent GRα-D3 and GRβ subtypes (cf. genes 1 and 2 in A–D). Height of arrows indicates magnitude of response

glucocorticoids and anti-glucocorticoids that selectively target one or certain combinations of the GR isoforms holds great promise for better patient care by reducing serious adverse effects associated with glucocorticoid therapy. Finally, other members of the steroid/thyroid/retinoic acid receptor family undergo alternative splicing and contain potential alternative translation initiation sites in their NTD, suggesting that the production of multiple receptor isoforms is a general mechanism for regulating cellular responsiveness to steroid hormones.

References

Bamberger CM, Bamberger AM, De Castro M, Chrousos GP. Glucocorticoid receptor beta, a potential endogenous inhibitor of glucocorticoid action in humans. *J Clin Invest* 1995; **95**: 2435–2441.

Barnes PJ. Anti-inflammatory actions of glucocorticoids: molecular mechanisms. *Clin Sci (Lond)* 1998; **94**: 557–572.

Beato M. Gene regulation by steroid hormones. *Cell* 1989; **56**: 335–344.

Beger C, Gerdes K, Lauten M et al. Expression and structural analysis of glucocorticoid receptor isoform gamma in human leukaemia cells using an isoform-specific real-time polymerase chain reaction approach. *Br J Haematol* 2003; **122**: 245–252.

Bledsoe RK, Montana VG, Stanley TB et al. Crystal structure of the glucocorticoid receptor ligand binding domain reveals a novel mode of receptor dimerization and coactivator recognition. *Cell* 2002; **110**: 93–105.

Bodwell JE, Orti E, Coull JM et al. Identification of phosphorylated sites in the mouse glucocorticoid receptor. *J Biol Chem* 1991; **266**: 7549–7555.

Breslin MB, Geng CD, Vedeckis WV. Multiple promoters exist in the human GR gene, one of which is activated by glucocorticoids. *Mol Endocrinol* 2001; **15**: 1381–1395.

Bronnegard M. Steroid receptor number. Individual variation and downregulation by treatment. *Am J Respir Crit Care Med* 1996; **154**: S28–32; discussion S32–23.

Charmandari E, Chrousos GP, Ichijo T et al. The human glucocorticoid receptor (hGR) beta isoform suppresses the transcriptional activity of hGRalpha by interfering with formation of active coactivator complexes. *Mol Endocrinol* 2005; **19**: 52–64.

Chikanza IC. Mechanisms of corticosteroid resistance in rheumatoid arthritis: a putative role for the corticosteroid receptor beta isoform. *Ann NY Acad Sci* 2002; **966**: 39–48.

Chrousos GP, Kino T. Intracellular glucocorticoid signaling: a formerly simple system turns stochastic. *Sci STKE* 2005; 48.

Cidlowski JA, Bellingham DL, Powell-Oliver FE et al. Novel antipeptide antibodies to the human glucocorticoid receptor: recognition of multiple receptor forms in vitro and distinct localization of cytoplasmic and nuclear receptors. *Mol Endocrinol* 1990; **4**: 1427–1437.

Dahlman-Wright K, Almlof T, Mcewan IJ et al. Delineation of a small region within the major transactivation domain of the human glucocorticoid receptor that mediates transactivation of gene expression. *Proc Natl Acad Sci USA* 1994; **91**: 1619–1623.

De Castro M, Elliot S, Kino T et al. The non-ligand binding beta-isoform of the human glucocorticoid receptor (hGR beta): tissue levels, mechanism of action, and potential physiologic role. *Mol Med* 1996; **2**: 597–607.

De Lange P, Segeren CM, Koper JW et al. Expression in hematological malignancies of a glucocorticoid receptor splice variant that augments glucocorticoid receptor-mediated effects in transfected cells. *Cancer Res* 2001; **61**: 3937–3941.

Dostert A, Heinzel T. Negative glucocorticoid receptor response elements and their role in glucocorticoid action. *Curr Pharm Des* 2004; **10**: 2807–2816.

Encio IJ, Detera-Wadleigh SD. The genomic structure of the human glucocorticoid receptor. *J Biol Chem* 1991; **266**: 7182–7188.

Evans RM. The steroid and thyroid hormone receptor superfamily. *Science* 1988; **240**: 889–895.

Francke U, Foellmer BE. The glucocorticoid receptor gene is in 5q31-q32 [corrected]. *Genomics* 1989; **4**: 610–612.

Freedman LP. Anatomy of the steroid receptor zinc finger region. *Endocr Rev* 1992; **13**: 129–145.

Fruchter O, Kino T, Zoumakis E et al. The human glucocorticoid receptor (GR) isoform {beta} differentially suppresses GR{alpha}-induced transactivation stimulated by synthetic glucocorticoids. *J Clin Endocrinol Metab* 2005; **90**: 3505–3509.

Gorovits R, Ben-Dror I, Fox LE et al. Developmental changes in the expression and compartmentalization of the glucocorticoid receptor in embryonic retina. *Proc Natl Acad Sci USA* 1994; **91**: 4786–4790.

Hamid QA, Wenzel SE, Hauk PJ et al. Increased glucocorticoid receptor beta in airway cells of glucocorticoid-insensitive asthma. *Am J Respir Crit Care Med* 1999; **159**: 1600–1604.

Hamilos DL, Leung DY, Muro S et al. GRbeta expression in nasal polyp inflammatory cells and its relationship to the anti-inflammatory effects of intranasal fluticasone. *J Allergy Clin Immunol* 2001; **108**: 59–68.

Hauk PJ, Goleva E, Strickland I et al. Increased glucocorticoid receptor Beta expression converts mouse hybridoma cells to a corticosteroid-insensitive phenotype. *Am J Respir Cell Mol Biol* 2002; **27**: 361–367.

Hauk PJ, Hamid QA, Chrousos GP, Leung DY. Induction of corticosteroid insensitivity in human PBMCs by microbial superantigens. *J Allergy Clin Immunol* 2000; **105**: 782–787.

Hollenberg SM, Weinberger C, Ong ES et al. Primary structure and expression of a functional human glucocorticoid receptor cDNA. *Nature* 1985; **318**: 635–641.

Holmstrom S, Van Antwerp ME, Iniguez-Lluhi JA. Direct and distinguishable inhibitory roles for SUMO isoforms in the control of transcriptional synergy. *Proc Natl Acad Sci USA* 2003; **100**: 15758–15763.

Honda M, Orii F, Ayabe T et al. Expression of glucocorticoid receptor beta in lymphocytes of patients with glucocorticoid-resistant ulcerative colitis. *Gastroenterology* 2000; **118**: 859–866.

Hsu SC, Defranco DB. Selectivity of cell cycle regulation of glucocorticoid receptor function. *J Biol Chem* 1995; **270**: 3359–3364.

Htun H, Barsony J, Renyi I et al. Visualization of glucocorticoid receptor translocation and intranuclear organization in living cells with a green fluorescent protein chimera. *Proc Natl Acad Sci USA* 1996; **93**: 4845–4850.

Kino T, De Martino MU, Charmandari E et al. Tissue glucocorticoid resistance/hypersensitivity syndromes. *J Steroid Biochem Mol Biol* 2003; **85**: 457–467.

Krett NL, Pillay S, Moalli PA et al. A variant glucocorticoid receptor messenger RNA is expressed in multiple myeloma patients. *Cancer Res* 1995; **55**: 2727–2729.

Kumar R, Thompson EB. Gene regulation by the glucocorticoid receptor: structure:function relationship. *J Steroid Biochem Mol Biol* 2005; **94**: 383–394.

Lamberts SW, Huizenga AT, De Lange P et al. Clinical aspects of glucocorticoid sensitivity. *Steroids* 1996; **61**: 157–160.

Le Drean Y, Mincheneau N, Le Goff P, Michel D. Potentiation of glucocorticoid receptor transcriptional activity by sumoylation. *Endocrinology,* 2002; **143**: 3482–3489.

Leung DY, Hamid Q, Vottero A et al. Association of glucocorticoid insensitivity with increased expression of glucocorticoid receptor beta. *J Exp Med* 1997; **186**: 1567–1574.

Lewis-Tuffin LJ, Cidlowski JA. The physiology of human glucocorticoid receptor beta (hGRbeta) and glucocorticoid resistance. *Ann NY Acad Sci* 2006; **1069**: 1–9.

Lewis-Tuffin LJ, Jewell CM, Bienstock RJ et al. The Human Glucocorticoid Receptor {beta} (hGR{beta}) Binds RU-486 and is Transcriptionally Active. *Mol Cell Biol* 2007; **27**: 2266–2282.

Lonard DM, O'Malley BW. Expanding functional diversity of the coactivators. *Trends Biochem Sci* 2005; **30**: 126–132.

Lu NZ, Cidlowski JA. The origin and functions of multiple human glucocorticoid receptor isoforms. *Ann NY Acad Sci* 2004; **1024**: 102–123.

Lu NZ, Cidlowski JA. Translational regulatory mechanisms generate N-terminal glucocorticoid receptor isoforms with unique transcriptional target genes. *Mol Cell* 2005; **18**: 331–342.

Lu NZ, Cidlowski JA. Glucocorticoid receptor isoforms generate transcription specificity. *Trends Cell Biol* 2006; **16**: 301–307.

Moalli PA, Pillay S, Krett NL, Rosen ST. Alternatively spliced glucocorticoid receptor messenger RNAs in glucocorticoid-resistant human multiple myeloma cells. *Cancer Res* 1993; **53**: 3877–3879.

Necela BM, Cidlowski JA. Mechanisms of glucocorticoid receptor action in noninflammatory and inflammatory cells. *Proc Am Thorac Soc* 2004; **1**: 239–246.

Oakley RH, Cidlowski JA. Homologous down regulation of the glucocorticoid receptor: the molecular machinery. *Crit Rev Eukaryot Gene Expr* 1993; **3**: 63–88.

Oakley RH, Cidlowski JA. The glucocorticoid receptor: expression, function, and regulation of glucocorticoid responsiveness. In: Goulding NJ, Flower RJ. (Eds) *Glucocorticoids.* Switzerland, Birkhauser Verlag, 2001.

Oakley RH, Jewell CM, Yudt MR et al. The dominant negative activity of the human glucocorticoid receptor beta isoform. Specificity and mechanisms of action. *J Biol Chem* 1999; **274**: 27857–27866.

Oakley RH, Sar M, Cidlowski JA. The human glucocorticoid receptor beta isoform. Expression, biochemical properties, and putative function. *J Biol Chem* 1996; **271**: 9550–9559.

Oakley RH, Webster JC, Sar M et al. Expression and subcellular distribution of the beta-isoform of the human glucocorticoid receptor. *Endocrinology* 1997; **138**: 5028–5038.

Orii F, Ashida T, Nomura M et al. Quantitative analysis for human glucocorticoid receptor alpha/beta mRNA in IBD. *Biochem Biophys Res Commun* 2002; **296**: 1286–1294.

Pratt WB. The role of heat shock proteins in regulating the function, folding, and trafficking of the glucocorticoid receptor. *J Biol Chem* 1993; **268**: 21455–21458.

Pratt WB, Toft DO. Steroid receptor interactions with heat shock protein and immunophilin chaperones. *Endocr Rev* 1997; **18**: 306–360.

Pujols L, Mullol J, Roca-Ferrer J et al. Expression of glucocorticoid receptor alpha- and beta-isoforms in human cells and tissues. *Am J Physiol Cell Physiol* 2002; **283**: C1324–1331.

Ray DW, Davis JR, White A, Clark AJ. Glucocorticoid receptor structure and function in glucocorticoid-resistant small cell lung carcinoma cells. *Cancer Res* 1996; **56**: 3276–3280.

Rhen T, Cidlowski JA. Antiinflammatory action of glucocorticoids – new mechanisms for old drugs. *N Engl J Med* 2005; **353**: 1711–1723.

Rivers C, Levy A, Hancock J et al. Insertion of an amino acid in the DNA-binding domain of the glucocorticoid receptor as a result of alternative splicing. *J Clin Endocrinol Metab* 1999; **84**: 4283–4286.

Sapolsky RM, Romero LM, Munck AU. How do glucocorticoids influence stress responses? Integrating permissive, suppressive, stimulatory, and preparative actions. *Endocr Rev* 2000; **21**: 55–89.

Shahidi H, Vottero A, Stratakis CA et al. Imbalanced expression of the glucocorticoid receptor isoforms in cultured lymphocytes from a patient with systemic glucocorticoid resistance and chronic lymphocytic leukemia. *Biochem Biophys Res Commun* 1999; **254**: 559–565.

Smoak KA, Cidlowski JA. Mechanisms of glucocorticoid receptor signaling during inflammation. *Mech Ageing Dev* 2004; **125**: 697–706.

Sousa AR, Lane SJ, Cidlowski JA et al. Glucocorticoid resistance in asthma is associated with elevated in vivo expression of the glucocorticoid receptor beta-isoform. *J Allergy Clin Immunol* 2000; **105**: 943–950.

Strickland I, Kisich K, Hauk PJ et al. High constitutive glucocorticoid receptor beta in human neutrophils enables them to reduce their spontaneous rate of cell death in response to corticosteroids. *J Exp Med* 2001; **193**: 585–593.

Theriault A, Boyd E, Harrap SB et al. Regional chromosomal assignment of the human glucocorticoid receptor gene to 5q31. *Hum Genet* 1989; **83**: 289–291.

Tian S, Poukka H, Palvimo JJ, Janne OA. Small ubiquitin-related modifier-1 (SUMO-1) modification of the glucocorticoid receptor. *Biochem J* 2002; **367**: 907–911.

Tliba O, Cidlowski JA, Amrani Y. CD38 expression is insensitive to steroid action in cells treated with tumor necrosis factor-alpha and interferon-gamma by a mechanism involving the up-regulation of the glucocorticoid receptor beta isoform. *Mol Pharmacol* 2006; **69**: 588–596.

Wallace AD, Cidlowski JA. Proteasome-mediated glucocorticoid receptor degradation restricts transcriptional signaling by glucocorticoids. *J Biol Chem* 2001; **276**: 42714–42721.

Wang Z, Frederick J, Garabedian MJ. Deciphering the phosphorylation "code" of the glucocorticoid receptor in vivo. *J Biol Chem* 2002; **277**: 26573–26580.

Webster JC, Jewell CM, Bodwell JE et al. Mouse glucocorticoid receptor phosphorylation status influences multiple functions of the receptor protein. *J Biol Chem* 1997; **272**: 9287–9293.

Webster JC, Oakley RH, Jewell CM, Cidlowski JA. Proinflammatory cytokines regulate human glucocorticoid receptor gene expression and lead to the accumulation of the dominant negative beta isoform: a mechanism for the generation of glucocorticoid resistance. *Proc Natl Acad Sci USA* 2001; **98**: 6865–6870.

Xu Q, Leung DY, Kisich KO. Serine-arginine-rich protein p30 directs alternative splicing of glucocorticoid receptor pre-mRNA to glucocorticoid receptor beta in neutrophils. *J Biol Chem* 2003; **278**: 27112–27118.

Yudt MR, Cidlowski JA. Molecular identification and characterization of a and b forms of the glucocorticoid receptor. *Mol Endocrinol* 2001; **15**: 1093–1103.

Yudt MR, Jewell CM, Bienstock RJ, Cidlowski JA. Molecular origins for the dominant negative function of human glucocorticoid receptor beta. *Mol Cell Biol* 2003; **23**: 4319–4330.

Zhang S, Liang X, Danielsen M. Role of the C terminus of the glucocorticoid receptor in hormone binding and agonist/antagonist discrimination. *Mol Endocrinol* 1996; **10**: 24–34.

4
Dissociated Glucocorticoids

Ian M. Adcock

4.1 Introduction

Endogenous glucocorticoids are important steroid hormones produced from the adrenal gland that control a number of key physiological functions in man, including glucose homeostasis (after which they are named), the regulation of metabolism, cell survival/death, development and the response to stress and infection (Barnes and Adcock, 2003). Synthetic glucocorticoid drugs are the most effective anti-inflammatory agents available and are used to treat a number of chronic diseases including inflammatory bowel disease, psoriasis, rheumatoid arthritis and asthma (Barnes, 1995). However the discovery of their clinical effectiveness in the early 1950s was followed by the realization that prolonged treatment with high doses of glucocorticoids leads to debilitating side effects such as osteoporosis, diabetogenesis, suppression of the hypothalamic-pituitary-adrenal (HPA) axis, reduction of growth velocity in children, weight gain, ocular symptoms and skin changes (Schacke et al., 2002). Thus, despite their impressive efficacy, these unwanted side effects have limited the dose and duration of systemic use of these topical and systemic glucocorticoids (Schacke et al., 2002).

This chapter will review the concept and potential of new glucocorticoid ligands that retain the beneficial aspects without possessing any of the detrimental side effects of conventional glucocorticoids.

4.2 Asthma and Chronic Obstructive Pulmonary Disease are Chronic Inflammatory Diseases of the Airways

Inflammation is a central feature of both asthma and chronic obstructive pulmonary disease (COPD) and is characterized by the recruitment and activation of

Overcoming Steroid Insensitivity in Respiratory Disease   Edited by Ian M. Adcock and Kian Fan Chung
© 2008 John Wiley & Sons, Ltd.

inflammatory cells and changes in the structural cells of the lung (Caramori et al., 2004; Di Stefano et al., 2004). This is associated with an increased expression of components of the inflammatory cascade, including cytokines, chemokines, growth factors, enzymes, receptors and adhesion molecules. As many of these genes are not expressed in normal cells but are induced in a cell-specific manner during the inflammatory process, the increased expression of these proteins is generally the result of enhanced gene transcription (Caramori et al., 2004; Di Stefano et al., 2004).

The exact infiltrating cells and their localization within the airway varies between asthma and COPD, with asthma being associated with infiltration of T-helper (Th) type 2 lymphocytes, eosinophils, macrophages/monocytes and mast cells into the bronchial airway wall (Busse and Lemanske, 2001). In addition, an "acute-on-chronic" inflammation may be observed during exacerbations, with an increase in eosinophils and sometimes neutrophils (Barnes, 1995). Increased transcription of inflammatory mediators under the control of transcription factors is again important in this aspect of the inflammatory response (Caramori et al., 2004). In contrast, the airway limitation in COPD is due to inflammation in the central and peripheral airways (bronchioles) and lung parenchyma (Barnes and Kleinert, 2004; Di Stefano et al., 2004; Hogg et al., 2004). Most patients with COPD have all three pathological conditions (chronic obstructive bronchitis/bronchiolitis, emphysema and mucus plugging), but the relative extent of emphysema and obstructive bronchitis within individual patients can vary widely (Barnes and Kleinet, 2004; Di Stefano et al., 2004; Hogg et al., 2004). Patients with COPD have infiltration of $CD8^+$ T cells, macrophages and an increased number of neutrophils within the bronchial mucosa and lung parenchyma, and eosinophils are not prominent except in patients with concomitant asthma or in some patients during exacerbations (Barnes and Kleinert, 2004; Di Stefano et al., 2004; Hogg et al., 2004). In addition, the bronchioles are obstructed by fibrosis and mucus plugging (as a consequence of an increased expression and secretion of MUC5AC and MUCB in the lumen) (Barnes and Kleinert, 2004; Di Stefano et al., 2004; Hogg et al., 2004).

4.3   Regulation of Inflammatory Gene Expression

Nuclear factor-κB (NF-κB) is considered the central driver of the inflammatory/ immune response in most diseases as it is activated by stimulation of cells by most inflammatory/noxious agents and can, in turn, activate the expression of many inflammatory mediators, receptors, enzymes, etc. (Baldwin, 2001; Perkins, 2007). NF-κB is ubiquitously expressed within cells and is able not only to control induction of inflammatory genes in its own right but also to enhance the activity of other cell- and signal-specific transcription factors (Baldwin, 2001b; Perkins, 2007). This leads to a feedforward inflammatory cascade under the control of this important factor (Perkins, 2007) and, importantly, enhanced activation of NF-κB and IKK2 has been implicated in asthma (Gagliardo et al., 2003; Hart et al., 1998) and COPD (Baldwin, 2001; Caramori et al., 2003).

It is important to realize, however, that NF-κB is not the only signalling pathway and/or transcription factor important in this inflammatory cascade and the activation of many other pathways can impinge upon, and modulate, the final response in asthma and COPD seen following NF-κB activation: for example, the transcription factor activator protein-1 (AP-1), the mitogen-activated protein kinases (MAPKs) and more signal-specific Janus kinase (JAKs)/signal transducer and activator of transcription (STAT) pathways (Eynott et al., 2003; Kumar et al., 2003; Pernis and Rothman, 2002). Although each pathway can activate specific downstream transcription factors there is considerable cross-talk between kinase pathways, at the membrane proximal and transcription factor proximal ends of each pathway, which allows signal integration. The importance of the NF-κB pathways has been shown by the ability of inhibitors to modulate the expression of many inflammatory mediators (such as IL-8, TNFα and GM-CSF) and adhesion molecules (such as ICAM-1), to control granulocyte apoptosis and chemotaxis and to control T-cell, macrophage and epithelial cell function (Bryan et al., 2000; Cosio et al., 2004; Holden et al., 2004; Koch et al., 2004; Kumar et al., 2003). Furthermore, NF-κB inhibitors have been reported to regulate airway smooth muscle proliferation and various other factors involved in airway remodelling in an animal model of asthma (Eynott et al., 2003).

Activation of the classic NF-κB p65–p50 heterodimer by cell surface receptors has been well described (Perkins, 2007) and involves phosphorylation of a specific kinase (inhibitor of NF-κB kinase, IKK) (Perkins, 2007). This, in turn, phosphorylates and targets for proteasomal degradation the inhibitor of κB (IκBα), resulting in nuclear translocation of the activated p65–p50 complex. Once in the nucleus, activated NF-κB binds to specific elements within the promoter regions of κB-responsive genes and recruits transcriptional coactivator molecules that can induce histone acetylation and other histone modifications in a temporal manner(Ito et al., 2000; Lee et al., 2006; Li et al., 2007), leading to recruitment of basal transcription factors and remodelling complexes and the induction of inflammatory gene expression (Perkins, 2007).

4.4 Effects on Inflammation

Inhaled glucocorticoids clearly reverse the specific chronic airway inflammation present in asthma (Adelroth et al., 1990; Jeffery et al., 1992; Laitinen et al., 1992; Laursen et al., 1988). As such there is a marked reduction in the number of eosinophils, mast cells, T-lymphocytes and macrophages in the sputum, bronchoalveolar lavage (BAL) and/or bronchial wall (Barnes, 1995; van Rensen et al., 1999). Furthermore, glucocorticoids reverse the goblet-cell hyperplasia and the basement-membrane thickening characteristically seen in biopsy specimens of bronchial epithelium from patients with asthma (Laitinen et al., 1992; Olivieri et al., 1997). In contrast, several large long-term studies have failed to show any beneficial effect of inhaled or oral steroids on the inexorable decline in lung function or any inflammatory parameters in COPD (Anon, 2006; Burge et al., 2000; Calverley et al., 2007; Pauwels et al., 1999; Soriano et al., 2007; Vestbo et al., 1999). At the same time this treatment, particularly when prolonged for many years, can produce systemic adverse effects, including skin bruising, adrenal suppression, cataracts and loss of bone density (Anon, 2006; Burge et al., 2000; Calverley et al., 2007; Pauwels et al., 1999; Soriano et al., 2007; Vestbo et al., 1999). The use of increasing doses that may potentially achieve significant effects on lung function and/or inflammatory indices is obviated by the increased risk of side effects that are evident in these more elderly subjects.

4.5 Mechanisms of Glucocorticoid Action

The glucocorticoid receptor (GR) is a ligand-activated transcription factor localized within the cytoplasm of virtually all cells (Ito et al., 2006a; Zhou and Cidlowski, 2005). Glucocorticoids freely diffuse from the circulation into the cell, bind to GR and induce a rapid translocation of the receptor into the nucleus. Within the nucleus the activated GR can have two major effects: it can bind directly to glucocorticoid response elements (GREs) in the promoter regions of responsive genes, thereby switching on the expression of anti-inflammatory genes, or it can interact with pro-inflammatory transcription factors such as NF-κB and suppress their actions (De Bosscher et al., 2006; Ito et al., 2006a; Zhou and Cidlowski, 2005). It is thought that the major anti-inflammatory effect of glucocorticoids is through actions on NF-κB and similar factors (Ito et al., 2006a; Zhou and Cidlowski, 2005).

Generally, the number of GREs and their position relative to the transcriptional start site are important determinants of the magnitude of the transactivation response to glucocorticoids (Ito et al., 2006a; Zhou and Cidlowski, 2005). Many genes, including liver-specific metabolic genes such as tyrosine aminotransferase (TAT) and stress response genes such as metallothionein, contain clearly identifiable GREs in their promoter regions, allowing activated GR to bind to DNA as a homodimer, to recruit transcriptional coactivators and to induce gene transcription (Ito et al., 2006a; Zhou and Cidlowski, 2005)(Figure 4.1). In a few cases, e.g. prolactin and osteocalcin where the GRE overlaps with the transcriptional start site, GR–GRE binding can suppress gene expression.

However, most pro-inflammatory genes, including IL-1β, IL-6, IL-8, TNFα, inducible nitric oxide synthase (NOS2) and intercellular adhesion molecule-1 (ICAM-1) whose activity is suppressed by glucocorticoids, do not contain discernible GREs (De Bosscher et al., 2006; Ito et al., 2006a). Inflammatory gene expression generally requires that a number of transcription factors, including AP-1 and NF-κB, act together in a coordinated manner and it is now established that GR, acting as a

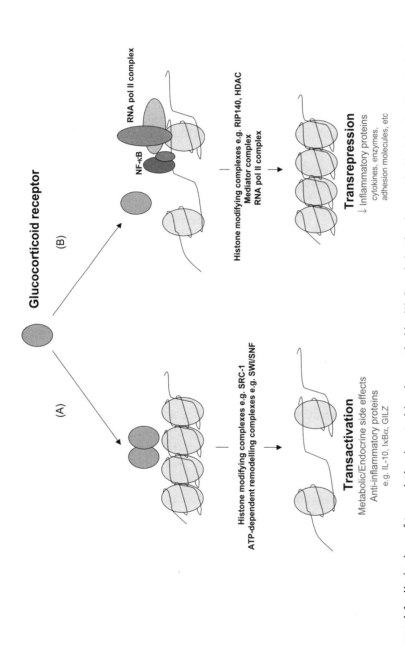

Figure 4.1 Mechanisms of transcriptional control by glucocorticoids. (A) Gene induction (transactivation) by the dimerized glucocorticoid receptor (GR) is mediated through a variety of interacting proteins, including the ATP-dependent chromatin remodelling enzymes that alter the packing of the nucleosomes and cofactors that either have histone-modifying activity or can recruit histone-modifying enzymes. Histone tails can be both methylated and acetylated, and the degree of modification of the histones regulates transcription rates. (B) Some of these processes are also targeted during GR-mediated transrepression of NF-κB activity. Thus, GR can engage with the transcriptional machinery through the mediator complex, which seems to function to integrate signals from the promoter and communicate with RNA polymerase II. In addition, differential recruitment of corepressor molecules by GR can reverse NF-κB-associated changes in histone modifications. Different genes in different cells are influenced by these activities to varying degrees, thus allowing considerable scope for pharmacological modulation. A full-colour version of this figure can be found in the colour plate section of this book.

monomer, binds directly to the activated NF-κB and AP-1 complexes and generally suppresses their transcriptional activity (Ito et al., 2006a) (Figure 4.1). The precise mechanism for this repression is still unclear and may include GR binding to, or recruiting, nuclear receptor corepressors (De Bosscher et al., 2006; Ito et al., 2006b; Rosenfeld et al., 2006), direct repression of coactivator complexes (Ito et al., 2000) or effects on RNA polymerase II phosphorylation (Luecke and Yamamoto, 2005; Nissen and Yamamoto, 2000). These effects are, however, context/gene dependent as some NF-κB-driven genes are not repressed by activated GR, such as IκBα. Moreover GR can combine with NF-κB to induce the expression of TLR2 and stem cell factor (SCF) (Da Silva et al., 2004; Hermoso et al., 2004).

Glucocorticoids also appear to exert anti-inflammatory actions that do not depend on the receptor's ability to regulate transcription in the nucleus. GR has been reported to regulate the levels of cell ribonucleases and mRNA-destabilizing proteins such as HuR and TTP, thereby reducing the levels of mRNA (Shim and Kapin, 2002; Smoak and Cidlowski, 2005) through a p38-MAPK-mediated pathway (Bergmann et al., 2004; Kassel et al., 2001; Lasa et al., 2001). However, significant modulation of these genes often appears at 10 nM dexamethasone rather than at the 1 nM concentrations associated with suppression of many inflammatory genes, although again these effects may be cell selective (Jalonen et al., 2005).

4.6   Dissociated Glucocorticoids

Whilst transrepression appears to be a major contributory mechanism to the anti-inflammatory effects of corticosteroids, the direct transactivation of genes appears to play a central role in many of the side effects (Belvisi et al., 2001; Schäcke et al., 2005). The upregulation of hepatic phosphoenolpyruvate carboxykinase and glucose-6-phosphatase are key events in the dysregulated glucose metabolism that ultimately result in insulin resistance and diabetes. Similarly, the induction of skeletal muscle glutamine synthetase is important in muscle wasting. However, the precise molecular events underlying glucocorticoid induction of osteoporosis and suppression of the HPA are complex and not fully understood (Schäcke et al., 2002, 2004). Thus, a novel glucocorticoid that shows selectivity for the transrepression pathway but does not transactivate might have an improved therapeutic index (Belvisi et al., 2001; Schäcke et al., 2005).

Support for this hypothesis comes from a series of elegant experiments in transgenic mice expressing mutated GRs that are unable to dimerize (GR^{dim}). In these mice, dexamethasone treatment has a reduced capacity to induce proopiomelanocort (POMC) transactivation but wild-type transrepression activity is maintained. In addition, dexamethasone inhibits both skin irritation caused by phorbol 12-myristate 13-acetate (PMA) and the systemic inflammatory response to lipopolysaccharides in GR^{dim} mice. Dexamethasone is also able to suppress the expression and release of numerous cytokines in these mice both *in vivo* and in isolated primary macrophages, thymocytes and CD4$^+$ splenocytes, probably through an effect on NF-κB activity (Reichardt et al., 2001). However, T-cell and thymocyte apoptosis are also impaired in these mice, suggesting a potential detrimental effect on immune function by preventing the resolution of the immune response (Reichardt et al., 2001).

Glucocorticoids generally appear to be more potent in assays of transrepression than transactivation (Adcock et al., 1999; Jaffuel et al., 2000). However the search for "dissociated" glucocorticoids that selectively transrepress without significant transactivation as a means of reducing the risk of systemic side effects has begun. In *in vitro* experiments RU24858 and similar compounds have a high affinity for GR and display a similar repression activity to dexamethasone but possess only 20–30% of the efficacy of dexamethasone in a transactivation assay (Vayssiere et al., 1997). Surprisingly, despite RU24858 showing comparable *in vivo* anti-inflammatory activity to prednisolone, there was no improvement in side-effect parameters such as osteoporosis, weight reduction or thymic involution (Belvisi et al., 2001). This may reflect RU24858 metabolism or problems inherent with differences between rodent and human GRs. Evidence for the latter effect comes from analysis of 17α-esters of beclomethasone and betamethasone, which show profound dissociation in rat systems, despite acting as classical corticosteroids in humans and mice (Tanigawa et al., 2002). In rats, these molecules have strong anti-inflammatory activity *in vivo* but fail to induce TAT and other liver enzymes.

More recently, researchers have moved away from classical steroidal molecules in favour of non-steroidal GR ligands because these molecules maintain a selective transrepression profile *in vivo* as well as in *in vitro* assays. AL-438, for example, maintains its anti-inflammatory activity *in vivo* and displays a reduced side-effect profile compared with prednisolone (Coghlan et al., 2003). Another drug from the same group, the non-terpenoid A276575, exhibits high affinity for GR and potently suppresses inflammatory gene expression in several cell types with a reduced induction of glucocorticoid-stimulated genes as compared with dexamethasone (Lin et al., 2002). The complexity of repression by GR is illustrated by the differential repression of RANTES and PGE$_2$ production in IL-1β-stimulated A549 cells by the two (−)-enantiomers of A276575 (Lin et al., 2002).

Similar results with other compounds containing non-steroidal backbones have also been reported from several laboratories (Kym et al., 2003; Shah and Scanlan, 2004; Smith et al., 2005; Thompson et al., 2007) and dissociated glucocorticoids have even been derived from natural products. Thus, a plant-derived phenyl aziridine precursor also shows clear dissociated properties at the GR in both *in vitro* and *in vivo* systems having good repression of NF-κB and lacking hyperglycaemic side effects (De Bosscher et al., 2005). In addition, ZK216348 is equipotent to prednisolone but has a reduced side-effect profile with respect to blood glucose levels and spleen involution compared to that of prednisolone *in vivo* (Schacke et al., 2004). Interestingly, however, ZK216348 exhibited similar suppression of adrenocorticotrophic hormone (ACTH) *in vivo* as prednisolone. This may suggest that dissociated glucocorticoids might not have an improved therapeutic index as far as HPA axis effects are concerned.

The recent resolution of the crystal structure of the GR (Bledsoe et al., 2002) has also helped in the better design of dissociated glucocorticoids (Barker et al., 2005, 2006), particularly when combined with data from directed mutagenesis studies. For example, modification of tyrosine 735 selectively impairs transactivation without affecting transrepression via the differential recruitment of NCoR1 rather than SRC-1, allowing a molecular switch to occur (Garside et al., 2004; Stevens et al., 2003).

Despite these efforts being to a certain extent in their infancy, preliminary data suggest that the development of glucocorticoids with a greater margin of safety is possible and may even lead to the development of oral glucocorticoids that do not have significant adverse effects. Many of these dissociated compounds show efficacy *in vivo* in some, but not all, animal models of disease perhaps due to metabolites being non-dissociated and results in man are imminent (Schäcke et al., 2007). For example, GlaxoSmithKline have a dissociated glucocorticoid in Phase IIa for asthma (http://www.abpi.org.uk/publications/publication_details/azResearch/a3.asp).

4.7 GR Cross-talk with Other Nuclear Receptors and Coactivators

Whilst the focus on the separation of transrepression from transactivation has resulted in the discovery of several novel GR ligands, these approaches have not explored the potential for tissue-specific regulation of the receptor. Interactions with tissue-specific cofactor proteins and cross-talk with other signalling pathways represent an additional opportunity to improve the therapeutic index (Lu and Cidlowski, 2005). Advances in gene expression profiling techniques have allowed the effects of mutations in GR that alter cofactor binding to be studied across a range of responsive genes in parallel. Such studies have revealed that different sets of genes are affected in different ways by each mutant (Lu and Cidlowski, 2005). For instance, the expression of some genes is dependent on the N-terminal AF-1 domain, while for others this activity is redundant. Since expression of some cofactor proteins, such as the peroxisome proliferator-activated receptor gamma (PPARγ) coactivator 1 (PGC-1), is controlled both temporally and spatially (Feingold et al., 2004), the opportunity for selective modulation of glucocorticoid response by the manipulation of GR's affinity for cofactors becomes apparent. Modulation of current compounds and screening of both steroidal and non-steroidal libraries for these properties is currently being undertaken.

In addition to the more classical modes of action, it is now clear that GR can bind to DNA as a heterodimer with other transcription factors, such as members of the signal transducer and activator of transcription (STAT) family (Biola et al., 2000; Stocklin et al., 1996) and the ETS transcription factors

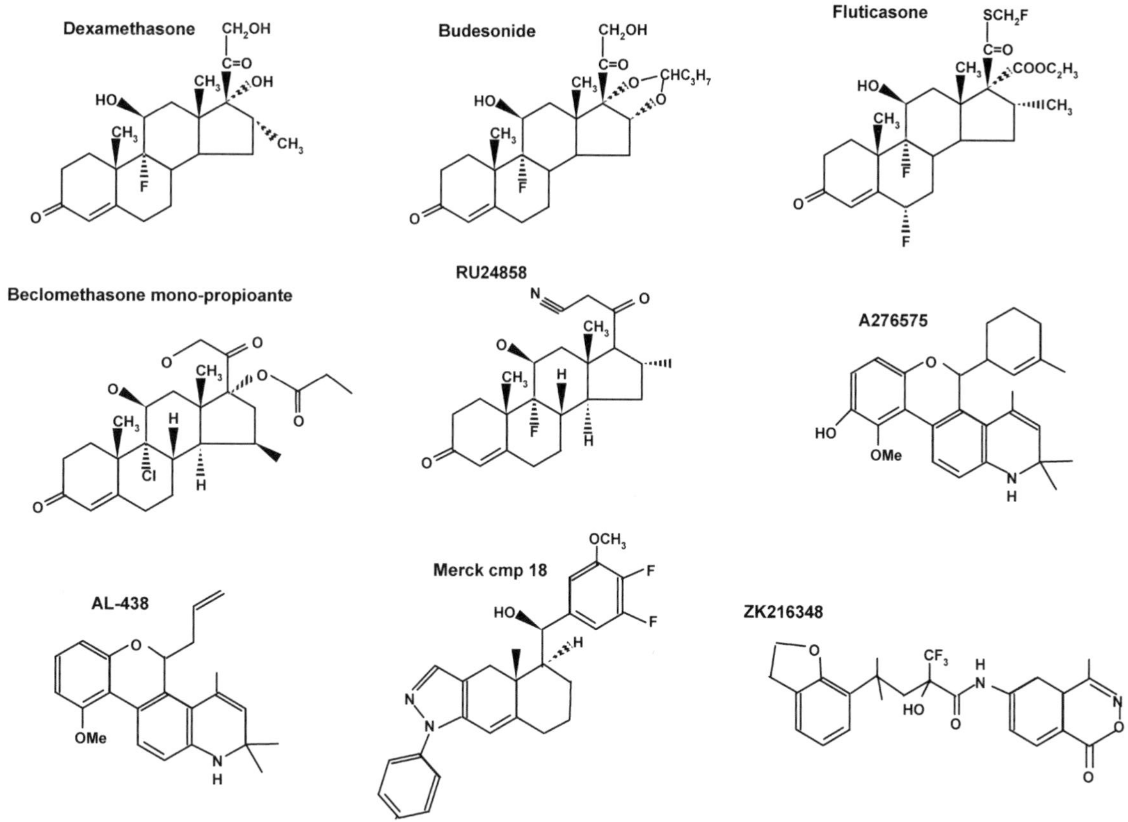

Figure 4.2 Structural modifications of dexamethasone that produce the clinically used corticosteroids dexamethasone, fluticasone and budesonide. The structures of representative non-steroidal glucocorticoid receptor modulators are also shown. RU24858 is a novel steroidal compound that showed evidence of novel pharmacology in some systems. Beclomethasone monopropionate (BMP), which is the active principle of the widely used drug BDP, is a classical corticosteroid in humans but is clearly a dissociated steroid in rats. Al-438, A276575, Merck cmp18 and ZK216348 are examples of novel non-steroidal ligands that selectively modulate the GR to generate unique pharmacological properties

(Mullick et al., 2001), leading to the recruitment of distinct coactivator (e.g. GRIP-1) or corepressor (e.g. RIP140 or HDAC) complexes (Barnes et al., 2004; Garside et al., 2004; Stevens et al., 2003). Recent evidence indicates that dexamethasone-activated GR represses a large set of functionally related inflammatory genes that are stimulated by p65–IRF-3 complexes (Ogawa et al., 2005). In contrast, PPARγ and (LXRs) repress a number of genes overlapping with GR transcriptional targets in a p65–IRF-3-independent manner and cooperate with GR to suppress additional distinct subsets of pattern recognition receptor (PRR)-responsive genes, thereby expanding the number/type of genes repressed by glucocorticoids (Ogawa et al., 2005).

The addition of other novel drugs to glucocorticoids may also affect the ratio of GR transactivation to transrepression. Thus, supraphysiological levels of vitamin B6 can reduce dexamethasone-stimulated GRE activity without affecting transrepression in a cell- and promoter-specific manner (Bamberger et al., 2004). In a similar manner, Combinatorix have developed a number of compounds (Crx-102, CRx-139 and CRx-191) that utilize different antidepressants to enhance the therapeutic window of either prednisolone or mometasone. CRx-102 has shown efficacy with no side effects in patients with osteoarthritis in the hand (Anon, 2006). Designing drugs with the capacity to activate both GR and other nuclear hormone receptors may, therefore, enhance the anti-inflammatory profile of glucocorticoids. Moreover, as the expression of many cofactors and nuclear receptors is tissue specific, there is the attractive possibility of designing tissue-specific ligands, although this approach will require a clearer understanding of the key tissue(s) targeted by glucocorticoids.

4.8 Overcoming Steroid Insensitivity

Despite their widespread utility, there remain certain conditions where glucocorticoids are less effective. In a very small number of cases this results from a polymorphism in the receptor that decreases the receptor's affinity for ligands. However, even without such links, there is a clear subpopulation of patients with severe asthma who appear clinically relatively insensitive to glucocorticoid therapy. Genetic analysis of such sensitive and resistant patients in an Icelandic population may have demonstrated a gene expression "fingerprint" that predicts clinical glucocorticoid responsiveness, although the utility of this work in a wider context has yet to be determined (Hakonarson et al., 2005). Other theories, such as increased expression of the alternative transcripts such as GRβ, have been proposed to explain such insensitivity but these have not been reported in all cases (Ito et al., 2006a).

COPD has become one of the commonest diseases worldwide and a major global healthcare problem, causing over 30 000 deaths a year in the UK alone. It is predicted to become the fifth most common cause of disability and the third commonest cause of death worldwide by 2020 (Lopez et al., 2006). It is now recognized that COPD involves a chronic inflammatory process affecting lower airways, with small airways representing the major site of airflow obstruction. Existing therapies for COPD are grossly inadequate and none have been shown to slow the relentless progression of the disease (Barnes and Kleinert, 2004). In sharp contrast to asthma, COPD appears to be relatively resistant to the anti-inflammatory actions of corticosteroids. By uncovering the reason for this paradox, it should be possible to implement treatment regimens that restore corticosteroid sensitivity.

In COPD there is a marked increase in local and systemic oxidative stress (Barnes et al., 2004; Macnee and Rahman, 2001), particularly during exacerbations (Barnes et al., 2004; Biernacki et al., 2003; Macnee and Rahman, 2001). Most striking are the increases in reactive oxygen and nitrogen species, such as 4-hydroxynonenal, nitrotyrosine, hydrogen peroxide (H_2O_2) and 8-isoprostane (Barnes et al., 2004; Macnee and Rahman, 2001). The relative lack of response to corticosteroids in COPD has been linked to oxidative stress and may reflect an effect on GR nuclear import (Okamoto et al., 1999) or on the activity of GR nuclear corepressors (Ito et al., 2005). Antioxidant therapy has been tried in COPD but has proved ineffective due to a failure to achieve sufficient efficacy at the site of the disease (Decramer et al., 2005). More potent antioxidants such as the SOD mimetic AEOL10150 should prove effective in COPD either alone or, more likely, by restoring steroid sensitivity (Orrell, 2006).

4.9   Glucorticoid-sparing Approaches to Anti-inflammatory Therapy

Advances in our understanding of molecular mechanisms of glucocorticoid actions may lead to the development of novel non-steroidal anti-inflammatory treatments that mimic some of the effects of glucocorticoids on inflammatory gene regulation. Potential therapeutic targets include specific coactivators activated by NF-κB, inhibition of which might also repress the action of other pro-inflammatory transcription factors (Turlais et al., 2001). Alternatively, corepressor molecules might be activated (Ito et al., 2002). Inhibition of the transcriptional effects of NF-κB appears to mediate many of the anti-inflammatory effects of glucocorticoids, and small-molecule inhibitors of IKK-2 (which activates NF-κB) are being developed. However the effects of glucocorticoids are also mediated via additional mechanisms, such as regulation of the AP-1 transcription factor and on mRNA stability. Therefore, it is not yet established whether IKK-2 inhibitors will parallel the clinical effectiveness of glucocorticoids. IKK-2 inhibitors may also have side effects, such as increased susceptibility to infections. However, it is worth noting that if glucocorticoids were discovered today their low therapeutic ratio and side-effect profile would be likely to prevent their use in humans.

4.10   Conclusion

Enormous progress has been made in improving glucocorticoid treatment since the introduction of hydrocortisone as the first clinically used corticosteroid. Extensive drug development has resulted in highly potent molecules, the pharmacokinetic profiles of which have been optimized in order to minimize systemic exposure and to target activity to the lung. Advances in delineating the fundamental mechanisms of glucocorticoid pharmacology, especially the concepts of transactivation and transrepression and cofactor recruitment, have resulted in a better understanding of the molecular mechanisms whereby glucocorticoids suppress inflammation. This knowledge has contributed to the rational design of drugs that target novel aspects of GR function in a cell- or tissue-specific manner and may additionally result in treatments that can restore glucocorticoid sensitivity in diseases such as COPD. Currently, we are awaiting the first clinical results of a dissociated glucocorticoid in man that will indicate whether the approach is sound. Future challenges are to address whether steroidal or non-steroidal structures are better, whether their properties are enhanced by combination with other therapeutic agents such as long-acting β_2-agonists and whether the properties can be maintained for a once-a-day treatment.

Acknowledgements

The literature in this area is extensive, and many important studies were omitted because of constraints on space, for which we apologize.

References

Adcock IM, Nasuhara Y, Stevens DA, Barnes PJ. Ligand-induced differentiation of glucocorticoid receptor (GR) trans-repression and transactivation: preferential targetting of NF-kappaB and lack of I-kappaB involvement. *Br J Pharmacol* 1999; **127**: 1003–1011.

Adelroth E, Rosenhall L, Johansson SA, Linden M, Venge P. Inflammatory cells and eosinophilic activity in asthmatics investigated by bronchoalveolar lavage. The effects of antiasthmatic treatment with budesonide or terbutaline. *Am Rev Respir Dis* 1990; **142**: 91–99.

Anon. Dipyridamole plus prednisolone [CRx 102] reduces pain in patients with hand osteoarthritis. *Inpharma* 2006; **1**: 8–8(1).

Baldwin AS, Jr. Series introduction: the transcription factor NF-kappaB and human disease. *J Clin Invest* 2001; **107**: 3–6.

Bamberger CM, Else T, Ellebrecht I, Milde-Langosch K et al. Vitamin B6 modulates glucocorticoid-dependent gene transcription in a promoter- and cell type-specific manner. *Exp Clin Endocrinol Diabetes* 2004; **112**: 595–600.

Barker M, Clackers M, Copley R, Demaine DA et al. Dissociated nonsteroidal glucocorticoid receptor modulators; discovery of the agonist trigger in a tetrahydronaphthalene-benzoxazine series. *J Med Chem* 2006; **49**: 4216–4231.

Barker M, Clackers M, Demaine DA, Humphreys D et al. Design and synthesis of new nonsteroidal glucocorticoid modulators through application of an "agreement docking" method. *J Med Chem* 2005; **48**: 4507–4510.

Barnes PJ. Inhaled glucocorticoids for asthma. *N Engl J Med* 1995; **332**: 868–875.

Barnes PJ, Adcock IM. How do corticosteroids work in asthma? *Ann Intern Med* 2003; **139**: 359–370.

Barnes PJ, Kleinert S. COPD – a neglected disease. *Lancet* 2004; **364**: 564–565.

Barnes PJ, Ito K, Adcock IM. Corticosteroid resistance in chronic obstructive pulmonary disease: inactivation of histone deacetylase. *Lancet* 2004; **363**: 731–733.

Belvisi MG, Wicks SL, Battram CH, Bottoms SE et al. Therapeutic benefit of a dissociated glucocorticoid and the relevance of in vitro separation of transrepression from transactivation activity. *J Immunol* 2001; **166**: 1975–1982.

Bergmann MW, Staples KJ, Smith SJ, Barnes PJ, Newto n R. Glucocorticoid inhibition of granulocyte macrophage-colony-stimulating factor from T cells is independent of control by nuclear factor-kappaB and conserved lymphokine element 0. *Am J Respir Cell Mol Biol* 2004; **30**: 555–563.

Biernacki WA, Kharitonov SA, Barnes PJ. Increased leukotriene B4 and 8-isoprostane in exhaled breath condensate of patients with exacerbations of COPD. *Thorax* 2003; **58**: 294–298.

Biola A, Andreau K, David M, Sturm M et al. The glucocorticoid receptor and STAT6 physically and functionally interact in T-lymphocytes. *FEBS Lett* 2000; **487**: 229–233.

Bledsoe RK, Montana VG, Stanley TB, Delves CJ et al. Crystal structure of the glucocorticoid receptor ligand binding domain reveals a novel mode of receptor dimerization and coactivator recognition. *Cell* 2002; **110**: 93–105.

Bryan SA, Leckie MJ, Hansel TT, Barnes PJ. Novel therapy for asthma. *Expert Opin Invest Drugs* 2000; **9**: 25–42.

Burge PS, Calverley PM, Jones PW, Spencer S et al. Randomised, double blind, placebo controlled study of fluticasone propionate in patients with moderate to severe chronic obstructive pulmonary disease: the ISOLDE trial. *BMJ* 2000; **320**: 1297–1303.

Busse WW, Lemanske RF Jr. Asthma. *N Engl J Med* 2001; **344**: 350–362.

Calverley PM, Anderson JA, Celli B, Ferguson GT et al. Salmeterol and fluticasone propionate and survival in chronic obstructive pulmonary disease. *N Engl J Med* 2007; **356**: 775–789.

Caramori G, Ito K, Adcock IM. Transcription factors in asthma and COPD. *IDrugs* 2004; **7**: 764–770.

Caramori G, Romagnoli M, Casolari P, Bellettato C et al. Nuclear localisation of p65 in sputum macrophages but not in sputum neutrophils during COPD exacerbations. *Thorax* 2003; **58**: 348–351.

Coghlan MJ, Jacobson PB, Lane B, Nakane M et al. A novel antiinflammatory maintains glucocorticoid efficacy with reduced side effects. *Mol Endocrinol* 2003; **17**: 860–869.

Cosio BG, Mann B, Ito K, Jazrawi E et al. Histone acetylase and deacetylase activity in alveolar macrophages and blood mononocytes in asthma. *Am J Respir Crit Care Med* 2004; **170**: 141–147.

Da Silva CA, Kassel O, Lebouquin R, Lacroix EJ, Frossard N. Paradoxical early glucocorticoid induction of stem cell factor (SCF) expression in inflammatory conditions. *Br J Pharmacol* 2004; **141**: 75–84.

De Bosscher K, Berghe WV, Beck IM, Van MW et al. A fully dissociated compound of plant origin for inflammatory gene repression. *Proc Natl Acad Sci USA* 2005; **102**: 15827–15832.

De Bosscher K, Vanden BW, Haegeman G. Cross-talk between nuclear receptors and nuclear factor kappaB. *Oncogene* 2006; **25**: 6868–6886.

Decramer M, Rutten-van MM, Dekhuijzen PN, Troosters T et al. Effects of N-acetylcysteine on outcomes in chronic obstructive pulmonary disease (Bronchitis Randomized on NAC

Cost-Utility Study, BRONCUS): a randomised placebo-controlled trial. *Lancet* 2005; **365**: 1552–1560.

Di Stefano A, Caramori G, Ricciardolo FL, Capelli A et al. Cellular and molecular mechanisms in chronic obstructive pulmonary disease: an overview. *Clin Exp Allergy* 2004; **34**: 1156–1167.

Eynott PR, Nath P, Leung SY, Adcock IM et al. Allergen-induced inflammation and airway epithelial and smooth muscle cell proliferation: role of Jun N-terminal kinase. *Br J Pharmacol* 2003; **140**: 1373–1380.

Feingold K, Kim MS, Shigenaga J, Moser A, Grunfeld C. Altered expression of nuclear hormone receptors and coactivators in mouse heart during the acute-phase response. *Am J Physiol Endocrinol Metab* 2004; **286**: E201–E207.

Gagliardo R, Chanez P, Mathieu M, Bruno A et al. Persistent activation of nuclear factor-kappaB signaling pathway in severe uncontrolled asthma. *Am J Respir Crit Care Med* 2003; **168**: 1190–1198.

Garside H, Stevens A, Farrow S, Normand C et al. Glucocorticoid ligands specify different interactions with NF-kappaB by allosteric effects on the glucocorticoid receptor DNA binding domain. *J Biol Chem* 2004; **279**: 50050–50059.

Hakonarson H, Bjornsdottir US, Halapi E, Bradfield J et al. Profiling of genes expressed in peripheral blood mononuclear cells predicts glucocorticoid sensitivity in asthma patients. *Proc Natl Acad Sci USA* 2005; **102**: 14789–14794.

Hart LA, Krishnan VL, Adcock IM, Barnes PJ, Chung KF. Activation and localization of transcription factor, nuclear factor-kappaB, in asthma. *Am J Respir Crit Care Med* 1998; **158**: 1585–1592.

Hermoso MA, Matsuguchi T, Smoak K, Cidlowski JA. Glucocorticoids and tumor necrosis factor alpha cooperatively regulate toll-like receptor 2 gene expression. *Mol Cell Biol* 2004; **24**: 4743–4756.

Hogg JC, Chu F, Utokaparch S, Woods R et al. The nature of small-airway obstruction in chronic obstructive pulmonary disease. *N Engl J Med* 2004; **350**: 2645–2653.

Holden NS, Catley MC, Cambridge LM, Barnes PJ, Newton R. ICAM-1 expression is highly NF-kappaB-dependent in A549 cells. No role for ERK and p38 MAPK. *Eur J Biochem* 2004; **271**: 785–791.

Ito K, Barnes PJ, Adcock IM. Glucocorticoid receptor recruitment of histone deacetylase 2 inhibits interleukin-1beta-induced histone H4 acetylation on lysines 8 and 12. *Mol Cell Biol* 2000; **20**: 6891–6903.

Ito K, Chung KF, Adcock IM. Update on glucocorticoid action and resistance. *J Allergy Clin Immunol* 2006a; **117**: 522–543.

Ito K, Ito M, Elliott WM, Cosio B et al. Decreased histone deacetylase activity in chronic obstructive pulmonary disease. *N Engl J Med* 2005; **352**: 1967–1976.

Ito K, Lim S, Caramori G, Cosio B et al. A molecular mechanism of action of theophylline: Induction of histone deacetylase activity to decrease inflammatory gene expression. *Proc Natl Acad Sci USA* 2002; **99**: 8921–8926.

Ito K, Yamamura S, Essilfie-Quaye S, Cosio B et al. Histone deacetylase 2-mediated deacetylation of the glucocorticoid receptor enables NF-kappaB suppression. *J Exp Med* 2006b; **203**: 7–13.

Jaffuel D, Demoly P, Gougat C, Balaguer P et al. Transcriptional potencies of inhaled glucocorticoids. *Am J Respir Crit Care Med* 2000; **162**: 57–63.

Jalonen U, Lahti A, Korhonen R, Kankaanranta H, Moilanen E. Inhibition of tristetraprolin expression by dexamethasone in activated macrophages. *Biochem Pharmacol* 2005; **69**: 733–740.

Jeffery PK, Godfrey RW, Adelroth E, Nelson F et al. Effects of treatment on airway inflammation and thickening of basement membrane reticular collagen in asthma. A quantitative light and electron microscopic study. *Am Rev Respir Dis* 1992; **145**: 890–899.

Kassel O, Sancono A, Kratzschmar J, Kreft B et al. Glucocorticoids inhibit MAP kinase via increased expression and decreased degradation of MKP-1. *EMBO J* 2001; **20**: 7108–7116.

Koch A, Giembycz M, Ito K, Lim S et al. Mitogen-activated protein kinase modulation of nuclear factor-kappaB-induced granulocyte macrophage-colony-stimulating factor release from human alveolar macrophages. *Am J Respir Cell Mol Biol* 2004; **30**: 342–349.

Kumar S, Boehm J, Lee JC. p38 MAP kinases: key signalling molecules as therapeutic targets for inflammatory diseases. *Nat Rev Drug Discov* 2003; **2**: 717–726.

Kym PR, Kort ME, Coghlan MJ, Moore JL et al. Nonsteroidal selective glucocorticoid modulators: the effect of C-10 substitution on receptor selectivity and functional potency of 5-allyl-2,5-dihydro-2,2,4-trimethyl-1H-[1]benzopyrano[3,4-f]quinolines. *J Med Chem* 2003; **46**: 1016–1030.

Laitinen LA, Laitinen A, Haahtela T. A comparative study of the effects of an inhaled corticosteroid, budesonide, and a beta 2-agonist, terbutaline, on airway inflammation in newly diagnosed asthma: a randomized, double- blind, parallel-group controlled trial. *J Allergy Clin Immunol* 1992; **90**: 32–42.

Laursen LC, Taudorf E, Borgeskov S, Kobayasi T et al. Fiberoptic bronchoscopy and bronchial mucosal biopsies in asthmatics undergoing long-term high-dose budesonide aerosol treatment. *Allergy* 1988; **43**: 284–288.

Lee KY, Ito K, Hayashi R, Jazrawi EP et al. NF-{kappa}B and activator protein 1 response elements and the role of histone modifications in IL-1{beta}-induced TGF-{beta}1 gene transcription. *J Immunol* 2006; **176**: 603–615.

Li B, Carey M, Workman JL. The role of chromatin during transcription. *Cell* 2007; **128**: 707–719.

Lin CW, Nakane M, Stashko M, Falls D et al. trans-Activation and repression properties of the novel nonsteroid glucocorticoid receptor ligand 2,5-dihydro-9-hydroxy-10-methoxy-2,2,4-trimethyl-5-(1-methylcyclohexen-3-y 1)-1H-[1]benzopyrano[3,4-f]quinoline (A276575) and its four stereoisomers. *Mol Pharmacol* 2002; **62**: 297–303.

Lopez AD, Mathers CD, Ezzati M, Jamison DT, Murray CJ. Global and regional burden of disease and risk factors, 2001: systematic analysis of population health data. *Lancet* 2006; **367**: 1747–1757.

Lu NZ, Cidlowski JA. Translational regulatory mechanisms generate N-terminal glucocorticoid receptor isoforms with unique transcriptional target genes. *Mol Cell* 2005; **18**: 331–342.

Luecke HF, Yamamoto KR. The glucocorticoid receptor blocks P-TEFb recruitment by NFkappaB to effect promoter-specific transcriptional repression. *Genes Dev* 2005; **19**: 1116–1127.

Macnee W, Rahman I. Is oxidative stress central to the pathogenesis of chronic obstructive pulmonary disease? *Trends Mol Med* 2001; **7**: 55–62.

Mullick J, Anandatheerthavarada HK, Amuthan G, Bhagwat SV et al. Physical interaction and functional synergy between glucocorticoid receptor and Ets2 proteins for transcription activation of the rat cytochrome P-450c27 promoter. *J Biol Chem* 2001; **276**: 18007–18017.

Nissen RM, Yamamoto KR. The glucocorticoid receptor inhibits NFkappaB by interfering with serine-2 phosphorylation of the RNA polymerase II carboxy-terminal domain. *Genes Dev* 2000; **14**: 2314–2329.

Ogawa S, Lozach J, Benner C, Pascual G et al. Molecular determinants of crosstalk between nuclear receptors and toll-like receptors. *Cell* 2005; **122**: 707–721.

Okamoto K, Tanaka H, Ogawa H, Makino Y et al. Redox-dependent regulation of nuclear import of the glucocorticoid receptor. *J Biol Chem* 1999; **274**: 10363–10371.

Olivieri D, Chetta A, Del Donno M, Bertorelli G et al. Effect of short-term treatment with low-dose inhaled fluticasone propionate on airway inflammation and remodeling in mild asthma: a placebo-controlled study. *Am J Respir Crit Care Med* 1997; **155**: 1864–1871.

Orrell RW. AEOL-10150 (Aeolus). *Curr Opin Invest Drugs* 2006; **7**: 70–80.

Pauwels RA, Lofdahl CG, Laitinen LA, Schouten JP et al. Long-term treatment with inhaled budesonide in persons with mild chronic obstructive pulmonary disease who continue smoking. European Respiratory Society Study on Chronic Obstructive Pulmonary Disease. *N Engl J Med* 1999; **340**: 1948–1953.

Perkins ND. Integrating cell-signalling pathways with NF-kappaB and IKK function. *Nat Rev Mol Cell Biol* 2007; **8**: 49–62.

Pernis AB, Rothman PB. JAK-STAT signaling in asthma. *J Clin Invest* 2002; **109**: 1279–1283.

Reichardt HM, Tuckermann JP, Gottlicher M, Vujic M et al. Repression of inflammatory responses in the absence of DNA binding by the glucocorticoid receptor. *EMBO J* 2001; **20**: 7168–7173.

Rosenfeld MG, Lunyak VV, Glass CK. Sensors and signals: a coactivator/corepressor/epigenetic code for integrating signal-dependent programs of transcriptional response. *Genes Dev* 2006; **20**: 1405–1428.

Schäcke H, Berger M, Rehwinkel H, Asadullah K. Selective glucocorticoid receptor agonists (SEGRAs): Novel ligands with an improved therapeutic index. *Mol Cell Endocrinol* 2007; **275**: 109–117.

Schäcke H, Docke WD, Asadullah K. Mechanisms involved in the side effects of glucocorticoids. *Pharmacol Ther* 2002; **96**: 23–43.

Schäcke H, Rehwinkel H, Asadullah K. Dissociated glucocorticoid receptor ligands: compounds with an improved therapeutic index. *Curr Opin Invest Drugs* 2005; **6**: 503–507.

Schäcke H, Schottelius A, Docke WD, Strehlke P et al. Dissociation of transactivation from transrepression by a selective glucocorticoid receptor agonist leads to separation of therapeutic effects from side effects. *Proc Natl Acad Sci USA* 2004; **101**: 227–232.

Shah N, Scanlan TS. Design and evaluation of novel nonsteroidal dissociating glucocorticoid receptor ligands. *Bioorg Med Chem Lett* 2004; **14**: 5199–5203.

Shim J, Karin M. The control of mRNA stability in response to extracellular stimuli. *Mol Cells* 2002; **14**: 323–331.

Smith CJ, Ali A, Balkovec JM, Graham DW et al. Novel ketal ligands for the glucocorticoid receptor: in vitro and in vivo activity. *Bioorg Med Chem Lett* 2005; **15**: 2926–2931.

Smoak KA, Cidlowski JA. A novel anti-inflammatory mechanism for glucocorticoids: regulation of TTP synthesis. *Am J Respir Crit Care Med* 2005; **171**: A74

Soriano JB, Sin DD, Zhang X, Camp PG et al. A pooled analysis of FEV1 decline in COPD patients randomized to inhaled corticosteroids or placebo. *Chest* 2007; **131**: 682–689.

Stevens A, Garside H, Berry A, Waters C et al. Dissociation of steroid receptor coactivator 1 and nuclear receptor corepressor recruitment to the human glucocorticoid receptor by modification of the ligand-receptor interface: the role of tyrosine 735. *Mol Endocrinol* 2003; **17**: 845–859.

Stocklin E, Wissler M, Gouilleux F, Groner B. Functional interactions between Stat5 and the glucocorticoid receptor. *Nature* 1996; **383**: 726–728.

Tanigawa K, Tanaka K, Nagase H, Miyake H et al. Cell type-dependent divergence of transactivation by glucocorticoid receptor ligand. *Biol Pharm Bull* 2002; **25**: 1619–1622.

Thompson CF, Quraishi N, Ali A, Mosley RT et al. Novel glucocorticoids containing a 6,5-bicyclic core fused to a pyrazole ring: Synthesis, in vitro profile, molecular modeling studies, and in vivo experiments. *Bioorg Med Chem Lett* 2007; **17**: 3354–3361.

Turlais F, Hardcastle A, Rowlands M, Newbatt Y et al. High-throughput screening for identification of small molecule inhibitors of histone acetyltransferases using scintillating microplates (FlashPlate). *Anal Biochem* 2001; **298**: 62–68.

Van Rensen EL, Straathof KC, Veselic-Charvat MA, Zwinderman AH et al. Effect of inhaled steroids on airway hyperresponsiveness, sputum eosinophils, and exhaled nitric oxide levels in patients with asthma. *Thorax* 1999; **54**: 403–408.

Vayssiere BM, Dupont S, Choquart A, Petit F et al. Synthetic glucocorticoids that dissociate transactivation and AP-1 transrepression exhibit antiinflammatory activity in vivo. *Mol Endocrinol* 1997; **11**: 1245–1255.

Vestbo J, Sorensen T, Lange P, Brix A et al. Long-term effect of inhaled budesonide in mild and moderate chronic obstructive pulmonary disease: a randomised controlled trial. *Lancet* 1999; **353**: 1819–1823.

Zhou J, Cidlowski JA. The human glucocorticoid receptor: one gene, multiple proteins and diverse responses. *Steroids* 2005; **70**: 407–417.

5

Generalized Glucocorticoid Insensitivity: Clinical Phenotype and Molecular Mechanisms

Evangelia Charmandari, Tomoshige Kino
and **George P. Chrousos**

5.1 Introduction

Glucocorticoid resistance is a rare, familial or sporadic condition characterized by generalized, partial end-organ insensitivity to glucocorticoids (Charmandari et al., 2004a; Chrousos, 2002; Chrousos et al., 1982, 1993; Kino and Chrousos, 2001; Kino et al., 2002, 2003; Vingerhoeds et al., 1976). Affected subjects have compensatory elevations in circulating cortisol and adrenocorticotrophic hormone (ACTH) concentrations, which maintain circadian rhythmicity and appropriate responsiveness to stressors, and resistance of the hypothalamic-pituitary-adrenal (HPA) axis to dexamethasone suppression, but no clinical evidence of hypercortisolism. The excess ACTH secretion results in increased production of adrenal steroids with mineralocorticoid activity, such as deoxycorticosterone (DOC) and corticosterone, and/or androgenic activity, such as androstenedione, dehydroepiandrosterone (DHEA) and DHEA sulphate (DHEAS) (Charmandari et al., 2004a; Chrousos, 2002; Chrousos et al., 1982, 1993; Kino and Chrousos, 2001; Kino et al., 2002, 2003; Vingerhoeds et al., 1976) (Figure 5.1). The former accounts for symptoms and signs of mineralocorticoid excess, such as hypertension and hypokalaemic alkalosis, and the latter accounts for manifestations of androgen excess, such as ambiguous genitalia and precocious puberty in children, acne, hirsutism and infertility in both sexes, male-pattern hair loss, menstrual irregularities and oligo-anovulation in

Overcoming Steroid Insensitivity in Respiratory Disease   Edited by Ian M. Adcock and Kian Fan Chung
© 2008 John Wiley & Sons, Ltd.

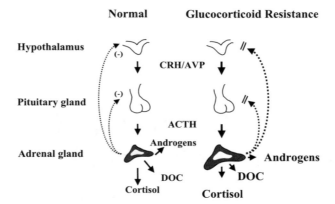

Figure 5.1 Alterations in the hypothalamic-pituitary-adrenal (HPA) axis in generalized glucocorticoid resistance. The impaired glucocorticoid feedback inhibition at the hypothalamic and anterior pituitary levels results in increased secretion of corticotrophin-releasing hormone (CRH) and adrenocorticotrophin hormone (ACTH), adrenal hyperplasia and increased secretion of adrenal steroids with mineralocorticoid and/or androgenic activity. AVP: arginine vasopressin; DOC: deoxycorticosterone

females and adrenal rests in the testes and oligospermia in males. The clinical spectrum of the condition is broad and a large number of subjects may be asymptomatic, displaying biochemical alterations only (Charmandari et al., 2004a; Chrousos et al., 1993; Kino et al., 2002, 2003) (Table 5.1).

Table 5.1　Clinical manifestations and diagnostic evaluation of syndromes of glucocorticoid resistance (adapted from Chrousos et al., 1993)

Clinical presentation
Apparently normal glucocorticoid function
　Asymptomatic
　Chronic fatigue (glucocorticoid deficiency?)
Mineralocorticoid excess
　Hypertension
　Hypokalaemic alkalosis
Androgen excess
　Females: Ambiguous genitalia at birth, acne, hirsutism, male-pattern hair loss, menstrual
　irregularities, oligo-anovulation, infertility, precocious puberty
　Males: Acne, hirsutism, oligospermia, infertility, precocious puberty
Diagnostic evaluation
Absence of clinical features of Cushing's syndrome
Normal or elevated plasma ACTH concentrations
Elevated plasma cortisol concentrations and increased 24-h urinary free cortisol excretion
Maintenance of a normal circadian and stress-induced pattern of cortisol and ACTH secretion
Resistance of the HPA axis to dexamethasone suppression
Thymidine incorporation assays
Dexamethasone binding assays
Molecular studies

The diagnosis of generalized glucocorticoid resistance is suggested by the elevated serum cortisol concentrations and 24-h urinary free cortisol excretion in the absence of clinical features of hypercortisolism. The plasma concentrations of ACTH may be normal or high. The circadian pattern of ACTH and cortisol secretion and their responsiveness to stressors is preserved, albeit at higher concentrations, and there is resistance of the HPA axis to dexamethasone suppression. The diagnosis is confirmed by thymidine incorporation and dexamethasone binding assays on peripheral blood mononuclear cells or cultured skin fibroblasts, and sequencing of the glucocorticoid receptor (GR) gene (Charmandari et al., 2004a; Chrousos et al., 1993; Kino et al., 2002, 2003) (Table 5.1).

The differential diagnosis includes: mild forms of Cushing's disease, in which hypercortisolism is accompanied by normal or mildly elevated ACTH concentrations; pseudo-Cushing's states, such as generalized anxiety disorder and melancholic depression; conditions associated with elevated serum concentrations of cortisol-binding globulin; other causes of mineralocorticoid-induced hypertension; and other causes of hyperandrogenism or virilization, such as idiopathic hirsutism, polycystic ovarian syndrome and congenital adrenal hyperplasia (Charmandari et al., 2004a; Chrousos et al., 1993; Kino et al., 2002, 2003).

The aim of treatment in generalized glucocorticoid resistance is to suppress the excess secretion of ACTH, thereby suppressing the increased production of mineralocorticoids and androgens from the adrenal cortex. Treatment involves administration of high doses of mineralocorticoid-sparing synthetic glucocorticoids such as dexamethasone (1–3 mg/day), which activate the mutant and/or wild-type human glucocorticoid receptor-alpha (hGRα) and suppress the endogenous secretion of ACTH in affected subjects (Charmandari et al., 2004a; Chrousos et al., 1993; Kino et al., 2002, 2003). Adequate suppression of the HPA axis is of particular importance in cases of severe impairment of hGRα action, given that longstanding corticotroph hyperstimulation in association with decreased glucocorticoid negative feedback inhibition may lead to the development of an ACTH-secreting adenoma (Karl et al., 1996). Long-term dexamethasone treatment should be carefully titrated based on the clinical manifestations and biochemical profile (Chrousos et al., 1982). Asymptomatic, normotensive subjects with primary glucocorticoid resistance do not require any treatment.

5.2 Molecular Mechanisms of Glucocorticoid Resistance

The molecular basis of generalized glucocorticoid resistance has been ascribed to mutations in the hGR gene, which impair one or more of the molecular mechanisms of GR action, thereby altering tissue sensitivity to glucocorticoids. Inactivating mutations within the ligand- and DNA-binding domains of the receptor and a four-base-pair deletion at the 3′ boundary of exon 6 of the gene have been described in five kindreds and five sporadic cases (Charmandari et al., 2005, 2007; Chrousos et al., 1982; Hurley et al., 1991; Karl et al., 1993, 1996; Kino et al., 2001; Malchoff et al., 1993; Mendonca et al., 2002; Ruiz et al., 2001; Vottero et al., 2002). The molecular mechanisms through which various natural GR mutants affect glucocorticoid signal transduction have been systematically investigated in all cases of generalized glucocorticoid resistance. These mechanisms included: the transcriptional activity of the mutant receptor; the ability of the mutant receptor to exert a dominant negative effect upon the wild-type receptor; the affinity of the mutant receptor for the ligand; the time required for nuclear translocation of the mutant receptor following exposure to the ligand; the ability of the mutant receptor to bind to glucocorticoid response elements (GREs); and the interaction of the mutant receptor with the glucocorticoid receptor interacting protein-1 (GRIP-1), which belongs to the p160 family of nuclear receptor coactivators and plays an important role in the formation of the transcription initiation complex and the hGRα-mediated transcriptional regulation of target genes (Figure 5.2).

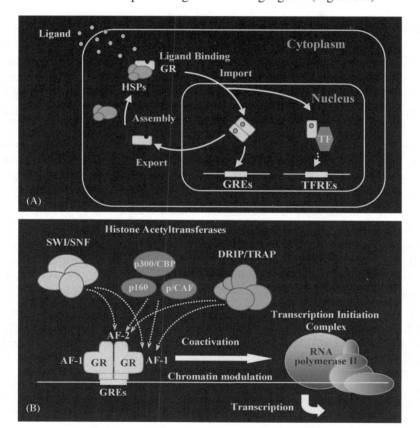

Figure 5.2 (A) Nucleocytoplasmic shuttling of the glucocorticoid receptor. Upon binding to the ligand, the activated hGRα dissociates from HSPs and translocates into the nucleus, where it homodimerizes and binds to GREs in the promoter region of target genes. (B) Schematic representation of the interaction of AF-1 and AF-2 of hGRα with coactivators. AF: activation function; DRIP/TRAP: vitamin D receptor-interacting protein/thyroid hormone receptor-associated protein; GR, glucocorticoid receptor; GREs, glucocorticoid response elements; HSP: heat shock protein; SWI/SNF: switching/sucrose non-fermenting; TF: transcription factor; TFRE: transcription factor response element. A full-colour version of this figure can be found in the colour plate section of this book.

The molecular defects elucidated in all reported cases of generalized glucocorticoid resistance are summarized in Table 5.2, while the corresponding mutations in
the hGR gene are shown in Table 5.2 and Figure 5.3. Finally, Figure 5.4 shows the
location of the known mutations of the hGR in the agonist- and antagonist-bound
form of the ligand-binding domain of the receptor. Mutations within the ligand-binding
domain of the receptor have been shown to affect mostly the affinity of the receptor for
the ligand and the interaction of the receptor with the p160 coactivators, while the
mutation identified in the DNA-binding domain of the receptor impaired its ability
to bind to GREs in the promoter region of target genes (Charmandari et al., 2004b,
2005, 2006, 2007; Chrousos et al., 1982; Hurley et al., 1991; Karl et al., 1993, 1996;
Kino et al., 2001; Malchoff et al., 1993; Mendonca et al., 2002; Ruiz et al., 2001;
Vottero et al., 2002) (Table 5.2).

The propositus of the original kindred was homozygous for a single, adenine to
thymine (A → T) substitution at nucleotide position 2054, which resulted in substitution of aspartic acid (D) by valine (V) at amino acid position 641 in the ligand-binding
domain of the receptor. This mutation resulted in a threefold reduction in the affinity
of the receptor for the ligand and caused a concomitant loss of the hGRα-mediated transactivation of the glucocorticoid-inducible mouse mammary tumour virus
(MMTV) promoter (Hurley et al., 1991). The mutant receptor hGRαD641V did
not exert a dominant negative effect upon the wild-type hGRα, showed a delay in
nuclear translocation (22 min), preserved its ability to bind to GREs and interacted
only with the amino-terminal fragment of GRIP-1 coactivator *in vitro* (Charmandari
et al., 2004b).

The proposita of the second kindred had a four-base-pair deletion at the 3′ boundary of exon 6 in one hGR allele, which removed a donor splice site. This deletion
resulted in complete ablation of expression of one hGR allele and a decrease in hGR
protein by 50% in affected members of the family (Karl et al., 1993).

The propositus of the third kindred had a single, homozygous, guanine to
adenine (G → A) substitution at nucleotide position 2317, resulting in valine (V)
to isoleucine (I) substitution at amino acid 729 in the ligand-binding domain of
the receptor (Malchoff et al., 1993). The mutant receptor hGRαV729I demonstrated a fourfold decrease in its transcriptional activity and a twofold reduction
in its affinity for the ligand. It showed a marked delay in nuclear translocation
(120 min) and interacted with the GRIP-1 coactivator *in vitro* only through its
activation function (AF)-1. Finally, it did not exert a dominant negative effect upon
the wild-type receptor and it preserved its ability to bind to GREs (Charmandari
et al., 2004b).

The first sporadic case of generalized glucocorticoid resistance was due to a
de novo, germ-line, heterozygous point mutation (T → A) at nucleotide position
1808, which resulted in isoleucine (I) to asparagine (N) substitution at amino acid
559 in the hinge region of the receptor (Karl et al., 1996; Kino et al., 2001). The
mutant receptor hGRαI559N had minimal transcriptional activity and undetectable
affinity for ligand. It exerted a potent dominant negative effect upon the wild-type
receptor, showed a marked delay in nuclear translocation (180 min), preserved its

Table 5.2 Mutations of the human glucocorticoid receptor gene causing generalized glucocorticoid resistance

Reference	Mutation position		Genotype	Molecular mechanisms	Phenotype
	cDNA	Amino acid			
Chrousos et al. (1982) Hurley et al. (1991) Charmandari et al. (2004b)	2054 (A→T)	641 (D→V)	Homozygous	Transactivation ↓ Affinity for ligand ↓ (×3) Nuclear translocation: 22 min Abnormal interaction with GRIP-1	Hypertension Hypokalaemic alkalosis
Karl et al. (1993)	4-bp deletion in exon–intron 6		Heterozygous	hGRα number: 50% of control Inactivation of the affected allele	Hirsutism Male-pattern hair loss Menstrual irregularities
Malchoff et al. (1993) Charmandari et al. (2004b)	2317 (G→A)	729 (V→I)	Homozygous	Transactivation ↓ Affinity for ligand ↓ (×2) Nuclear translocation: 120 min Abnormal interaction with GRIP-1	Precocious puberty Hyperandrogenism
Karl et al. (1996) Kino et al. (13)	1808 (T→A)	559 (I→N)	Heterozygous	Transactivation ↓ No affinity for ligand Transdominance (+) Nuclear translocation: 180 min Abnormal interaction with GRIP-1	Hypertension Oligospermia Infertility
Ruiz et al. (2001) Charmandari et al. (2006)	1430 (G→A)	477 (R→H)	Heterozygous	Transactivation ↓ No DNA binding Nuclear translocation: 20 min	Hirsutism Fatigue Hypertension
Ruiz et al. (2001) Charmandari et al. (2006)	2035 (G→A)	679 (G→S)	Heterozygous	Transactivation ↓ Affinity for ligand ↓ (×2) Nuclear translocation: 30 min Abnormal interaction with GRIP-1	Hirsutism Fatigue Hypertension

Reference	Nucleotide	Amino acid	Molecular effects	Zygosity	Clinical features
Mendonca et al. (2002) Charmandari et al. (2004b)	1844 (C→T)	571 (V→A)	Transactivation ↓ Affinity for ligand ↓ (×6) Nuclear translocation: 25 min Abnormal interaction with GRIP-1	Homozygous	Ambiguous genitalia Hypertension Hypokalaemia Hyperandrogenism
Vottero et al. (2002)	2373 (T→G)	747 (I→M)	Transactivation ↓ Transdominance (+) Affinity for ligand ↓ (×2) Nuclear translocation → Abnormal interaction with GRIP-1	Heterozygous	Cystic acne Hirsutism Oligo-amenorrhoea
Charmandari et al. (2005)	2318 (T→C)	773 (L→P)	Transactivation ↓ Transdominance (+) Affinity for ligand ↓ (×2.6) Nuclear translocation: 30 min Abnormal interaction with GRIP-1	Heterozygous	Fatigue Anxiety Acne Hirsutism Hypertension
Charmandari et al. (2007)	2209 (T→C)	737 (F→L)	Transactivation ↓ Transdominance (conditional) (+) Affinity for ligand ↓ (×1.5) Nuclear translocation: 180 min	Heterozygous	Hypertension Hypokalaemia

(A)

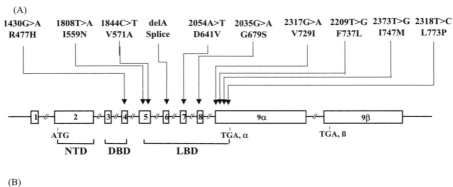

(B)

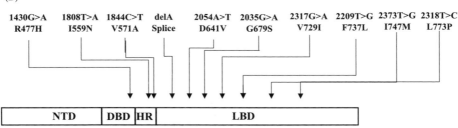

Figure 5.3 Location of the known mutations of the glucocorticoid receptor (hGR) gene (*upper panel*) and protein (*lower panel*). The lack of continuity in terms of increasing order in the nucleotide positions reported for various mutations is likely to be due to the fact that various authors may have included or not included the 183 nucleotides preceding the coding sequence. DBD: DNA-binding domain; LBD: ligand-binding domain; NTD: amino-terminal domain

ability to bind to DNA and did not interact with the GRIP-1 coactivator *in vitro* (Charmandari et al., 2004b; Kino et al., 2001). This mutant receptor was associated with the development of Cushing's disease due to an ACTH-secreting adenoma, which was attributed to chronic corticotroph hyperstimulation and ACTH hypersecretion (Karl et al., 1996).

The fifth case of generalized glucocorticoid resistance (sporadic) was due to a single, heterozygous nucleotide substitution (G → A) at position 1430, which resulted in arginine (R) to histidine (H) substitution at amino acid 477 in the second zinc finger of the DNA binding domain of the receptor (Ruiz et al., 2001). The mutant receptor hGRαR477H had no transcriptional activity due to lack of binding to GREs. Furthermore, it did not exert a dominant negative effect upon the wild-type hGRα, had normal affinity for the ligand, showed mild delay in nuclear translocation (20 min) and displayed a normal interaction with the GRIP-1 coactivator *in vitro* (Charmandari et al., 2006).

The sixth case (sporadic) was due to a single, heterozygous nucleotide substitution (G → A) at position 2035, which resulted in glycine (G) to serine (S) substitution at amino acid position 679 in the ligand-binding domain of the receptor (Ruiz et al., 2001). The mutant receptor hGRαG679S showed a 55% reduction in its ability to

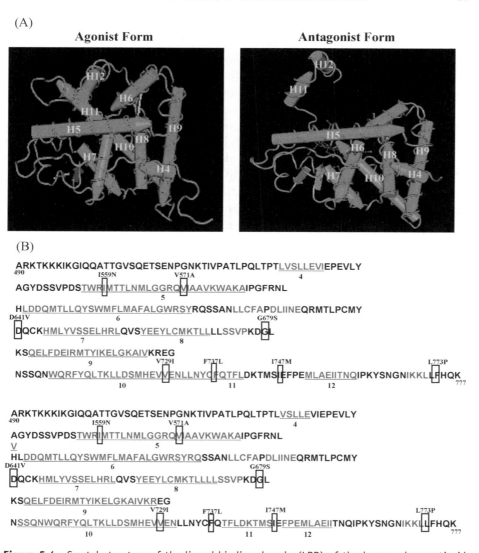

Figure 5.4 Crystal structure of the ligand-binding domain (LBD) of the human glucocorticoid receptor (hGR). (A) Stereotactic conformation of the agonist (*left*) and antagonist (*right*) form of the LBD of hGRα. The α-helices (H4–H12) are depicted as cylinders, whereas broad arrows represent the β-turn. (B) Location of the known mutations of hGR in the agonist (*upper panel*) and antagonist (*lower panel*) form of the LBD of hGRα. Helices are indicated in red and are underlined, while β-sheets are indicated in green. Two mutations (I559 and V571A) are located within H5, while four mutations (V729I, F737L, I747M and L773P) are located within or close to helices 11 and 12. The ligand-binding pocket is formed by helices 3, 5, 11 and 12. Upon ligand binding, the receptor undergoes major conformational changes, which alter the position of H11 and H12 and generate an interaction surface that allows coactivators to bind to the LBD through their LXXLL motifs. Helix 12 plays a critical role in the formation of both the ligand-binding pocket and the AF-2 surface that facilitates interaction with coactivators. The fact that most hGR mutations are clustered around H5, H11 and H12 indicates that these helices play an important role in glucocorticoid signal transduction. A full-colour version of this figure can be found in the colour plate section of this book.

stimulate the transcription of the MMTV promoter in response to dexamethasone, displayed a twofold reduction in its affinity for ligand, had delayed nuclear translocation (30 min) and interacted with the GRIP-1 coactivator only through its AF-1. The mutant receptor did not exert a dominant negative effect upon the wild-type hGRα and showed normal binding to GREs (Charmandari et al., 2006).

The proposita of the fourth kindred had a single, homozygous, cytocine to thymine (C → T) substitution at nucleotide position 1844, resulting in valine (V) to alanine (A) substitution at amino acid 571 in the ligand-binding domain of the receptor (Mendonca et al., 2002). The mutant receptor hGRαV571A demonstrated a 50-fold decrease in its transcriptional activity, a sixfold reduction in its affinity for the ligand and a delay in nuclear translocation (25 min). It did not exert a dominant negative effect upon the wild-type receptor, it preserved its ability to bind to GREs and showed a weak interaction with the amino-terminal fragment of GRIP-1 coactivator *in vitro* (Charmandari et al., 2004b). This was the first case of generalized glucocorticoid resistance reported in which the affected female presented with ambiguous genitalia at birth.

The propositus of the fifth kindred had a homozygous, thymine to guanine (T → G) substitution at nucleotide position 2373, which resulted in isoleucine (I) to methionine (M) substitution at amino acid position 747 in the ligand-binding domain of the receptor (Vottero et al., 2002). The mutant receptor hGRαI747M showed a 20–30-fold reduction in its ability to stimulate the transcription of the MMTV promoter in response to dexamethasone and a twofold reduction in its affinity for the ligand. It exerted dominant negative activity upon the wild-type receptor and interacted with the GRIP-1 coactivator only through its AF-1 domain. Overexpression of GRIP1 restored the transcriptional activity and reversed the negative dominant activity of the mutant receptor. The mutant receptor displayed a mild delay in translocating into the nucleus and formed coarser nuclear speckles compared with the wild-type hGRα but preserved normal binding to GREs (Charmandari et al., 2004b; Vottero et al., 2002).

We have recently identified two new cases of glucocorticoid resistance caused by novel, heterozygous, point mutations in the hGR gene and investigated the molecular mechanisms of action of these natural hGRα mutants.

The first patient was a 29-year-old female who presented with a longstanding history of fatigue, profound anxiety, acne, hirsutism, menstrual irregularities and hypertension. She had been treated with calcium channel-blockers and contraceptives with no improvement for 3 years. On clinical examination, she was noted to have acne, hirsutism and elevated blood pressure despite adherence to anti-hypertensive treatment (BP: 140/90 mmHg), but no clinical signs suggestive of Cushing's syndrome. Biochemical and endocrinological evaluation at presentation revealed elevated 08:00 h serum cortisol concentrations (56.2 μg/dl; normal range (nr): 8–19 μg/dl), increased 24-h urinary free cortisol excretion (187.6 μg/day; nr: 10–34 μg/day) and elevated 08:00 h plasma ACTH (80 pg/ml; nr: 10–60 pg/ml), and serum testosterone (93 ng/dl; nr: 10–55 ng/dl), androstenedione (209 ng/dl;

nr: 85-275 ng/dl) and DHEAS (458 ng/dl; nr: 60–255 ng/dl) concentrations. A low-dose dexamethasone suppression test (0.5 mg of dexamethasone every 6h for 48h) revealed resistance of the HPA axis to dexamethasone suppression (08:00 h serum cortisol: 13.9 µg/dl, 08:00 h plasma ACTH: 53 pg/ml). Additional investigations excluded Cushing's disease, hyperaldosteronism and other causes of hypertension (Charmandari et al., 2005).

Thymidine incorporation assays performed on fresh peripheral lymphocytes revealed increased resistance to dexamethasone-induced suppression of phytohaemagglutinin-stimulated thymidine incorporation in the patient compared to an age-matched control, while whole-cell dexamethasone-binding assays performed on Epstein-Barr virus (EBV)-transformed lymphocytes showed that the affinity of the glucocorticoid receptor for the ligand was 2.7-fold lower in the patient than in the control cells (K_d: 23.6 vs. 8.8 nM). Genomic DNA was obtained from peripheral lymphocytes and the entire coding region of the hGR gene was amplified by polymerase-chain reaction (PCR) and sequenced. A single, heterozygous, thymine to cytosine (T → C) substitution was identified at nucleotide position 2318 (exon 9α), which resulted in leucine (L) to proline (P) substitution (CTG → CCG) at amino acid position 773 in the ligand-binding domain of the receptor. RNA extraction from peripheral lymphocytes, reverse transcription (RT)-PCR amplification of the coding region of the gene and sequencing confirmed these findings (Charmandari et al., 2005).

We systematically investigated the molecular mechanisms through which the mutant receptor hGRαL773P affects glucocorticoid signal transduction (Figures 5.2). In transient transfection assays performed on CV-1 embryonic African green monkey kidney cells, which are devoid of endogenous GR expression, the mutant receptor hGRαL773P demonstrated a twofold reduction in its ability to transactivate the glucocorticoid-responsive MMTV promoter in response to dexamethasone compared to the wild-type receptor. The concentration of dexamethasone required to achieve 50% of transactivation was 10^{-9} M for the wild-type and 10^{-8} M for the mutant receptor. In the same reporter assays performed on CV-1 cells, co-transfection with a constant amount of hGRα and five progressively increasing concentrations of hGRαL773P (so that the ratio between wild-type and mutant receptor would range from 1:0 to 1:10) showed a dose-dependent inhibition of hGRα-mediated transactivation of the MMTV promoter, which ranged from 23% at the 1:1 hGRα/hGRαL773P ratio to 59% at the 1:10 hGRα/hGRαL773P ratio. These findings suggest that the mutant receptor exerts a dominant negative effect upon the wild-type receptor (Charmandari et al., 2005).

Dexamethasone-binding studies performed on COS-7 cells (which are also devoid of endogenous GR expression) transfected with either hGRα or hGRαL773P showed that the apparent dissociation constant (K_d) of hGRαL773P was significantly higher than that of the wild-type receptor (mean ± SE: 24.4 ± 5.0 vs. 9.4 ± 0.8 nM, $P = 0.03$), suggesting that the affinity of the mutant receptor hGRαL773P for the ligand was 2.6-fold lower than that of the wild-type hGRα (Charmandari et al., 2005).

We next studied the subcellular localization and nuclear translocation of the wild-type and mutant receptors in HeLa human cervical carcinoma cells in the absence or presence of dexamethasone, by creating green fluorescent protein (GFP)-fused constructs of the two receptors. In the absence of dexamethasone, hGRα was primarily localized in the cytoplasm of cells. Addition of dexamethasone (10^{-6} M) resulted in translocation of the wild-type receptor into the nucleus within 12 min (mean ± SE: 12.00 ± 0.71 min). The pathological mutant receptor hGRαL773P was also observed predominantly in the cytoplasm of cells in the absence of ligand. Exposure to the same concentration of dexamethasone induced a slow translocation of this receptor into the nucleus, which required 30 min (mean ± SE: 30.00 ± 1.18 min). These findings suggest that the mutant receptor shows a 2.5-fold delay in nuclear translocation compared to the wild-type receptor. Coexpression of both receptors at a 1:1 ratio had no apparent effect on the nuclear translocation of the wild-type hGRα (Charmandari et al., 2005).

We investigated the ability of the mutant receptor to bind DNA in a chromatin immunoprecipitation (ChIP) assay. HCT-116 human colon carcinoma cells stably transfected with MMTV-luc were transiently transfected with the wild-type, the mutant receptor or a control plasmid. Both the wild-type and mutant receptor were co-precipitated with MMTV GREs similarly in a ligand-dependent fashion, suggesting that the mutant receptor preserves its ability to bind to DNA (Charmandari et al., 2005).

To determine whether the mutant receptor hGRαL773P has an abnormal interaction with the p160 coactivators, we investigated the interaction between this receptor and the GRIP-1 coactivator. GRIP-1 contains two sites that bind to steroid receptors: one site, the nuclear receptor-binding (NRB) site, is located at the amino-terminus of the protein (between amino acids 542 and 745) and interacts with the AF-2 of hGRα in a ligand-dependent fashion through multiple LXXLL motifs (McKenna and O'Malley, 2002). The other site is located at the carboxyl-terminus of the protein (between amino acids 1121 and 1250) and binds to the AF-1 of hGRα in a ligand-independent fashion (McKenna and O'Malley, 2002). *In vitro* translated and ^{35}S-radiolabelled hGRα and hGRαL773P were tested for binding to bacterially produced and purified GST-fused full-length GRIP-1 [GRIP-1(1–1462)], NRB fragment of GRIP-1 [GRIP-1(559–774)] and carboxyl-terminal fragment of GRIP-1 [GRIP-1(740–1217)] in a glutathione-*S*-transferase (GST) pull-down assay. Both the wild-type and mutant receptors bound to full-length GRIP-1 and the carboxyl-terminal fragment of GRIP-1. However, unlike the wild-type hGRα, the mutant receptor did not interact with the NRB fragment of GRIP-1, suggesting that the mutant receptor interacts with the GRIP-1 coactivator *in vitro* only through its AF-1.

The above findings suggest that the mutant receptor hGRαL773P causes generalized glucocorticoid resistance because of a dominant negative effect upon the wild-type receptor, decreased affinity for the ligand, delayed nuclear translocation and an abnormal interaction with the GRIP-1 and possibly other p160 coactivators and components of the vitamin D receptor-interacting protein (DRIP)/thyroid hormone receptor-associated protein (TRAP) complex. The abnormal interaction between the mutant receptor and the GRIP-1 coactivator *in vitro* might have been predicted by the location of the mutation 13 amino acids downstream of helix 12 of the ligand-binding domain of the receptor (Figures 5.3 and 5.4). Helix 12 plays an important role in protein–protein interactions between nuclear receptors and p160 coactivators, and it is likely that the mutant receptor forms a partially ineffective complex with GRIP-1, given that one site of their interaction is either weak or non-existent (Bledsoe et al., 2002; Bourguet et al., 2000; Kauppi et al., 2003).

The second patient with generalized glucocorticoid resistance was a 7-year-old boy who presented with hypertension and hypokalaemia. Endocrinological evaluation at presentation showed elevated 08:00 h serum cortisol (160 μg/dl) and ACTH (425 pg/ml) concentrations, which maintained circadian rhythmicity and resistance of the HPA axis to dexamethasone suppression. Sequencing of the coding region of the hGR gene revealed a single, heterozygous thymine to cytosine (T → C) substitution at nucleotide position 2209 (exon 9α) of the gene, which resulted in phenylalanine (F) to leucine (L) substitution (TTC → CTC) at amino acid position 737 in the ligand-binding domain of the receptor. Using the three-dimensional crystal structure of the ligand-binding domain of hGRα, we determined that the F737L mutation is located in helix 11 of the agonist bound form of the receptor (Charmandari et al., 2007) (Figures 5.3 and 5.4).

Once again we investigated the molecular mechanisms through which this mutant receptor affects glucocorticoid signal transduction. In transient transfection assays, the mutant receptor hGRαF737L displayed a 1.7-fold reduction in its ability to transactivate the MMTV promoter in response to dexamethasone compared to the wild-type receptor, it exerted a time-dependent dominant negative effect upon the wild-type hGRα and had a 1.9-fold lower affinity for the ligand compared to the wild-type hGRα. Western blot analyses demonstrated no differences in the expression of hGRα and hGRαF737L proteins in CV-1 or COS-7 cells. Subcellular localization and nuclear translocation studies showed that in the absence of ligand the mutant receptor hGRαF737L was localized both in the cytoplasm and nucleus of the cells, while exposure to dexamethasone resulted in a 12-fold delay in nuclear translocation compared to the wild-type receptor. Chromatin immunoprecipitation assays demonstrated that the mutant receptor preserves its ability to bind to GREs. Finally, GST pull-down assays confirmed that the mutant receptor hGRαF737L interacted with the GRIP-1 coactivator *in vitro* only through its AF-1 (Charmandari et al., 2007).

5.3 Conclusions

Mutations in the human glucocorticoid receptor gene impair one or more of the molecular mechanisms of glucocorticoid action, thereby altering tissue sensitivity to glucocorticoids. A subsequent increase in the activity of the HPA axis compensates for the reduced sensitivity of peripheral tissues to glucocorticoids, however, at the expense of ACTH hypersecretion-related pathology. The study of the functional defects of natural hGR mutants sheds light on the mechanisms of hGR action and highlights the importance of integrated cellular and molecular signalling mechanisms for maintaining homeostasis and preserving normal physiology.

Acknowledgements

This work was funded by the Intramural Research Program of the National Institute of Child Health and Human Development, National Institutes of Health, Bethesda, Maryland 20892, USA.

References

Bledsoe RK, Montana VG, Stanley TB, Delves CJ et al. Crystal structure of the glucocorticoid receptor ligand binding domain reveals a novel mode of receptor dimerization and coactivator recognition. *Cell* 2002; **110**: 93–105.

Bourguet W, Germain P, Gronemeyer H. Nuclear receptor ligand-binding domains: three-dimensional structures, molecular interactions and pharmacological implications. *Trends Pharmacol Sci* 2000; **21**: 381–388.

Charmandari E, Kino T, Chrousos GP. Familial/sporadic glucocorticoid resistance: clinical phenotype and molecular mechanisms. *Ann NY Acad Sci* 2004a; **1024**: 168–181.

Charmandari E, Kino T, Ichijo T, Jubiz W, Mejia L, Zachman K, Chrousos GP. A novel point mutation in helix 11 of the ligand-binding domain of the human glucocorticoid receptor gene causing generalized glucocorticoid resistance. *J Clin Endocrinol Metab* 2007; **92(10)**: 3986–3990.

Charmandari E, Kino T, Ichijo T, Zachman K, Alatsatianos A, Chrousos GP. Functional characterization of the natural human glucocorticoid receptor (hGR) mutants hGRalphaR477H and hGRalphaG679S associated with generalized glucocorticoid resistance. *J Clin Endocrinol Metab* 2006; **91**: 1535–1543.

Charmandari E, Kino T, Vottero A, Souvatzoglou E, Bhattacharyya N, Chrousos GP. Natural glucocorticoid receptor mutants causing generalized glucocorticoid resistance: Molecular genotype, genetic transmission and clinical phenotype. *J Clin Endocrinol Metab* 2004b; **89**: 1939–1949.

Charmandari E, Raji A, Kino T, Ichijo T, Tiulpakov A, Zachman K, Chrousos GP. A novel point mutation in the ligand-binding domain (LBD) of the human glucocorticoid receptor (hGR) causing generalized glucocorticoid resistance: the importance of the C terminus of hGR LBD in conferring transactivational activity. *J Clin Endocrinol Metab* 2005; **90**: 3696–3705.

Chrousos GP. Hormone resistance and hypersensitivity states. In: Chrousos GP, Olefsky JM, Samols E (eds). Modern Endocrinology Series. Philadelphia, PA: Lippincott, Williams & Wilkins; 2002; p. 542.

Chrousos GP, Detera-Wadleigh SD, Karl M. Syndromes of glucocorticoid resistance. *Ann Intern Med* 1993; **119**: 1113–1124.

Chrousos GP, Vingerhoeds A, Brandon D, Eil C et al. Primary cortisol resistance in man. A glucocorticoid receptor-mediated disease. *J Clin Invest* 1982; **69**: 1261–1269.

Hurley DM, Accili D, Stratakis CA, Karl M et al. Point mutation causing a single amino acid substitution in the hormone binding domain of the glucocorticoid receptor in familial glucocorticoid resistance. *J Clin Invest* 1991; **87**: 680–686.

Karl M, Lamberts SW, Detera-Wasdleigh SD, Encio IJ et al. Familial glucocorticoid resistance caused by a splice site deletion in the human glucocorticoid receptor gene. *J Clin Endocrinol Metab* 1993; **76**: 683–689.

Karl M, Lamberts SW, Koper JW, Katz DA et al. Cushing's disease preceded by generalized glucocorticoid resistance: clinical consequences of a novel, dominant-negative glucocorticoid receptor mutation. *Proc Assoc Am Physicians* 1996; **108**: 296–307.

Kauppi B, Jakob C, Farnegardh M, Yang J et al. The three-dimensional structures of antagonistic and agonistic forms of the glucocorticoid receptor ligand-binding domain: RU-486 induces a transconformation that leads to active antagonism. *J Biol Chem* 2003; **278**: 22748–22754.

Kino T, Chrousos GP. Glucocorticoid and mineralocorticoid resistance/ hypersensitivity syndromes. *J Endocrinol* 2001; **169**: 437–445.

Kino T, De Martino MU, Charmandari E, Mirani M, Chrousos GP. Tissue glucocorticoid resistance/hypersensitivity syndromes. *J Steroid Biochem Mol Biol* 2003; **85**: 457–467.

Kino T, Stauber RH, Resau JH, Pavlakis GN, Chrousos GP. Pathologic human GR mutant has a transdominant negative effect on the wild-type GR by inhibiting its translocation into the nucleus: importance of the ligand-binding domain for intracellular GR trafficking. *J Clin Endocrinol Metab* 2001; **86**: 5600–5608.

Kino T, Vottero A, Charmandari E, Chrousos GP. Familial/sporadic glucocorticoid resistance syndrome and hypertension. *Ann NY Acad Sci* 2002; **970**: 101–111.

Malchoff DM, Brufsky A, Reardon G , McDermott P et al. A mutation of the glucocorticoid receptor in primary cortisol resistance. *J Clin Invest* 1993; **91**: 1918–1925.

McKenna NJ, O'Malley BW. Combinatorial control of gene expression by nuclear receptors and coregulators. *Cell* 2002; **108**: 465–474.

Mendonca BB, Leite MV, de Castro M, Kino T et al. Female pseudohermaphroditism caused by a novel homozygous missense mutation of the GR gene. *J Clin Endocrinol Metab* 2002; **87**: 1805–1809.

Ruiz M, Lind U, Gafvels M, Eggertsen G et al. Characterization of two novel mutations in the glucocorticoid receptor gene in patients with primary cortisol resistance. *Clin Endocrinol (Oxf)* 2001; **55**: 363–371.

Vingerhoeds AC, Thijssen JH, Schwarz F. Spontaneous hypercortisolism without Cushing's syndrome. *J Clin Endocrinol Metab* 1976; **43**: 1128–1133.

Vottero A, Kino T, Combe H, Lecomte P, Chrousos GP. A novel, C-terminal dominant negative mutation of the GR causes familial glucocorticoid resistance through abnormal interactions with p160 steroid receptor coactivators. *J Clin Endocrinol Metab* 2002; **87**: 2658–2667.

6

Corticosteroid Responsiveness in Asthma: Clinical Aspects

Kian Fan Chung

6.1   Introduction

When corticosteroids were first used for the treatment of asthma over 60 years ago in the form of cortisone, the clinical effects observed in the first patients were dramatic (Carey et al., 1950; Schwartz, 1951). However, with increasing experience of its use in treating this condition, patients who responded less well were reported. The responsiveness of patients with asthma to corticosteroids appears to follow a unimodal distribution with patients at both ends of the spectrum of responsiveness. Therefore, there is a variation in the therapeutic response to corticosteroids. The most important question is to what extent this response is determined genetically, and to what extent this responsiveness can be modulated by disease processes such as asthma.

6.2   Effects of Corticosteroids in Asthma

The introduction of inhaled corticosteroid (ICS) therapy in asthma has been one of the most effective advances in the therapy of this condition. The topical route of administration has ensured that the benefit/risk ratio is improved, since this results in minimal absorption of corticosteroids into the systemic circulation and hence reduces the risk of systemic side effects. ICS therapy is now the therapy of choice for all asthmatic patients who need regular therapy to control asthma symptoms or to prevent exacerbations of asthma. In the patient with more severe disease, the combination of inhaled corticosteroid therapy with a long-acting β-adrenergic agonist

Overcoming Steroid Insensitivity in Respiratory Disease   Edited by Ian M. Adcock and Kian Fan Chung
© 2008 John Wiley & Sons, Ltd.

provides greater control of asthma than using an inhaled corticosteroid agent alone (Greening et al., 1994; Pauwels et al., 1997).

ICS therapy improves asthma control, with a reduction in the need for reliever medication such as short-acting β-adrenergic agonists, and lung function levels are measured in terms of peak expiratory flow rates or forced expiratory volume in one second (FEV_1) (Barnes et al., 1998). In part the efficacy of ICS lies in improving bronchial hyper-responsiveness and in reducing the eosinophilic and lymphocytic inflammation in the airway wall (Djukanovic et al., 1992; van Essen-Zandvliet et al., 1992; Vathenen et al., 1991). There is some evidence that ICS may also reverse certain features of airway wall remodelling, such as the thickness of the sub-basement membrane (Olivieri et al., 1997; Sont et al., 1999).

Corticosteroid therapy via the oral or systemic route is usually reserved for the treatment of acute severe exacerbations of asthma, where they speed the time of recovery. Typically, the treatment is provided over a period of 1–2 weeks until the exacerbation shows signs of recovery. Short bursts of corticosteroid therapy such as prednisolone administered to a patient with stable asthma at a dose of 40 mg/day for 2 weeks are sometimes used to determine the responsiveness of airflow obstruction; an excellent response from significant airflow obstruction to absence of airflow obstruction would provide support for a diagnosis of asthma that would be useful to the clinician in planning the treatment of the patient. Alternatively, a dose of a more potent corticosteroid, triamcinolone, is administered intramuscularly, and this may overcome any issue of non-adherence to oral corticosteroid therapy (ten Brinke et al., 2004).

6.3   Definition of Corticosteroid Insensitivity

While the majority of patients with asthma demonstrate a good therapeutic response to corticosteroid (CS) therapy, there is a proportion of patients who appear to have a lesser response. This was first noted with the response to systemic CS therapy, which was the initial form of therapy with CS. Our idea of CS insensitivity in asthma has been very much influenced by the initial publication of Schwartz and colleagues who described CS resistance in asthmatic patients with poorly controlled asthma who demonstrated bronchodilator responses to inhaled β-agonists but no airway responses to large oral doses of CS (Schwartz et al., 1968). They also observed that the reduction of blood eosinophil count caused by corticosteroids was much less while the patients showed evidence of Cushingoid side effects similar to those patients who responded well to CS therapy. Carmichael et al described 58 subjects with chronic asthma based on a strict definition of reversal of airflow obstruction in response to CS therapy (Carmichael et al., 1981). Corticosteroid-resistant (CSR) asthma was defined as changes in baseline FEV_1 after a 14-day course of oral prednisolone of 40 mg/day of <15% of the baseline measurement, while demonstrating a >15% improvement in FEV_1 following inhaled β_2-agonist, salbutamol. Patients who showed improvements of FEV_1 of $\geq 30\%$ were considered as corticosteroid sensitive (CSS). This definition was used in subsequent studies and reiterated later by other authors, particularly for studies investigating the mechanisms of CS resistance (Woolcock, 1996).

This definition of CSR asthma is likely to represent one end of the extreme spectrum of CS responsiveness, the least responsive, and an arbitrary cut-off response of $<15\%$ response was chosen empirically without knowledge of the distribution of responses to oral or inhaled CS. The arbitrary cut-off point of $>30\%$ response that defines the CSS patient was taken to represent an extremely good response to CS. From the point of view of investigating the mechanisms of CS resistance, a comparison of these two extreme groups of asthmatics would be useful to provide mechanistic clues.

The definition of CSR asthma has been based on the reversibility of airflow obstruction to pharmacological agents without accompanying indication as to whether this group of patients is characterized by a particular clinical type or pattern of asthma. The study of Carmichael et al. (1981) reported that in the 58 patients defined as CSR there was a longer duration of asthma (>5 years), a more frequent family history of asthma, poorer morning lung function and a greater degree of non-specific bronchial hyper-responsiveness. The latter two features suggest that these may represent a more severe group of patients with asthma. In a study of 34 children with CS insensitivity, an association with significantly poorer quality of life at a 2-year follow-up and with a worse form of asthma with a more fixed pattern of airflow obstruction was reported (Wamboldt et al., 1999).

In studies of CSR asthma only a few patients have been described, usually ranging from 6 to 12 subjects recruited from patients attending hospital asthma clinics and who have satisfied the physiological criteria set out in the definition of Carmichael et al (1981) (Table 6.1). Very few details have been provided as to the type of asthma these patients were suffering from, apart from their baseline FEV_1 and their response to oral prednisolone. One may surmise that these patients may have fixed airflow obstruction, without necessarily having uncontrolled asthma or falling into the category of "severe" asthma (see section 6.6).

6.4   Oral CS Responsiveness in Asthma

It is interesting that a definition for CS resistance based on response of airflow obstruction was first suggested on the basis of a given cut-off level of improvement or lack of improvement in airflow obstruction. It is also clear that using this method of diagnosing CS resistance, patients who start with no evidence of airflow obstruction would theoretically not be diagnosed using this procedure, since there cannot be any further response with a "normal" set of lung function measures. The cut-off point of an improvement or a lack of improvement by 15% was made arbitrarily without any knowledge of the CS responsiveness of asthma patients to CS therapy.

Table 6.1 Summary of studies of corticosteroid-insensitive asthma in the literature

Reference	Number of patients	FEV$_1$ (% predicted)	Study objective
Wilkinson et al. (1989)	8	47.2	Monocyte-derived neutrophil activating factor
Corrigan et al. (1991a)	13	49.2	Glucocorticoid pharmacokinetics
Corrigan et al. (1991b)	12	NA	Lymphocyte proliferation
Brown et al. (1991)	15	NA	Skin blanching
Sousa et al. (1996)	6	71	Skin tuberculin response
Sousa et al. (1999)	6	71	c-jun N-terminal kinase activation
Sousa et al. (2000)	6	71	GRβ
Adcock et al. (1995a)	9	71	GR–AP-1 interaction
Adcock et al. (1995b)	9	71	GR–GRE interactions
Lane et al. (1993)	8	68	Monocyte-derived cytokines
Lane et al. (1996b)	8	NA	Bone turnover
Sher et al. (1994)	17	58	Glucocorticoid receptor binding (PBMC)
Leung et al. (1995)	12	56	IL-4 and IL-5 expression in bronchial biopsies
Leung et al. (1997)	8	NA	GRβ
Hamid et al. (1999)	7	56	GRβ
Chan et al. (1998)	21	NA	Clinical characteristics
Wamboldt et al. (1999)	34	NA	Clinical outcomes
Chakir et al. (2002)	11	56	Bronchial inflammation

NA: Not available

There is only one report of oral prednisolone response in a sizeable number of patients with asthma. In 784 patients with mild to moderate asthma who responded by >15% improvement of baseline peak expiratory flow rate (PEFR) after inhaled β-agonist, the improvement in morning PEF rate following a 7–12-day course of prednisone or prednisolone at a dose of 30 mg/day showed a normal distribution with responses of 0–40% increase and a median increase of 20% in 23% of the cohort (Figure 6.1) (Colice et al., 2005). This distribution indicates that there are some patients who respond poorly to oral prednisolone. Using a cut-off point of 15% improvement is likely to be too generous, and perhaps a cut-off point of <5% would be most appropriate as a definition of CSR asthma, although an equivalence

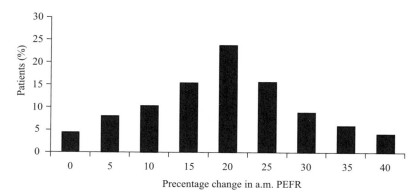

Figure 6.1 Frequency distribution of change in morning peak expiratory flow rate (PEFR) after oral prednisolone or prednisone 30 mg/day for 7–12 days. Reproduced from Colice et al., *J Allergy Clin Immunol* 2005; **115(1)**:200-201, with permission from Elsevier

of FEV_1 to PEFR is assumed. If CS resistance is defined by a threshold increase in morning PEF of <15%, then 26% of the patients would have been CSR, making the condition of CSR fairly common within the asthmatic population of mild to moderate asthma. The study would also support the view that the clinical features of the CSR asthmatics are not different from the rest of the cohort since the patients were all within a mild to moderate category of severity. However, there was no comparison of the non-responders (CSR) to the responders (CSS) in this study, in terms of their clinical features.

PEFR measurements are usually more variable and less reproducible than FEV_1, and a study using FEV_1 as a measure of airflow limitation would be more useful. Studies with smaller numbers have been published in this regard, and two recent examples are reviewed. In 26 "unselected" patients with mild to moderate non-smoking asthma with a baseline FEV_1 of 69% predicted and responding with an 18.9% increase after inhalation of salbutamol, a course of 40 mg/day of prednisolone for 14 days increased FEV_1 by 0.237 L, i.e. an increase of 9.2% (Chaudhuri et al., 2003). This would place these patients in the CSR category as defined by Carmichael et al. (1981), underlying the use of a 15% cut-off point as being unusually high. In the same report, the effect of prednisolone on FEV_1 in a comparable group of asthmatics who were chronic smokers was reported to cause a 0.047 L (+2.15%) increase, which is significantly lower compared to the asthmatics who did not smoke (Chaudhuri et al., 2003) (Table 6.2). Chakir et al. (2002) presented selected patients (according to their CS response) who were clearly responsive to oral prednisolone (an improvement of 39% in 10 asthmatic patients, compared to a small reduction in FEV_1 of –1.6% in 11 patients labelled as CSR asthmatics (Table 6.3). Because this study looked specifically at CSR and CSS patients, they were chosen as such to represent the two ends of the spectrum

Table 6.2 Definition of corticosteroid-sensitive and corticosteroid-resistant asthma (adapted from Chakir et al., *Clin Experimental Allergy* 2004; **32**: 578, with permission from Wiley-Blackwell Publishing Ltd)

FEV$_1$	Corticosteroid-sensitive (n=10)	Corticosteroid-resistant (n=11)
Litres	1.91	2.02
% predicted	62 (5)	56 (5)
After prednisolone		
Litres	2.60	1.97
% Change	+39 (6)	−1.6 (3)
After salbutamol		
% Change	48 (4)	48 (6)

of CS responsiveness for the investigation of inflammatory differences in the groups.

The variability of prednisolone responsiveness with time is not known, although one study has indicated in a small group of patients that CSR may become CSS with time (Demoly et al., 1998). Certainly the availability of such information should lead to a review of the definition of CS resistance in asthma according to response to oral prednisolone. Another issue is whether the chronic use of ICS may influence the response of the airways to oral prednisolone; this question also applies to the chronic use of oral prednisolone.

6.5   ICS Responsiveness in Asthma

Of greater interest is the recent availability of data on the responsiveness of asthmatics to ICS since this is the most commonly-used treatment for asthmatic patients, although we very rarely measure responsiveness to ICS. Although there have been many studies that examine the response of airway function to ICS therapy,

Table 6.3   FEV$_1$ response to prednisolone (40 mg/day for 14 days) in smoking and non-smoking asthmatics (adapted with permission from Chaduri et al., *Am J Resp Crit Care Med* [Official Journal of the American Thoracic Society] 2003; **168(11)**:1308–1311. © American Thoracic Society)

FEV$_1$	Smokers (n=14)	Ex-smokers (n=10)	Never-smokers (n=26)
Litres (SEM)	2.23 (0.5)	2.21 (0.55)	2.57 (0.49)
% predicted	70.5	68.4	69
ΔFEV$_1$ (l) after prednisolone	0.047 (+2.1%)	0.143 (+6.5%)	0.237 (+9.2%)
ΔFEV$_1$ (l) after salbutamol	0.423 (+17.3%)	0.640 (+22.6%)	0.615 (+18.9%)

most have reported results in terms of mean changes and very few have reported the results in terms of distribution of responses. Two studies have shown that there is a unimodal distribution in terms of FEV_1 response to a low dose of inhaled beclomethasone, with a median response (~40% of patients) of >0.0–0.4 L of FEV_1 (Baumgartner et al., 2003; Israel et al., 2002). In 304 patients with mild to moderate asthma (mean FEV_1 65.9% predicted; β-agonist reversal 29.8%) there was a normal distribution of responsiveness to 400 μg beclomethasone per day, with responses of 0.4–1.0 L change in FEV_1 (Figures 6.2 and 6.3). The most frequent responses were 4%, 12% and 20% increases in FEV_1 above baseline at 6 weeks in 20%, 19.6% and 17.5% of the cohort, respectively (Baumgartner et al., 2003). We clearly need further data in large asthmatic cohorts to get a truer picture of ICS responsiveness in asthma. Interestingly, the unimodal distribution was also mimicked by a comparative asthmatic cohort treated with the leukotriene receptor antagonist montelukast in both studies (Figures 6.2 and 6.3) (Baumgartner et al., 2003; Israel et al., 2002).

The significant intersubject variability in a limited dose–response to ICS in terms of improvement in FEV_1 was also noted in a smaller study (Szefler et al., 2002). A good FEV_1 response of >15% in contrast to a poor response of <5% was found to be associated with high exhaled NO, high bronchodilator reversibility and low

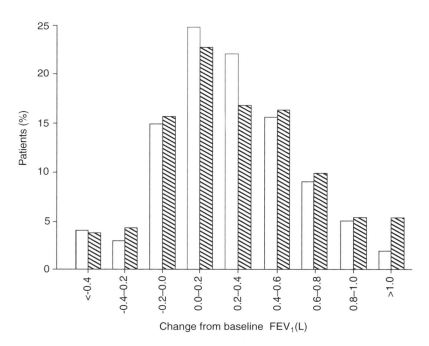

Figure 6.2   Frequency distribution of change in FEV_1 (L) from baseline in asthmatic patients receiving inhaled beclomethasone 200 μg twice daily (hatched bars) or montelukast (open bars). Reproduced from Baumgartner et al., *Eur Respir J* 2003; **21(1)**:123-128, with permission from European Respiratory Society Journals Ltd

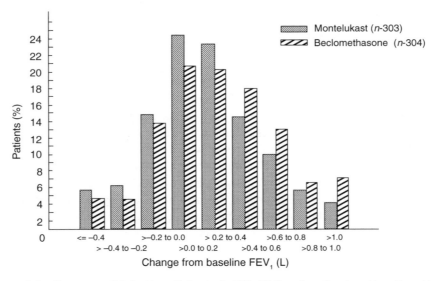

Figure 6.3   Frequency distribution of change in FEV_1 (L) from baseline in asthmatic patients receiving inhaled beclomethasone (hatched bars) or montelukast (stippled bars). Reproduced from Israel et al., *J Allergy Clin Immunol* 2002; **110(6)**:847-8, with permission from Elsevier

FEV_1/FVC ratio measured before treatment with ICS. Because of the difficulty of performing a dose–response to ICS, it would not be possible to determine whether the differences between the relative non-responders and responders represent a shift of the curve or changes of the maximal response. It is not known whether chronic treatment with inhaled CS alters the responsiveness to ICS. This issue has not been broached, since control of inflammation or pharmacological downregulation of ICS effects may both modulate ICS responsiveness.

One of the major drawbacks to understanding this distribution of CS responsiveness in asthmatics is the lack of information on the distribution of CS responsiveness in a normal non-diseased population. Of course, in the normal population one would use a measure that would be possible in normal subjects, such as the skin blanching effect of topical CS, the suppression of peripheral blood lymphocyte proliferation or the cortisol suppression test. However, there are no studies of large cohorts that could provide an idea of their distribution. Another way of approaching this issue would be to measure these responses in the asthma cohorts and determine whether the distribution of these responses is similar to that of the airway responses to CS therapy. This would indicate how much the CS responsiveness of asthma may be genetically determined.

The unimodal distribution of responses of the asthmatics to both oral and inhaled CS therapy may support a genetic component. A variant of TBX21 that encodes for the transcription factor T-bet has been associated with an improvement in airway responsiveness in asthmatic patients treated with ICS (Tantisira et al., 2004).

Analysis of 31 single nucleotide polymorphisms in 14 candidate genes in the CS activation pathway has identified a specific polymorphism in the corticotrophhin-releasing hormone (CRH) receptor gene that is associated with FEV_1 improvement after ICS therapy (Weiss et al., 2004). Further studies in this area are bound to pick up other genetic determinants of the CS response in asthma.

The unimodal distribution of the responses observed in the mild to moderate asthmatics also raises the issue as to whether the asthmatic patients defined as CSR are those who fall within the less responsive population and those defined as CSS fall within the most responsive. Therefore, the mechanisms that have been found regarding CS insensitivity in the studies of CSR asthma patients (Table 6.1) may pertain to differences at the two extremes of this unimodal distribution.

There has been no comparison of CS responsiveness measured with ICS compared to that using oral prednisolone. One potential difference in responsiveness may be due to the lack of penetration of ICS into the distal airways, where the site of obstruction or inflammation may be most prominent and will be amenable to oral or systemically administered CS. Use of oral prednisolone overcomes this possibility.

6.6   CS Responsiveness in Severe Asthma

CS responsiveness in patients with severe asthma may be impaired because these patients do not acquire control of asthma with high doses of ICS, often administered together with oral prednisolone therapy. In many definitions of severe asthma, this condition is recognized as being therapy resistant, particularly to inhaled plus oral CS therapies. These patients are also often labelled as corticosteroid-dependent asthmatics, which is usually defined as the need for oral (in addition to inhaled) CS therapy to maintain their asthma under reasonable control (Chung et al., 1999; Stirling and Chung, 2001); any reduction in the dose of oral CS particularly may lead to a deterioration in asthma control. Such a definition, in contrast to the definition for CSR asthma, is less precise, and is dependent on changes in asthma control that have not been precisely set out. Patients with severe asthma have frequent episodes of asthma attacks, or suffer from chronic symptoms, only partly controlled by systemic CS. The dose of oral corticosteroids needed to satisfactorily control asthma contributes to significant side effects such as osteoporosis, skin bruising, diabetes and obesity, but may not completely reverse chronic airflow limitation. These patients may also present as difficult-to-control asthma, but before determining that these patients have severe asthma it must be established that the diagnosis of asthma is ascertained, the patient is adequately and appropriately treated and that he/she is taking asthma medications as prescribed. Patients labelled as severe asthmatics represent a different cohort from patients with CSR asthma.

There are several such cohorts described in the literature that emphasize the lack of control of asthma despite the use of adequate asthma therapies, particularly CS (ENFUMOSA, 2003; Moore et al., 2007; Robinson et al., 2003). The clinical presentation of severe asthma can be varied, and many recognize patients with un-controlled chronic symptoms at one end and, at the other extreme, those presenting with frequent eposides of acute severe asthma needing systemic CS treatment and sometimes mechanical ventilation.

In a study of difficult-to-control asthma, 24% of adolescents were deemed to be CSR according to a definition of <15% improvement in morning FEV_1 following a burst of prednisone for poor asthma control (Chan et al., 1998); the CSR asthmatics required oral corticosteroids at a younger age, a larger maintenance oral dose on admission and were likely to be Afro-American, compared to those with CSS asthma. In a multi-centre European study (ENFUMOSA, 2003), up to 70% of a cohort of 153 severe asthma patients was defined as CS-dependent, and there were no differences in terms of the severity of airflow obstruction between the severe asthma patients who were CS-dependent and those not on oral prednisolone therapy. Persistent symptoms and abnormal lung function despite high-dose regular use of controller and reliever medications were accompanied by a component of irrevers-ible airflow obstruction, neutrophilic inflammation, ongoing mediator release and a reduced association with atopy. A more recent cohort from the US (SARP) described 204 patients with severe asthma defined according to the criteria of the American Thoracic Society workshop (Moore et al., 2007). In addition to using high-dose cor-ticosteroids, these patients used multiple controller medications and yet remained symptomatic and required high levels of healthcare utilization. Of these patients, 32% needed the use of oral corticosteroids for at least 50% of the year. The criteria that best separated severe from mild and moderate asthma were frequent and severe asthma exacerbations. Of the severe subjects, 80% had persistent airflow obstruc-tion (FEV_1 <80%) and nearly half had a baseline of <60% when bronchodilators were withheld before spirometry. Patients with severe asthma and irreversible air-flow obstruction had longer disease duration, a greater inflammatory process and more evidence of airway wall remodelling and airway hyper-responsiveness (Bum-bacea et al., 2004; ten Brinke et al., 2001).

There are very few studies that have examined the effect of a course of pred-nisolone in patients with severe asthma, and certainly the definition of CSR asthma according to response to prednisolone has not been applied to severe asthma patients. One potential reason is that many patients with severe asthma are already on regular oral CS therapy and, in addition, it is unclear what dose of additional CS should be given to assess CS responsiveness. In addition, it is unclear what the effect of chronic oral (and inhaled) CS therapy has on CS responsiveness. However, there are small studies that have demonstrated that in patients with poorly controlled severe asthma there is improved control of asthma and inflammatory markers when these patients are treated with a high dose of parenteral triamcinolone (ten Brinke et al., 2001). These observations indicate that there is relative CS resistance in severe asthma, although it would be unclear as to whether this is a shift of the dose–response or an effect seen with only the maximal doses of CS.

Therefore, the true distribution of CS responsiveness as defined by airway response to inhaled or oral CS in severe asthma is not known, but if there is an impairment of CS responsiveness it is relative. The question that arises is whether any abnormal CS responsiveness in severe asthma is genetically determined or acquired through the asthmatic disease process or is a mixture of both. CS insensitivity can certainly be reproduced in inflammatory cells *in vitro*, e.g. through incubation with inflammatory T-cell cytokines such as a combination of IL-2 and IL-4, or IL-13 (Irusen et al., 2002; Kam et al., 1993; Spahn et al., 1996).

6.7   Surrogates for CS Responsiveness in Asthma

The lack of airway CS responsiveness in CSR asthma is also reflected by a loss of suppression of mediators released from peripheral blood mononuclear cells (Wilkinson et al., 1989) or of peripheral blood T-cell proliferation stimulated *in vitro* (Corrigan et al., 1991b). CSR asthmatics also demonstrate a lack of skin blanching response to topical CS application, indicating that the resistance is not only localized to the airway effects (Brown et al., 1991). Also demonstrated in the skin of CSR patients is the lack of suppression of inflammatory cell infiltrate caused by tuberculin reaction (Sousa et al., 1996). Prednisolone treatment also did not lead to inhibition of $CD3^+$ T-cells or in MBP^+-eosinophils in biopsies taken from patients with CSR asthma, while in CSS asthma patients the number of these cells was significantly inhibited (Chakir et al., 2002). More specifically, the expression of IL-4 and IL-5 mRNA in the airways is also not inhibited by a course of prednisolone (Leung et al., 1995). In previous studies, no effect of hydrocortisone was observed on blood monocytes exposed to lipopolysaccharides regarding the release of $TNF\alpha$, IL-1 and GM-CSF from CSR patients (Lane et al., 1993).

Studies in CS-dependent asthma also demonstrate a persistent eosinophilic inflammation, with activated mast cells and T cells, and in others a persistent neutrophilia and release of IL-8, despite the use of oral CS therapy (Jatakanon et al., 1999; Wenzel et al., 1999). Similarly, levels of exhaled nitric oxide may remain persistently elevated in CS-dependent asthma (Stirling et al., 1998). However, side effects such as adrenocortical suppression or osteoporosis are also experienced by the CSR patient (Lane et al., 1996a).

These studies indicate that it would be possible to assess the degree of CS responsiveness by examining the *ex vivo* responsiveness of lung cells or even circulating cells. The release of the cytokines GM-CSF, IFNγ and IL-6 from peripheral blood mononuclear cells of patients with severe asthma induced by lipopolysaccharide was less suppressible by dexamethasone than from those with moderate asthma (Hew et al., 2006). In nocturnal asthma, steroid responsiveness of peripheral blood mononuclear cells measured as CS inhibition of proliferation was found to be reduced at 4 a.m. compared to 4 p.m., indicating a diurnal variation that parallels with the period of bronchoconstriction; this diurnal responsiveness of mononuclear cells was not observed in asthmatics without nocturnal asthma (Kraft et al., 1999). In alveolar macrophages from patients with severe asthma, there was less suppressibility by dexamethasone particularly for the lipopolysaccharide-stimulated release of cytokines IL-1β, IL-6, IL-8, MCP-1 and MIP-1α (Bhavsar et al., 2005). This may provide a convenient way of quantifying CS responsiveness in asthma, but more work will be needed to develop this test. Perhaps the most accessible marker would be to use the response in terms of a non-invasive surrogate marker for inflammation, such as exhaled nitric oxide or sputum eosinophils. Very little is known about the responsiveness of bronchial hyper-responsiveness to CS in CSR or severe asthma. Currently, there are no generally accepted methods for determining the degree of CS responsiveness in the target tissue for asthma.

6.8   Pharmacokinetics of Systemic CS in Severe Asthma

The pharmacokinetics of oral and intravenous CS used to treat asthma have been studied in normal subjects and small groups of mild asthmatics; "normal" values for clearance, half-life and volume of distribution of several CS are available (Szefler, 1991). Prednisone and prednisolone are both absorbed rapidly and achieve peak concentrations within 2 h. Methylprednisolone is more slowly absorbed. While prednisolone is bound primarily to transcortin, methylprednisolone binds primarily to albumin. Greater penetration of methylprednisolone with longer retention in lung tissue has been reported, probably due to its lower volume of distribution. Erythromycin and troleandomycin, and the newer macrolides, can delay the clearance of methylprednisolone and therefore increase the activity of methylprednisolone (Pauwels et al., 1999; Szefler et al., 1980). Is there any evidence for abnormal pharmacokinetics in patients with CSR asthma or in patients with severe CS-dependent asthma? In a subset of patients with asthma, rapid clearance of prednisolone or methylprednisolone has been described (Hill et al., 1990). In these patients, changing to another CS may provide better therapeutic effects. Mortimer et al. (1987) and others have found that orally administered prednisolone was rapidly absorbed with complete bioavailability in CSR asthmatics compared to healthy volunteers and other non-CSR asthmatic patients (Corrigan et al., 1991a; Hill et al., 1990). They also found that there was a decrease in the number of eosinophils after oral or intravenous prednisolone in these patients, perhaps querying the validity of the CSR label of these patients (Mortimer et al., 1987). However, there is little evidence that CSR is explained by abnormal pharmacokinetics of oral CS. There are few data regarding CS-dependent asthmatics.

The pharmacokinetics of ICS in CSR or in severe asthma has not been studied. The presence of airflow obstruction would limit the deposition of inhaled drugs to the central airways and may be contributory to a reduced effect of ICS therapy. Nebulized corticosteroids may achieve a greater deposition in the airways.

6.9   CS Responsiveness in Cigarette Smokers and Chronic Obstructive Pulmonary Disease

CS responsiveness has been assessed in asthmatic patients who smoke; both responses to ICS and to oral CS are attenuated in these asthmatic patients compared to those who do not smoke (Chaudhuri et al., 2003, 2004). However, the differences reported between those who smoke and those who do not are not as wide as those reported between CSR and CSS asthmatics. There is no long-term follow-up of these patients as to whether there is a worse outcome in the smoking asthmatics.

The FEV_1 response of 524 patients with chronic obstructive pulmonary disease (COPD) with a predicted mean baseline FEV_1 of 43.1% to a 2-week course of prednisolone (0.6 mg/kg for 14 days) has been recently published, and this also shows a unimodal response (Burge et al., 2003). The mean post-bronchodilator response was 60 ml (95% CI 46–74) and these were distributed around the mean value. Using a definition of steroid responders as being >20% of baseline, 62 patients were responders and 462 were non-responders. These patients with COPD had a pre-entry requirement of a bronchodilator response of <10% of predicted FEV_1 values. Age, atopy, gender, baseline FEV_1 and bronchodilator response were not related to the response to prednisolone. These data indicate, as previously shown in patients with asthma, that the response to oral CS in COPD (i.e. responder or non-responder) cannot predict the response to inhaled CS.

A trial period with oral corticosteroids and measurement of FEV_1 is used to identify "responders" who would be suitable for long-term inhaled CS therapy. However, there was also no correlation between the response to prednisolone and the subsequent decline in FEV_1. Thus, use of CS responsiveness measure would not predict those who may benefit from long-term inhaled CS therapy, although this test may point to an alternative diagnosis in those who have a marked improvement in FEV_1. Very good response to oral CS therapy in COPD patients is usually associated with the presence of lung eosinophilia (Chanez et al., 1997). Another study has shown that those who respond well to oral CS also have a better response to ICS at one year (Davies et al., 1999).

Studies of ICS in COPD indicate that it has no effect on modifying the rate of decline in lung function in 3-year studies (Bourbeau et al., 1998; Burge et al., 2000; Pauwels et al., 1999; Vestbo et al., 1999); however, ICS may reduce exacerbation rates of COPD in more severely affected patients (Burge et al., 2000). The lack of effect of ICS in COPD could reflect a relative resistance to corticosteroids (Adcock and Chung, 2002). Indeed, oral or inhaled corticosteroids do not suppress inflammatory cells, cytokines or proteases in airway secretions (Culpitt et al., 1999; Keatings et al., 1997), although a small significant inhibitory effect on sputum neutrophilia of

ICS has been reported (Confalonieri et al., 1998). Dexamethasone failed to inhibit induced release of IL-8 from alveolar macrophages of COPD patients (Culpitt et al., 2003).

6.10   Other Diseases of CS Insensitivity

A classification of CS resistance syndromes has been proposed. Generalized glucocorticoid resistance is a rare hormonal condition characterized by a generalized reduced sensitivity of end-organs to CS (Huizenga et al., 2000). This is typified by increased serum cortisol levels and relative resistance of adrenal cortisol suppression to dexamethasone and the absence of any signs of hypercortism, i.e. Cushing's syndrome. The increased serum cortisol levels are due to the activation of the hypothalamic-pituitary-adrenal axis with increased adrenocorticotrophic hormone (ACTH) due to increased sensitivity to cortisol. Overproduction of mineralocorticoids and of adrenal androgens may lead to hypertension and hypokalaemic acidosis, or to acne, hirsutism, menstrual irregularity and infertility in women.

The CS resistance or insensitivity found in asthma is classified within a separate group of inflammatory diseases that encompasses asthma, inflammatory bowel disease and rheumatoid arthritis. Failure to respond to CS therapy has been described in 20% of patients with Crohn's disease, with 36% described as CS-dependent (Munkholm et al., 1994). Steroid dependency occurs in 28% of Crohn's and 22% of ulcerative colitis patients, and steroid resistance in 16% of both Crohn's and ulcerative colitis patients (Faubion et al., 2001). Bioavailability of oral CS therapy may be impaired in patients with inflammatory bowel disease, particularly those with severe diarrhoea, and these may add to the lack of response to CS in uncontrolled disease. However, these patients may respond to intravenous CS. Rheumatoid arthritis is a chronic autoimmune inflammatory disease often treated with CS. A proportion of patients fail to respond adequately to CS therapy. Clinical resistance has been correlated with *in vitro* inhibition of induced T-cell proliferation by CS *ex vivo* (Chikanza and Kozaci, 2004).

6.11   Conclusions

The data available indicate that the response to CS therapy in asthma and in COPD is a continuum response with a unimodal distribution. Whether this mimics similar distribution of CS responsiveness in the normal population is not known. There are no definite clinical features that distinguish the very sensitive from the least sensitive asthmatic patient, and CS side effects may be acquired irrespective of CS sensitivity. The genetic factors that govern CS responsiveness in asthma need to be determined, and the issue is whether these genes would be the same genes that govern CS responsiveness in the normal population.

It is not known at present whether the reduced CS responsiveness seen in severe asthma may be genetically determined or acquired or both. Measurement of CS responsiveness is not easy in this condition. However, it is also of interest that in COPD, which is relatively resistant to CS, the distribution of CS responsiveness is also unimodal, although this would not exclude a potential for acquiring CS resistance. If inflammatory factors in severe asthma were to modulate or cause CS insensitivity, then it is plausible to postulate that CS responsiveness may be a reflection of disease severity. This is certainly a hypothesis worth testing with the proviso that a good test of CS responsiveness is available and that the effect of concomitant CS treatment on CS responsiveness is assessed. The corollary of this is that treatment aimed at improving CS responsiveness may be effective in controlling asthma when it is severe.

References

Adcock IM, Chung KF. Overview: why are corticosteroids ineffective in COPD? *Curr Opin Invest* Drugs 2002; **3**: 58–60.

Adcock IM, Lane SJ, Brown CR, Lee TH, Barnes PJ. Abnormal glucocorticoid receptor–activator protein 1 interaction in steroid-resistant asthma. *J Exp Med* 1995a; **182**: 1951–1958.

Adcock IM, Lane SJ, Brown CR, Peters MJ, Lee TH, Barnes PJ. Differences in binding of glucocorticoid receptor to DNA in steroid-resistant asthma. *J Immunol* 1995b; **154**: 3500–3505.

Barnes PJ, Pedersen S, Busse WW. Efficacy and safety of inhaled corticosteroids: new developments. *Am J Respir Crit Care Med* 1998; **157**: S1–S53.

Baumgartner RA, Martinez G, Edelman JM, Rodriguez Gomez GG et al. Distribution of therapeutic response in asthma control between oral montelukast and inhaled beclomethasone. *Eur Respir J* 2003; **21**: 123–128.

Bhavsar PK, Hew M, Torrego A, Barnes PJ, Adcock I, Chung KF. Increased release of cytokines and reduced corticosteroid suppression in alveolar macrophages from severe compared to moderate asthmatics. *Proc Am Thorac Soc* 2005; **2**: A370.

Bourbeau J, Rouleau MY, Boucher S. Randomised controlled trial of inhaled corticosteroids in patients with chronic obstructive pulmonary disease. *Thorax* 1998; **53**: 477–482.

Brown PH, Teelucksingh S, Matusiewicz SP, Greening AP, Crompton GK, Edwards CRW. Cutaneous vasoconstrictor response to glucocorticoids in asthma. *Lancet* 1991; **337**: 576–580.

Bumbacea D, Campbell D, Nguyen L, Carr D et al. Parameters associated with persistent airflow obstruction in chronic severe asthma. *Eur Respir J* 2004; **24**: 122–128.

Burge PS, Calverley PM, Jones PW, Spencer S, Anderson JA. Prednisolone response in patients with chronic obstructive pulmonary disease: results from the ISOLDE study. *Thorax* 2003; **58**: 654–658.

Burge PS, Calverley PM, Jones PW, Spencer S, Anderson JA, Maslen TK. Randomised, double blind, placebo controlled study of fluticasone propionate in patients with moderate to severe chronic obstructive pulmonary disease: the ISOLDE trial. *Br Med J* 2000; **320**: 1297–1303.

Carey RA, Harvey AM, Howard JE, Winkenwerder WL. The effect of adrenocorticotrophic hormone (ACTH) and cortisone on the course of chronic bronchial asthma. *Bulle John Hopkins Hospi* 1950; **87**: 387–414.

Carmichael J, Paterson IC, Diaz P, Crompton GK, Kay AB, Grant IWB. Corticosteroid resistance in asthma. *Br Med J* 1981; **282**: 1419–1422.

Chakir J, Hamid Q, Bosse M, Boulet LP, Laviolette M. Bronchial inflammation in corticosteroid-sensitive and corticosteroid-resistant asthma at baseline and on oral corticosteroid treatment. *Clin Exp Allergy* 2002; **32**: 578–582.

Chan MT, Leung DY, Szefler SJ, Spahn JD. Difficult-to-control asthma: clinical characteristics of steroid-insensitive asthma. *J Allergy Clin Immunol* 1998; **101**: 594–601.

Chanez P, Vignola AM, O'Shaugnessy T, Enander I et al. Corticosteroid reversibility in COPD is related to features of asthma. *Am J Respir Crit Care Med* 1997; **155**: 1529–1534.

Chaudhuri R, Livingston E, McMahon AD, Thomson L, Borland W, Thomson NC. Cigarette smoking impairs the therapeutic response to oral corticosteroids in chronic asthma. *Am J Respir Crit Care Med* 2003; **168**: 1308–1311.

Chaudhuri R, McMahon AD, Thomson LJ, MacLeod KJ et al. Effect of inhaled corticosteroids on symptom severity and sputum mediator levels in chronic persistent cough. *J Allergy Clin Immunol* 2004; **113**: 1063–1070.

Chikanza IC, Kozaci DL. Corticosteroid resistance in rheumatoid arthritis: molecular and cellular perspectives. *Rheumatology (Oxf)* 2004; **43**: 1337–1345.

Chung KF, Godard P, Adelroth E, Ayres J et al. Difficult/therapy-resistant asthma: the need for an integrated approach to define clinical phenotypes, evaluate risk factors, understand patho-physiology and find novel therapies. ERS Task Force on Difficult/Therapy-Resistant Asthma. *Eur Respir J* 1999; **13**: 1198–1208.

Colice GL, Stampone P, Leung DY, Szefler SJ. Oral corticosteroids in poorly controlled asthma. *J Allergy Clin Immunol* 2005; **115**: 200–201.

Confalonieri M, Mainardi E, Della PR, Bernorio S et al. Inhaled corticosteroids reduce neu-trophilic bronchial inflammation in patients with chronic obstructive pulmonary disease [see comments]. *Thorax* 1998; **53**: 583–585.

Corrigan CJ, Brown PH, Barnes NC, Tsai J-J, Frew AJ, Kay AB. Glucocorticoid resistance in chronic asthma. Glucocorticoid pharmacokinetics, glucocorticoid receptor characteristic, and inhibition of peripheral blood T cell proliferation by glucocorticoids *in vitro*. *Am Rev Respir Dis* 1991a; **144**: 1016–1025.

Corrigan CJ, Brown PH, Barnes NC, Tsai JJ, Frew AJ, Kay AB. Glucocorticoid resistance in chronic asthma. Peripheral blood T lymphocyte activation and comparison of the T lym-phocyte inhibitory effects of glucocorticoids and cyclosporin A. *Am Rev Respir Dis* 1991b; **144**: 1026–1032.

Culpitt SV, Maziak W, Loukidis S, Nightingale JA, Matthews JL, Barnes PJ. Effect of high dose inhaled steroid on cells, cytokines, and proteases in induced sputum in chronic obstructive pulmonary disease. *Am J Respir Crit Care Med* 1999; **160**: 1635–1639.

Culpitt SV, Rogers DF, Shah P, De Matos C et al. Impaired inhibition by dexamethasone of cytokine release by alveolar macrophages from patients with chronic obstructive pulmonary disease. *Am J Respir Crit Care Med* 2003; **167**: 24–31.

Davies L, Nisar M, Pearson MG, Costello RW, Earis JE, Calverley PM. Oral corticosteroid trials in the management of stable chronic obstructive pulmonary disease. *QJM* 1999; **92**: 395–400.

Demoly P, Jaffuel D, Mathieu M, Sahla H et al. Glucocorticoid insensitive asthma: a one year clinical follow up pilot study. *Thorax* 1998; **53**: 1063–1065.

Djukanovic R, Wilson JW, Britten KM, Wilson SJ et al. The effect of an inhaled corticosteroid on airway inflammation and symptoms in asthma. *Am Rev Respir Dis* 1992; **145**: 669–674.

ENFUMOSA. Cross-sectional European multicentre study of the clinical phenotype of chronic severe asthma. *Eur Respir J* 2003; **22**: 470–477.

Faubion WA Jr, Loftus EV Jr, Harmsen WS, Zinsmeister AR, Sandborn WJ. The natural history of corticosteroid therapy for inflammatory bowel disease: a population-based study. *Gastro-enterology* 2001; **121**: 255–260.

Greening AP, Ind PW, Northfield M, Shaw G. Added salmeterol versus higher-dose corticosteroid in asthma patients with symptoms on existing inhaled corticosteroid. *Lancet* 1994; **344**: 219–224.

Hamid QA, Wenzel SE, Hauk PJ, Tsicopoulos A et al. Increased glucocorticoid receptor beta in airway cells of glucocorticoid-insensitive asthma. *Am J Respir Crit Care Med* 1999; **159**: 1600–1604.

Hew M, Bhavsar P, Torrego A, Meah S et al. Relative corticosteroid insensitivity of peripheral blood mononuclear cells in severe asthma. *Am J Respir Crit Care Med* 2006; **174**: 134–141.

Hill MR, Szefler SJ, Ball BD, Bartoszek M, Brenner AM. Monitoring glucocorticoid therapy: a pharmacokinetic approach. *Clin Pharmacol Ther* 1990; **48**: 390–398.

Huizenga NA, de Lange P, Koper JW, de Herder WW et al. Five patients with biochemical and/or clinical generalized glucocorticoid resistance without alterations in the glucocorticoid receptor gene. *J Clin Endocrinol Metab* 2000; **85**: 2076–2081.

Irusen E, Matthews JG, Takahashi A, Barnes PJ, Chung KF, Adcock IM. p38 Mitogen-activated protein kinase-induced glucocorticoid receptor phosphorylation reduces its activity: role in steroid-insensitive asthma. *J Allergy Clin Immunol* 2002; **109**: 649–657.

Israel E, Chervinsky PS, Friedman B, van Bavel J et al. Effects of montelukast and beclomethasone on airway function and asthma control. *J Allergy Clin Immunol* 2002; **110**: 847–854.

Jatakanon A, Uasuf C, Maziak W, Lim S, Chung KF, Barnes PJ. Neutrophilic inflammation in severe persistent asthma. *Am J Respir Crit Care Med* 1999; **160**: 1532–1539.

Kam JC, Szefler SJ, Surs W, Sher ER, Leung DY. Combination IL-2 and IL-4 reduces glucocorticoid receptor- binding affinity and T cell response to glucocorticoids. *J Immunol* 1993; **151**: 3460–3466.

Keatings VM, Jatakanon A, Worsdell YM, Barnes PJ. Effects of inhaled and oral glucocorticoids on inflammatory indices in asthma and COPD. *Am J Respir Crit Care Med* 1997; **155**: 542–548.

Kraft M, Vianna E, Martin RJ, Leung DM. Nocturnal asthma is associated with reduced glucocorticoid receptor binding affinity and decreased steroid responsiveness at night. *J Allergy Clin Immunol* 1999; **103**: 66–71.

Lane SJ, Atkinson BA, Swaminathan R, Lee TH. Hypothalamic-pituitary-adrenal axis in corticosteroid-resistant bronchial asthma. *Am J Respir Crit Care Med* 1996a; **153**: 557–560.

Lane SJ, Vaja S, Swaminathan R, Lee TH. Effects of prednisolone on bone turnover in patients with corticosteroid resistant asthma. *Clin Exp Allergy* 1996b; **26**: 1197–1201.

Lane SJ, Wilkinson JR, Cochrane GM, Lee TH, Arm JP. Differential in vitro regulation by glucocorticoids of monocyte- derived cytokine generation in glucocorticoid-resistant bronchial asthma. *Am Rev Respir Dis* 1993; **147**: 690–696.

Leung DY, Hamid Q, Vottero A, Szefler SJ et al. Association of glucocorticoid insensitivity with increased expression of glucocorticoid receptor beta. *J Exp Med* 1997; **186**: 1567–1574.

Leung DY, Martin RJ, Szefler SJ, Sher ER et al. Dysregulation of interleukin 4, interleukin 5, and interferon gamma gene expression in steroid-resistant asthma. *J Exp Med* 1995; **181**: 33–40.

Moore WC, Bleecker ER, Curran-Everett D, Erzurum SC et al. Characterisation of the severe asthma phenotype by teh NHLBI severe asthma reserach program. *J Allergy Clin Immunol* 2007; **119**: 405–413.

Mortimer O, Grettve L, Lindstrom B, Lonnerholm G, Zetterstrom O. Bioavailability of prednisolone in asthmatic patients with a poor response to steroid treatment. *Eur J Respir Dis* 1987; **71**: 372–379.

Munkholm P, Langholz E, Davidsen M, Binder V. Frequency of glucocorticoid resistance and dependency in Crohn's disease. *Gut* 1994; **35**: 360–362.

Olivieri D, Chetta A, Del Donno M, Bertorelli G et al. Effect of short-term treatment with low-dose inhaled fluticasone propionate on airway inflammation and remodeling in mild asthma: a placebo-controlled study. *Am J Respir Crit Care Med* 1997; **155**: 1864–1871.

Pauwels RA, Lofdahl CG, Laitinen LA, Schouten JP et al. Long-term treatment with inhaled budesonide in persons with mild chronic obstructive pulmonary disease who continue smoking. European Respiratory Society Study on Chronic Obstructive Pulmonary Disease [see comments]. *N Engl J Med* 1999; **340**: 1948–1953.

Pauwels RA, Lofdahl C, Postma D, Tattersfield A et al. Effect of inhaled formoterol and budesonide on exacerbations of asthma. *New Engl J Med* 1997; **337**: 1405–1411.

Robinson DS, Campbell DA, Durham SR, Pfeffer J, Barnes PJ, Chung KF. Systematic assessment of difficult-to-treat asthma. *Eur Respir J* 2003; **22**: 478–483.

Schwartz E. Oral cortisone in intractable bronchial asthma. *J Allergy* 1951; **22**: 164–166.

Schwartz HJ, Lowell FC, Melby JC. Steroid resistance in bronchial asthma. *Ann Intern Med* 1968; **69**: 493–499.

Sher ER, Leung DY, Surs W, Kam JC et al. Steroid-resistant asthma. Cellular mechanisms contributing to inadequate response to glucocorticoid therapy. *J Clin Invest* 1994; **93**: 33–39.

Sont JK, Willems LN, Bel EH, van Krieken JH, Vandenbroucke JP, Sterk PJ. Clinical control and histopathologic outcome of asthma when using airway hyperresponsiveness as an additional guide to long-term treatment. The AMPUL Study Group. *Am J Respir Crit Care Med* 1999; **159**: 1043–1051.

Sousa AR, Lane SJ, Atkinson BA, Poston RN, Lee TH. The effects of prednisolone on the cutaneous tuberculin response in patients with corticosteroid-resistant bronchial asthma. *J Allergy Clin Immunol* 1996; **97**: 698–706.

Sousa AR, Lane SJ, Cidlowski JA, Staynov DZ, Lee TH. Glucocorticoid resistance in asthma is associated with elevated in vivo expression of the glucocorticoid receptor beta-isoform. *J Allergy Clin Immunol* 2000; **105**: 943–950.

Sousa AR, Lane SJ, Soh C, Lee TH. In vivo resistance to corticosteroids in bronchial asthma is associated with enhanced phosyphorylation of JUN N-terminal kinase and failure of prednisolone to inhibit JUN N-terminal kinase phosphorylation. *J Allergy Clin Immunol* 1999; **104**: 565–574.

Spahn JD, Szefler SJ, Surs W, Doherty DE, Nimmagadda SR, Leung DY. A novel action of IL-13: induction of diminished monocyte glucocorticoid receptor-binding affinity. *J Immunol* 1996; **157**: 2654–2659.

Stirling RG, Chung KF. Severe asthma: definition and mechanisms. *Allergy* 2001; **56**: 825–840.

Stirling RG, Kharitonov SA, Campbell D, Robinson DS et al. Increase in exhaled nitric oxide levels in patients with difficult asthma and correlation with symptoms and disease severity despite treatment with oral and inhaled corticosteroids. Asthma and Allergy Group. *Thorax* 1998; **53**: 1030–1034.

Szefler SJ. Glucocorticoid therapy for asthma: Clinical pharmacology. *J Allergy Clin Immunol* 1991; **88**: 147–165.

Szefler SJ, Martin RJ, King TS, Boushey HA et al. Significant variability in response to inhaled corticosteroids for persistent asthma. *J Allergy Clin Immunol* 2002; **109**: 410–418.

Szefler SJ, Rose JQ, Ellis EF, Spector SL, Green AW, Jusko WJ. The effect of troleandomycin on methylprednisolone elimination. *J Allergy Clin Immunol* 1980; **66**: 447–451.

Tantisira KG, Hwang ES, Raby BA, Silverman ES et al. TBX21: a functional variant predicts improvement in asthma with the use of inhaled corticosteroids. *Proc Natl Acad Sci USA* 2004; **101**: 18099–18104.

Ten Brinke A, Zwinderman AH, Sterk PJ, Rabe KF, Bel EH. Factors associated with persistent airflow limitation in severe asthma. *Am J Respir Crit Care Med* 2001; **164**: 744–748.

Ten Brinke A, Zwinderman AH, Sterk PJ, Rabe KF, Bel EH. "Refractory" eosinophilic airway inflammation in severe asthma: effect of parenteral corticosteroids. *Am J Respir Crit Care Med* 2004; **170**: 601–605.

Van Essen-Zandvliet EE, Hughes MD, Waalkens HJ, Duiverman EJ et al. Effects of 22 months of treatment with inhaled corticosteroids and/or beta-2-agonists on lung function, airway responsiveness, and symptoms in children with asthma. *Am Rev Respir Dis* 1992; **146**: 547–554.

Vathenen AS, Knox AJ, Wisniewski A, Tattersfield AE. Time course of change in bronchial reactivity with an inhaled corticosteroid in asthma. *Am Rev Respir Dis* 1991; **143**: 1317–1321.

Vestbo J, Sorensen T, Lange P, Brix A, Torre P, Viskum K. Long-term effect of inhaled budesonide in mild and moderate chronic obstructive pulmonary disease: a randomised controlled trial. *Lancet* 1999; **353**: 1819–1823.

Wamboldt FS, Spahn JD, Klinnert MD, Wamboldt MZ et al. Clinical outcomes of steroid-insensitive asthma. *Ann Allergy Asthma Immunol* 1999; **83**: 55–60.

Weiss ST, Lake SL, Silverman ES, Silverman EK et al. Asthma steroid pharmacogenetics: a study strategy to identify replicated treatment responses. *Proc Am Thorac Soc* 2004; **1**: 364–367.

Wenzel SE, Schwartz LB, Langmack EL, Halliday JL et al. Evidence that severe asthma can be divided pathologically into two inflammatory subtypes with distinct physiologic and clinical characteristics. *Am J Respir Crit Care Med* 1999; **160**: 1001–1008.

Wilkinson JRW, Crea AEG, Clark TJH, Lee TH. Identification and characterization of a monocyte-derived neutrophil-activating factor in corticosteroid-resistant bronchial asthma. *J Clin Invest* 1989; **84**: 1930–1941.

Woolcock AJ. Corticosteroid-resistant asthma. Definitions. *Am J Respir Crit Care Med* 1996; **154**: S45–S48.

7

Glucocorticoid-insensitive Asthma: Molecular Mechanisms

John W. Bloom

7.1   Introduction

Immune activation and tissue inflammation play a critical role in the pathogenesis of chronic allergic and autoimmune diseases. The anti-inflammatory corticosteroids (CSs) are the most effective agents for the treatment of these diseases. Although the majority of patients respond to CS therapy, some demonstrate persistent tissue inflammation despite treatment with high-dose CS (Ito et al., 2006). CS insensitivity has been widely recognized as complicating the management of chronic inflammatory diseases such as asthma, autoimmune diseases and inflammatory bowel disease (Leung and Bloom, 2003). Knowledge of the molecular mechanisms responsible for CS insensitivity is crucial for the development of more effective therapies.

In patients with asthma there is a range of responsiveness, with CS insensitivity at one extreme of this spectrum. Although complete resistance to therapy with CS is rare in asthma, reduced responsiveness to CS in patients with severe asthma is more common. These CS-dependent asthma patients require chronic oral CS or large doses of inhaled CS for asthma control but in clinical practice are a relatively small group (10% or less of asthmatics) (Wenzel and Busse, 2007). Another potentially large group of CS-insensitive asthmatics are those who smoke cigarettes (Thomson et al., 2006). Surprisingly, cigarettes smoking rates among asthmatics are similar to the rates in the general population in developed countries (Silverman et al., 2003; Siroux et al., 2000; Turner et al., 1998). Accumulating evidence suggests that asthmatic patients who smoke are less sensitive to the anti-inflammatory effects of CS than non-smoking asthmatics (Chalmers et al., 2001; Chaudhuri et al., 2003).

Overcoming Steroid Insensitivity in Respiratory Disease   Edited by Ian M. Adcock and Kian Fan Chung
© 2008 John Wiley & Sons, Ltd.

This chapter is a review of the studies investigating the molecular mechanisms producing CS insensitivity in asthma. Much of the cited work has been performed utilizing specimens from patients with severe asthma that was clinically determined as either CS resistant or CS dependent. CS resistance is defined as failure of lung function to improve by 15% after 1–2 weeks of high-dose oral CS (Sher et al., 1994).

The anti-inflammatory effects of CS are mediated through the glucocorticoid receptor (GR), which is a ligand-activated transcription factor that modulates inflammatory and anti-inflammatory gene expression by a variety of molecular signalling pathways (Leung and Bloom, 2003). The details of the molecular mechanism of GR action are reviewed in Chapter 1 and are outlined only briefly here. CSs are extremely lipophilic and enter the cell cytoplasm from the extracellular space, primarily by means of passive diffusion. Prior to ligand binding, GRs exist as a large multiunit complex in the cytoplasm that includes two molecules of heat shock protein (hsp) 90 (Cheung and Smith, 2000). After activation by binding of CS, the GR dissociates from the chaperone proteins and rapidly translocates to the nucleus. Within the nucleus, the GRs bind as a dimer to specific glucocorticoid response elements (GREs) on DNA within the promoter region of CS-responsive genes to enhance transcription of anti-inflammatory genes. GRs can also repress transcription of pro-inflammatory genes by interaction with inflammatory transcription factors, such as activator protein 1 (AP-1) and nuclear factor kappa B (NF-κB). Both activation of anti-inflammatory genes and repression of pro-inflammatory genes by GR involve modification of histones and alteration of chromatin structure (Adcock et al., 2005).

Insensitivity to CS may develop at multiple points in anti-inflammatory signalling pathways, including GR abnormalities (e.g. reduced GR number and ligand binding affinity), decreased translocation of the GR from the cytoplasm to the nucleus, altered GR interactions with other transcription factors and abnormalities of histone-modifying enzymes. Here, the putative molecular mechanisms of CS insensitivity are reviewed in relation to these critical points in the CS signalling pathway (Ito et al., 2006a).

7.2   GR Abnormalities

The glucocorticoid (GC) insensitivity in asthma must be distinguished from the rare familial GC resistance syndrome (see Chapter 5), which is caused by inactivating polymorphisms in the gene encoding the GR that produce generalized GC insensitivity associated with abnormalities of cortisol secretion and hypothalamic-pituitary-adrenal (HPA) axis sensitivity (Bray and Cotton, 2003; Chrousos et al., 1993). In CS-insensitive asthma, no GR polymorphisms responsible for resistance have been identified (Lane et al., 1994). In addition, endogenous cortisol secretion and HPA axis sensitivity are not altered as in familial CS resistance (Lane et al., 1996).

Initial ligand binding studies utilizing peripheral blood mononuclear cells (PBMCs) from CS-insensitive patients failed to demonstrate any significant abnormalities (Corrigan et al., 1991a, b; Lane and Lee, 1991). However, Sher and co-workers subsequently were able to demonstrate two types of ligand binding abnormalities in PBMCs from CS-insensitive asthmatics (Sher et al., 1994). The most important defect was a significant decrease in the ligand binding affinity of GR in the nuclear cell fraction. This defect was reversible with *in vitro* culture of the cells and could be induced by culture with a combination of IL-2 and IL-4 or by IL-13 alone. Importantly, bronchoalveolar lavage (BAL) cells from patients with GC-insensitive asthma express more IL-2 and IL-4 mRNA than patients with GC-sensitive asthma, and the IL-4 expression was decreased after systemic CS therapy only in the CS-sensitive asthmatics (Leung et al., 1995).

Irusen and co-workers investigated the mechanism of the decrease in GR affinity resulting from treatment of PBMCs with the combination of IL-2 and IL-4 or IL-13 (Irusen et al., 2002). They hypothesized that phosphorylation of the GR in the nucleus was responsible for the altered binding affinity. Inhibition of the p38 mitogen-activated protein kinase (MAPK) blocked the decrease in GR binding affinity resulting from IL-2/IL-4 or IL-13. In addition, the ability of CS to modulate IL-10 release from PBMCs was inhibited by IL-2/IL-4 treatment and restored by inhibition of p38 MAPK. Activation of p38 MAPK by IL-2 and IL-4, as shown by means of phosphorylation of activated transcription factor 2, resulted in GR phosphorylation. Although there is clearly an association between p38 MAPK activity and GR ligand binding affinity, further investigation will be required to determine if the altered GR binding is due to a direct effect of p38 MAPK producing phosphorylation of the GR protein. Nonetheless, the therapeutic implication is that p38-MAPK inhibitors might have a beneficial effect on steroid insensitivity (Adcock et al., 2006a).

Increased expression of an alternatively spliced form of the GR, termed GRβ, has been extensively studied and proposed as a mechanism for CS insensitivity (Lu and Cidlowski, 2004). GRβ binds DNA but not CS and may act as a dominant negative inhibitor by competing with the active GRα for binding to GREs (Oakley et al., 1999) or by forming transcriptionally inactive GRα–GRβ heterodimers (Charmandari et al., 2005) (Figure 7.1). The expression of GRβ is enhanced by pro-inflammatory cytokines and has been associated with CS insensitivity in several cell types, including BAL cells (Goleva et al., 2006; Hamid et al., 1999; Kraft et al., 2001; Strickland et al., 2001). The physiological role of GRβ in CS-insensitivity has been controversial (Brogan et al., 1999; Carlstedt-Duke, 1999; Gagliardo et al., 2000). The debate stems from studies demonstrating that GR-α is much more abundant than GRβ, suggesting that it is unlikely that GRβ has an important inhibitory effect. Also, GRβ has no ability to inhibit expression of pro-inflammatory genes by interaction with inflammatory transcription factors. The role of GR-β in CS-insensitive asthma is discussed in detail in Chapter 3.

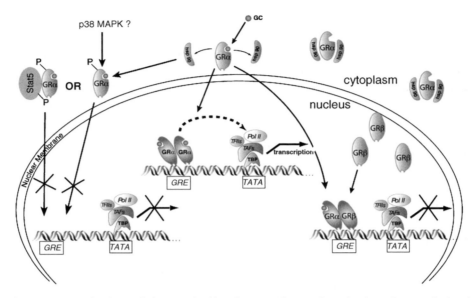

Figure 7.1 Mechanisms of glucocorticoid resistance. The usual mechanism of transcriptional activation through the GR is shown (centre). In IL-2-treated cells, the interaction of the GR with the STAT5 protein in the cytoplasm (left) prevents translocation of the GR to the nucleus, thus blocking transcriptional activation. The GR/STAT5 interaction appears to require phosphorylation of the GR and STAT5. Also shown on the left of the figure is defective GR nuclear translocation, possibly due to phosphorylation of GR by p38 MAPK (Matthews et al., 2004; see text). An alternative, non-exclusive mechanism of resistance results from enhanced expression of the GRβ isoform (right). GRβ does not bind glucocorticoid hormone, but in contrast to the GR it is located in the nucleus of cells independent of hormone treatment. GRβ can bind as a heterodimer with the GR at GREs and inhibit GR-mediated transcription by means of a dominant negative effect

7.3   GR Nuclear Translocation

Because the initial step in the classical CS signalling pathway is GR translocation from the cytoplasm to the nucleus, decreased nuclear localization is a particularly plausible molecular mechanism of CS insensitivity. Findings from several studies investigating mechanisms of CS insensitivity have identified altered nuclear translocation as a potential mechanism.

Matthews and co-workers investigated the responses to CS in PBMCs from patients with CS-resistant and CS-dependent asthma (Matthews et al., 2004). Ligand binding studies demonstrated similar decreased affinity for CS as described above. But, in addition, nuclear localization of the GR was impaired in the peripheral blood mononuclear cells (PBMCs) from a subgroup of these patients with CS-insensitive asthma. These data suggested an explanation for earlier results from electrophoretic mobility shift assays that demonstrated a reduction in GR binding to DNA in PBMCs from CS-insensitive asthma patients (Adcock et al., 1995b). Scathard analysis of the binding data demonstrated a decrease in the number but not the affinity of the GRs available in the CS-insensitive cells, consistent with a defect in nuclear translocation of the receptor (Figure 7.1). Although the mechanism underlying the abnormality of nuclear localization was not investigated directly in the study, in light of the work by Irusen et al. in PBMCs from CS-insensitive asthma the possibility of alterations in GR phosphorylation by p38 MAPK was raised as a potential mechanism. In the remainder of the patients, nuclear translocation was normal but there was a defect in histone acetylation (see section 7.5).

Goleva and co-workers identified a potential molecular mechanism altering GR nuclear translocation in studies investigating CS insensitivity in murine T cells (Goleva et al., 2002). Incubation with IL-2 alone produced CS insensitivity in the murine T-cell line HT-2, and the insensitivity to dexamethasone treatment was associated with inability of GR to translocate to the nucleus. The IL-2-induced effects on GR nuclear translocation occurred within 30 min and were not blocked by cyclohexamide, suggesting the possibility of a post-translational modification. Pre-incubation of the cells with a Janus-associated kinase (JAK) 3 inhibitor restored GR nuclear translocation even in the presence of IL-2. Immunoprecipitation experiments demonstrated that GR and phosphorylated signal transducer and activator of transcription 5 (STAT5) formed complexes, suggesting a potential mechanism for altered nuclear translocation of GR (Figure 7.1). The essential role of STAT5 was demonstrated by the inability of IL-2 to induce CS insensitivity in splenocytes from STAT5 knockout mice. Also of interest is that a p38-MAPK inhibitor blocked the effect of IL-2 on GR nuclear translocation in a manner similar to the JAK 3 inhibitor. Suppressor of cytokine signalling (SOCS), a natural regulator of the JAK-STAT pathway, has been proposed to play a role in treatment-insensitive allergy (Ito et al., 2006a). Interestingly, IL-4 induction of SOCS3 is blocked by inhibitors of both the c-jun N-terminal kinase (JNK) and p38-MAPK pathways. This finding suggests a link between MAPK activation and SOCS induction and potentially to CS insensitivity.

Li and co-workers have reported studies of a mechanism of staphylococcal superantigen-induced CS resistance in T cells from normal subjects (Li et al., 2004). T-cell proliferation induced by anti-cluster of differentiation 3 (anti-CD3) activation of the T-cell receptor (TCR) was sensitive to inhibition by the CS dexamethasone, but T-cell proliferation induced by superantigen was insensitive to inhibition by CS. The development of CS resistance following superantigen stimulation required the presence of antigen-presenting cells or additional stimulation of CD28. Superantigen, compared to anti-CD3, initiated a more rapid and sustained phosphorylation of the MAPK extracellular signal-related kinase (ERK), and ERK was able to phosphorylate GR in an *in vitro* kinase assay. Specific inhibitors of the ERK pathway, but not other kinase inhibitors, blocked the development of superantigen-induced steroid resistance in the proliferation assay. Importantly, CS insensitivity was associated with a decrease in GR nuclear localization following CS treatment, and this effect was reversed with ERK pathway inhibitors. These findings suggest the possibility that development of superantigen-induced CS resistance in T cells is mediated by phosphorylation of GR (or proteins that interact with GR) and is associated with decreased localization of GR in the nucleus. Although the authors do not directly demonstrate the mechanism for the development of resistance, blockade of ERK signalling in their system reversed resistance as well as restored GR translocation.

Tsitoura and Rothman examined murine and human T cells for responsiveness to CS *in vitro* and found that dexamethasone suppressed TCR-induced proliferation of naive $CD4^+$ T cells through a mechanism involving inhibition of the pro-inflammatory transcription factor AP-1, nuclear factor of activated T cells (NF-AT) and NFκB (Tsitoura and Rothman, 2004). Enhancement of TCR signalling by CD28- or IL-2-mediated co-stimulation produced resistance to the suppressive effect of dexamethasone and restored cellular proliferation. Although the effect of MAPK signalling on GR nuclear translocation was not examined in these studies, ERK signalling was essential for the development of T-cell CS resistance. Thus, these findings demonstrate that ERK signalling is a potential therapeutic target for patients with CS resistance.

Taken together, the above studies demonstrate that signalling through MAPK pathways may produce CS insensitivity and suggest that inhibition of GR nuclear translocation is associated with the GR phosphorylation state. Studies with cell lines support the hypothesis that post-translational modification of GR by phosphorylation modulates receptor function and subcellular localization (Ismaili and Garabedian, 2004). The GR is a phosphoprotein and is phosphorylated in the absence of ligand, but further phosphorylation occurs with CS binding. Data from *in vitro* studies suggest that phosphorylation sites in the amino-terminal region of GR (at serines 203, 211 and 226) play a crucial role in GR function (Krstic et al., 1997; Rogatsky et al., 1998; Wang et al., 2002). In the absence of CS, the GR is phosphorylated primarily at the serine 203 site. Treatment with the GR agonist results in increased phosphorylation at serine 211 relative to serine 203. Localization studies showed that after CS treatment, the serine-203-phosphorylated GR is predominantly in the cytoplasm, whereas the serine-211-phosphorylated form is found in the nucleus. Of particular interest, the transcriptional activity of the GR correlated with the degree of phosphorylation at serine 211. Also, phosphorylation at serine 226 has been shown to inhibit GR-mediated transcriptional activation. Phosphorylation of the GR at serine 226 by the MAPK JNK enhances GR nuclear export and likely contributes to termination of GR-mediated transcription (Itoh et al., 2002). In summary, post-translational modification of the GR by means of phosphorylation induces a distinct receptor conformation and influences the association with coregulatory proteins that modulate the GR subcellular location and transcriptional activation.

7.4 Cross-talk with Transcription Factors

Adcock and colleagues were the first to demonstrate an abnormal GR interaction with another transcription factor as a molecular mechanism of CS-insensitive asthma (Adcock et al., 1995a). They investigated the ability of several transcription factors to bind to their DNA response elements and to interact with GR in PBMCs from CS-insensitive patients. Compared with CS-sensitive patients, the interaction between GR and AP-1 was reduced in PBMCs from CS-insensitive patients. Notably, the interaction with NF-κB was not affected. In addition, the basal level of AP-1 was increased in PBMC nuclei of CS-insensitive asthmatics. These data suggest that in CS-insensitive asthma either GR binding to its GRE and AP-1 is altered or increased AP-1 levels inhibit GR binding to DNA.

AP-1 is a heterodimer of a combination of related transcription factors belonging to the fos and jun families of oncoproteins, but the most common stable heterodimer is formed by c-fos and c-jun (Shaulian and Karin, 2002). Activation of AP-1 is mediated primarily by transcriptional regulation of c-fos and the post-translational phosphorylation of c-jun by JNK. The expression of c-fos is increased in PBMCs from patients with CS-insensitive asthma compared to those from patients with CS-sensitive asthma and healthy control subjects (Lane et al., 1998). Because CSs have been shown to block AP-1 activation by inhibition of phosphorylation and activation of JNK (Gonzalez et al., 2000; Swantek et al., 1997), this pathway was investigated in two studies involving CS-insensitive asthma patients. First, using a model of tuberculin-induced inflammatory responses in the skin, Sousa and co-workers demonstrated that a therapeutically effective dose of oral prednisolone suppressed inflammatory cell infiltration into the skin of CS-sensitive but not CS-insensitive subjects (Sousa et al., 1996). In subsequent studies using the same cutaneous tuberculin-induced model of inflammation, these investigators demonstrated an increase in the expression of c-fos, JNK and activated phosphorylated c-jun in CS-insensitive versus CS-sensitive asthmatics. Prednisolone reduced the levels of both phosphorylated c-jun and phosphorylated JNK in the CS-sensitive asthmatics but not in the CS-insensitive group (Sousa et al., 1999). In a more recent study, these investigators determined the levels of total and phosphorylated c-jun and JNK and the expression of c-fos in bronchial mucosal biopsies in CS-insensitive and CS-sensitive patients. In CD45$^+$ mucosal leukocytes they found increased expression of c-fos in the CS-insensitive subjects but no differences in the total cells expressing phosphorylated c-jun or JNK between the groups. Following systemic CS treatment, cells expressing phosphorylated c-jun and JNK decreased in the CS-sensitive subjects but not in subjects with CS insensitivity (Loke et al., 2006).

Thus, there is a complex relationship between the expression of AP-1 and inhibitory effects of CS in asthma. The data suggest that increased levels of c-fos and enhanced phosphorylation of c-jun from JNK activation lead to an increase in AP-1 activity, explaining at least some of the resistance in CS-insensitive asthma. In addition to the inhibitory cross-talk between AP-1 and GR, either *c*-jun or JNK may also suppress GR function by downregulating GR transcription or altering function through phosphorylation of GR (Cabral et al., 2001; Itoh et al., 2002; Rogatsky et al., 1998).

7.5 NF-κB, GR, Histones and Chromatin Remodelling

Although numerous pathways are activated during the inflammatory response in asthma, NF-κB is thought to be of particular importance because it is activated by numerous extracellular stimuli involved in lung inflammation (Baldwin, 1996; Barnes and Adcock, 1997). NF-κB is a dimer most frequently composed of two subunits, p65 and p50, and in inactive cells it resides in the cytoplasm. Following activation, NF-κB translocates to the nucleus where it associates with sequence-specific DNA binding elements in the promoter region of responsive genes (Ghosh and Karin, 2002). NF-κB induces inflammatory gene expression via recruitment of coactivator proteins that remodel chromatin through specific histone modifications (Ito et al., 2000; Lee et al., 2006).

The basic structural unit of chromatin is the nucleosome, which consists of approximately 146 bp of DNA wrapped approximately two turns around an octamer consisting of two molecules each of the four core histone proteins (H2A, H2B, H3, H4) (Kornberg and Lorch, 1999). Histones package all chromosomal DNA into chromatin, and the packaging of DNA into chromatin performs a critical role in regulating gene expression. In the resting cell, nucleosome assembly into chromatin inhibits the ability of the general transcription factors (such as the RNA polymerase II holoenzyme) to interact with promoter sequences. Transcriptional coactivator proteins have intrinsic histone acetyltransferase (HAT) activity and act as molecular switches to regulate gene expression. Acetylation of histones occurs at lysine (K) residues located on the amino-terminal tails of the histone. As a consequence of acetylation of the histone tails, the nucleosomal conformation is more relaxed, and the DNA becomes accessible to the binding of transcriptional regulators. The acetylation is reversible and removal of the acetyl groups by histone deacetylases (HDACs) is associated with restoration of a dense closed chromatin structure and gene silencing (Agarwal et al., 1999; Tyler and Kadonaga, 1999). Thus, gene-specific transcription factors such as NF-κB and GR, which regulate gene expression, must recruit not only the required basal transcription machinery but also the specialized enzymes required to acetylate or deacetylate histones and remodel chromatin (Figure 7.2). In addition to recruitment of the histone-modifying enzymes to the promoter at the right time, an additional level of complexity and gene regulation involves the specificity of the enzyme for the tails of a particular histone (e.g. H3 versus H4) and a specific lysine residue in that tail (Ito and Adcock, 2002).

Because histone acetylation is essential for chromatin remodelling and gene activation, defects in histone acetylation could produce insensitivity to

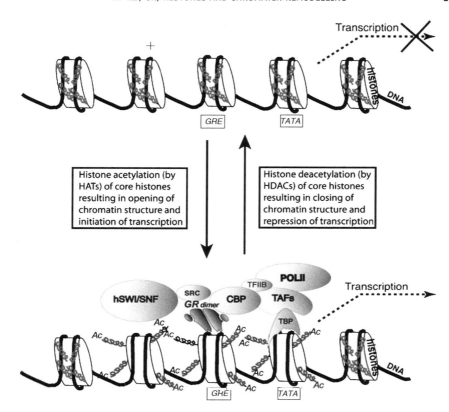

Figure 7.2 GR-mediated transcriptional activation: role of coactivators HATs and HDACs and chromatin remodelling. The bound GR homodimer interacts with the basal transcriptional machinery shown bound to the TATA box (bottom). The interaction of the GR with the basal transcription complex through the coactivator proteins SRC (steroid receptor coactivator) and CBP (CREB binding protein) is depicted. The ATP-dependent chromatin remodelling factor *(hSWI/SNF)* is also shown as part of the complex. The basal transcription complex includes TATA binding protein, associated transcription factors *(TAFs* and *TFIIs)* and RNA polymerase II *(pol II)*. The interaction between GR and the basal transcription complex enhances transcription of the GR target gene. DNA is shown packaged into chromatin by histones. SRC and CBP, as well as some proteins in the basal transcription complex, have intrinsic HAT activity and are able to acetylate histones. Acetylation of histone tails produces an allosteric change in the nucleosome conformation, destabilizes the interaction between the histone tails and DNA and allows the nucleosomal DNA to become more accessible to transcription factors. In contrast, condensed deacetylated (by HDAC activity) chromatin is shown (top), which is transcriptionally inactive. Because histone acetylation is essential for chromatin remodelling and gene activation, defects in histone acetylation could produce insensitivity to CS-mediated activation of anti-inflammatory genes (see text). *Ac,* hyperacetylation of the histone tails

CS-mediated activation of anti-inflammatory genes (Adcock et al., 2005). In steroid-sensitive asthmatic patients, CSs induce nuclear translocation of GR, which interact with H4 resulting in acetylation of lysine residues K5 and K16 and gene activation (Matthews et al., 2004). As described in section 7.3 Matthews and co-workers studied CS insensitivity in mononuclear cells from resistant patients and found defective histone acetylation (Matthews et al., 2004). In one subgroup, nuclear translocation was impaired, possibly due to phosphorylation of GR by p38 MAPK. This finding was not surprising because there is a direct correlation between nuclear localization and histone acetylation. However, in the other subgroup, despite normal nuclear translocation, there was defective histone acetylation of H4 at K5. This defect probably results in faulty CS-mediated activation of anti-inflammatory genes, which could explain the CS insensitivity in these patients (Figure 7.2).

Despite the ability of CS to induce transcription of anti-inflammatory genes, the major anti-inflammatory effects of CS are thought to occur via repression of immune and inflammatory genes induced primarily by NF-κB (Leung and Bloom, 2003). Initial studies suggested that GR blocked NF-κB activity by inhibiting NF-κB binding to DNA by protein–protein interaction. An important finding by Hart and co-workers led to our current understanding of GR repression of NF-κB activity. Treatment of asthmatic patients with doses of inhaled CS that suppressed airway inflammation did not reduce NF-κB binding to DNA but did turn off NF-κB regulated inflammatory genes (Hart et al., 2000). In subsequent studies, Ito and coworkers further defined the mechanism of CS repression of NF-κB-mediated inflammation (Ito et al., 2000). At low concentrations of CS that are therapeutically relevant in asthma therapy, GR recruited HDAC2 to the NF-κB transcriptional complex, resulting in deacetylation of histones and repression of NF-κB-mediated inflammatory gene transcription but not genes involved in basic cell function (Figure 7.3). This critical finding guided these investigators to studies essential to the current understanding of a central mechanism of CS insensitivity. They clearly demonstrated that decreased HDAC2 levels play a central role in CS insensitivity (Ito et al., 2001, 2002a).

Recent studies demonstrate that transcription factors as well as histones are targets for HATS (Adcock et al., 2006b). For example, the p65 component of NF-κB and GR can be acetylated, resulting in modification of their transcriptional activity (Ito et al., 2006b). GR is acetylated upon CS binding and deacetylation by HDAC2 is essential for interaction with and repression of NF-κB. Of particular importance is that knockdown of HDAC2 by RNA interference prevented GR association with NF-κB and reduced suppression of IL-1-stimulated GM-CSF release from cells. In addition, overexpression of HDAC2 in CS-insensitive alveolar macrophages from patients with COPD restored CS sensitivity (Ito et al., 2006b). Together, these data demonstrate that HDAC2 plays a critical role in GR regulation of NF-κB-mediated gene expression and suggest that decreases in HDAC2 levels are an important mechanism of CS insensitivity (Figure 7.3).

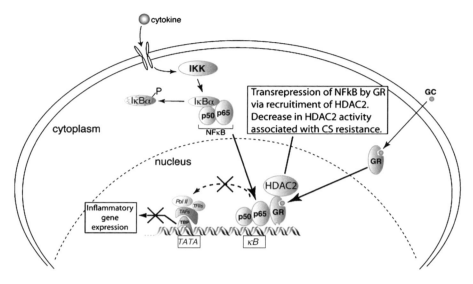

Figure 7.3 GR, HDAC2 and repression of NF-κB activity. In the inactive state, NF-κB (heterodimer of p65 and p50) is anchored in the cytoplasm by IκBα. Activation signals through cell-surface receptors result in activation of IκB kinase, which phosphorylates IκBα. After phosphorylation, IκBα undergoes proteolytic degradation and the NF-κB heterodimer (p65–p50) is free to pass into the nucleus, where it binds to sites in the promoter regions of inflammatory mediator genes and enhances transcription. Repression of NF-κB-mediated gene expression by GR requires recruitment of HDAC2. Insufficient levels/activity of HDAC2 appear to play a critical role in CS insensitivity (see text)

7.6 Epigenetics and Asthma

As described above, histone acetylation status is a critical factor in the regulation of inflammatory gene transcription and a potential mechanism of CS insensitivity. In bronchial biopsies from patients with mild asthma there is a marked increase in HAT and a small reduction in HDAC activity compared to normal airways (Ito et al., 2002a). Interestingly, treatment with inhaled CS decreased HAT activity and increased HDAC activity. Similar changes are found in alveolar macrophages obtained by BAL from patients with asthma (Cosio et al., 2004a). Although PBMCs appeared to have normal HAT and HDAC activity, treatment with oral CS for 1 week increased HDAC activity and expression of PBMCs in subjects with mild asthma but not in subjects with more severe asthma, suggesting a potential role for HDACs in CS insensitivity (Cosio et al., 2004a).

Accumulating evidence demonstrates that cigarette smoking and oxidative stress have an inhibitory effect on HDAC function (Ito et al., 2001, 2004). Oxidative stress is increased in patients with severe asthma and amplified during exacerbations (Caramori and Papi, 2004; Katsoulis et al., 2003; Kharitonov and Barnes, 2003;

Montuschi et al., 1999). In addition, asthmatic patients who smoke cigarettes have more severe disease and are resistant to the anti-inflammatory effects of CS (Chalmers et al., 2001; Chaudhuri et al., 2003; Thomson and Spears, 2005). Thus, in severe asthma patients and asthmatic smokers, a reasonable explanation for CS insensitivity is the effect of asthma and cigarette smoking resulting in a marked decrease in HDAC activity (Cosio et al., 2004a) (Figure 7.3). Oxidative stress along with increased nitric oxide production results in peroxynitrite formation in the lung (Ito et al., 2004). Peroxynitrite reduces the anti-inflammatory effect of CS, possibly by nitration of certain tyrosine residues on HDAC2 resulting in decreased activity and protein levels (Barnes, 2006). This suggests that antioxidants or nitric oxide synthase inhibitors, by decreasing the formation of peroxynitrite, may be effective in restoring responsiveness in severe asthma and asthmatic subjects who smoke (Adcock et al., 2006b; Cosio et al., 2004b). In addition, theophylline has been shown to activate HDAC and to potentiate the anti-inflammatory effects of CS (Cosio et al., 2004b; Ito et al., 2002b). In macrophages from patients with chromic obstructive pulmonary disease (COPD) low concentrations of theophylline restore HDAC function and CS sensitivity *in vitro*. Thus, in addition to patients with COPD, patients with severe asthma or asthmatics who smoke may benefit from low-dose theophylline therapy (Barnes, 2006).

7.7   Conclusions

CSs produce anti-inflammatory effects through a variety of signalling pathways. Recent studies have further characterized the mechanisms of CS-mediated repression of inflammatory gene expression, particularly those involving inhibition of HATs and recruitment of HDACs to inflammatory gene transcriptional complexes. These findings have expanded our understanding of how specific histone abnormalities and alterations in chromatin remodelling could lead to CS resistance in patients. This knowledge has led not only to an enhanced understanding of the mechanisms of CS insensitivity but also to the potential development of novel and effective therapies for severe CS-insensitive asthma.

References

Adcock IM, Chung KF, Caramori G, Ito K. Kinase inhibitors and airway inflammation. *Eur J Pharmacol* 2006a; **533**: 118–132.

Adcock IM, Ford P, Barnes PJ, Ito K. Epigenetics and airways disease. *Respir Res* 2006b; **7**: 21.

Adcock IM, Ito K, Barnes PJ. Histone deacetylation: an important mechanism in inflammatory lung diseases. *COPD* 2005; **2**: 445–455.

Adcock IM, Lane SJ, Brown CR et al. Abnormal glucocorticoid receptor-activator protein 1 interaction in steroid-resistant asthma. *J Exp Med* 1995a; **182**: 1951–1958.

Adcock IM, Lane SJ, Brown CR et al. Differences in binding of glucocorticoid receptor to DNA in steroid-resistant asthma. *J Immunol* 1995b; **154**: 3500–3505.

Agarwal S, Viola JP, Rao A. Chromatin-based regulatory mechanisms governing cytokine gene transcription. *J Allergy Clin Immunol* 1999; **103**: 990–999.

Baldwin AS, Jr. The NF-kappa B and I kappa B proteins: new discoveries and insights. *Annu Rev Immunol* 1996; **14**: 649–683.

Barnes, PJ. Corticosteroids: the drugs to beat. *Eur J Pharmacol* 2006; **533**: 2–14.

Barnes PJ, Adcock IM. NF-kappa B: a pivotal role in asthma and a new target for therapy. *Trends Pharmacol Sci* 1997; **18**: 46–50.

Bray PJ, Cotton RG. Variations of the human glucocorticoid receptor gene (NR3C1): pathological and in vitro mutations and polymorphisms. *Hum Mutat* 2003; **21**: 557–568.

Brogan IJ, Murray IA, Cerillo G et al. Interaction of glucocorticoid receptor isoforms with transcription factors AP-1 and NF-kappaB: lack of effect of glucocorticoid receptor beta. *Mol Cell Endocrinol* 1999; **157**: 95–104.

Cabral AL, Hays AN, Housley PR et al. Repression of glucocorticoid receptor gene transcription by c-Jun. *Mol Cell Endocrinol* 2001; **175**: 67–79.

Caramori G, Papi A. Oxidants and asthma. *Thorax* 2004; **59**: 170–173.

Carlstedt-Duke J. Glucocorticoid Receptor beta: View II. *Trends Endocrinol Metab* 1999; **10**: 339–342.

Chalmers GW, MacLeod KJ, Thomson L et al. Smoking and airway inflammation in patients with mild asthma. *Chest* 2001; **120**: 1917–1922.

Charmandari E, Chrousos GP, Ichijo T et al. The human glucocorticoid receptor (hGR) beta isoform suppresses the transcriptional activity of hGRalpha by interfering with formation of active coactivator complexes. *Mol Endocrinol* 2005; **19**: 52–64.

Chaudhuri R, Livingston E, McMahon AD et al. Cigarette smoking impairs the therapeutic response to oral corticosteroids in chronic asthma. *Am J Respir Crit Care Med* 2003; **168**: 1308–1311.

Cheung J, Smith DF. Molecular chaperone interactions with steroid receptors: an update. *Mol Endocrinol* 2000; **14**: 939–946.

Chrousos GP, Detera-Wadleigh SD, Karl M. Syndromes of glucocorticoid resistance. *Ann Intern Med* 1993; **119**: 1113–1124.

Corrigan CJ, Brown PH, Barnes NC et al. Glucocorticoid resistance in chronic asthma. Glucocorticoid pharmacokinetics, glucocorticoid receptor characteristics, and inhibition of peripheral blood T-cell proliferation by glucocorticoids in vitro. *Am Rev Respir Dis* 1991a; **144**: 1016–1025.

Corrigan CJ, Brown PH, Barnes NC et al. Glucocorticoid resistance in chronic asthma. Peripheral blood T lymphocyte activation and comparison of the T lymphocyte inhibitory effects of glucocorticoids and cyclosporin A. *Am Rev Respir Dis* 1991b; **144**: 1026–1032.

Cosio BG, Mann B, Ito K et al. Histone acetylase and deacetylase activity in alveolar macrophages and blood mononocytes in asthma. *Am J Respir Crit Care Med* 2004a; **170**: 141–147.

Cosio BG, Tsaprouni L, Ito K et al. Theophylline restores histone deacetylase activity and steroid responses in COPD macrophages. *J Exp Med* 2004b; **200**: 689–695.

Gagliardo R, Chanez P, Vignola AM et al. Glucocorticoid receptor alpha and beta in glucocorticoid dependent asthma. *Am J Respir Crit Care Med* 2000; **162**: 7–13.

Ghosh S, Karin M. Missing pieces in the NF-kappaB puzzle. *Cell* 2002; **109**: S81–96.

Goleva E, Kisich KO, Leung DY. A role for STAT5 in the pathogenesis of IL-2-induced glucocorticoid resistance. *J Immunol* 2002; **169**: 5934–5940.

Goleva E, Li LB, Eves PT et al. Increased glucocorticoid receptor beta alters steroid response in glucocorticoid-insensitive asthma. *Am J Respir Crit Care Med* 2006; **173**: 607–616.

Gonzalez MV, Jimenez B, Berciano MT et al. Glucocorticoids antagonize AP-1 by inhibiting the Activation/phosphorylation of JNK without affecting its subcellular distribution. *J Cell Biol* 2000; **150**: 1199–1208.

Hamid QA, Wenzel SE, Hauk PJ et al. Increased glucocorticoid receptor beta in airway cells of glucocorticoid-insensitive asthma. *Am J Respir Crit Care Med* 1999; **159**: 1600–1604.

Hart L, Lim S, Adcock I et al. Effects of inhaled corticosteroid therapy on expression and DNA-binding activity of nuclear factor kappaB in asthma. *Am J Respir Crit Care Med* 2000; **161**: 224–231.

Irusen E, Matthews JG, Takahashi A et al. p38 Mitogen-activated protein kinase-induced glucocorticoid receptor phosphorylation reduces its activity: role in steroid-insensitive asthma. *J Allergy Clin Immunol* 2002; **109**, 649–657.

Ismaili N, Garabedian MJ. Modulation of glucocorticoid receptor function via phosphorylation. *Ann NY Acad Sci* 2004; **1024**: 86–101.

Ito K, Adcock IM. Histone acetylation and histone deacetylation. *Mol Biotechnol* 2002; **20**: 99–106.

Ito K, Barnes PJ, Adcock IM. Glucocorticoid receptor recruitment of histone deacetylase 2 inhibits interleukin-1beta-induced histone H4 acetylation on lysines 8 and 12. *Mol Cell Biol* 2000; **20**: 6891–6903.

Ito K, Caramori G, Lim S et al. Expression and activity of histone deacetylases in human asthmatic airways. *Am J Respir Crit Care Med* 2002a; **166**: 392–396.

Ito K, Chung KF, Adcock IM. Update on glucocorticoid action and resistance. *J Allergy Clin Immunol* 2006a; **117**: 522–543.

Ito K, Hanazawa T, Tomita K et al. Oxidative stress reduces histone deacetylase 2 activity and enhances IL-8 gene expression: role of tyrosine nitration. *Biochem Biophys Res Commun* 2004; **315**: 240–245.

Ito K, Lim S, Caramori G et al. Cigarette smoking reduces histone deacetylase 2 expression, enhances cytokine expression, and inhibits glucocorticoid actions in alveolar macrophages. *FASEB J* 2001; **15**: 1110–1112.

Ito K, Lim S, Caramori G et al. A molecular mechanism of action of theophylline: Induction of histone deacetylase activity to decrease inflammatory gene expression. *Proc Natl Acad Sci USA* 2002b; **99**: 8921–8926.

Ito K, Yamamura S, Essilfie-Quaye S et al. Histone deacetylase 2-mediated deacetylation of the glucocorticoid receptor enables NF-kappaB suppression. *J Exp Med* 2006b; **203**: 7–13.

Itoh M, Adachi M, Yasui H et al. Nuclear export of glucocorticoid receptor is enhanced by c-jun N-terminal kinase-mediated phosphorylation. *Mol Endocrinol* 2002; **16**: 2382–2392.

Katsoulis K, Kontakiotis T, Leonardopoulos I et al. Serum total antioxidant status in severe exacerbation of asthma: correlation with the severity of the disease. *J Asthma* 2003; **40**: 847–854.

Kharitonov SA, Barnes PJ. Nitric oxide, nitrotyrosine, and nitric oxide modulators in asthma and chronic obstructive pulmonary disease. *Curr Allergy Asthma Rep* 2003; **3**: 121–129.

Kornberg RD, Lorch Y. Twenty-five years of the nucleosome, fundamental particle of the eukaryote chromosome. *Cell* 1999; **98**: 285–294.

Kraft M, Hamid Q, Chrousos GP et al. Decreased steroid responsiveness at night in nocturnal asthma. Is the macrophage responsible? *Am J Respir Crit Care Med* 2001; **163**: 1219–1225.

Krstic MD, Rogatsky I, Yamamoto KR, Garabedian MJ. Mitogen-activated and cyclin-dependent protein kinases selectively and differentially modulate transcriptional enhancement by the glucocorticoid receptor. *Mol Cell Biol* 1997; **17**: 3947–3954.

Lane SJ, Lee TH. Glucocorticoid receptor characteristics in monocytes of patients with corticosteroid-resistant bronchial asthma. *Am Rev Respir Dis* 1991; **143**: 1020–1024.

Lane SJ, Adcock IM, Richards D et al. Corticosteroid-resistant bronchial asthma is associated with increased c-fos expression in monocytes and T lymphocytes. *J Clin Invest* 1998; **102**: 2156–2164.

Lane SJ, Arm JP, Staynov DZ, Lee TH. Chemical mutational analysis of the human glucocorticoid receptor cDNA in glucocorticoid-resistant bronchial asthma. *Am J Respir Cell Mol Biol* 1994; **11**: 42–48.

Lane SJ, Atkinson BA, Swaminathan R, Lee TH. Hypothalamic-pituitary-adrenal axis in corticosteroid-resistant bronchial asthma. *Am J Respir Crit Care Med* 1996; **153**: 557–560.

Lee KY, Ito K, Hayashi R et al. NF-kappaB and activator protein 1 response elements and the role of histone modifications in IL-1beta-induced TGF-beta1 gene transcription. *J Immunol* 2006; **176**: 603–615.

Leung DY, Bloom JW. Update on glucocorticoid action and resistance. *J Allergy Clin Immunol* 2003; **111**: 3–23.

Leung DY, Martin RJ, Szefler SJ et al. Dysregulation of interleukin 4, interleukin 5, and interferon gamma gene expression in steroid-resistant asthma. *J Exp Med* 1995; **181**: 33–40.

Li LB, Goleva E, Hall CF et al. Superantigen-induced corticosteroid resistance of human T cells occurs through activation of the mitogen-activated protein kinase kinase/extracellular signal-regulated kinase (MEK-ERK) pathway. *J Allergy Clin Immunol* 2004; **114**: 1059–1069.

Loke TK, Mallett KH, Ratoff J et al. Systemic glucocorticoid reduces bronchial mucosal activation of activator protein 1 components in glucocorticoid-sensitive but not glucocorticoid-resistant asthmatic patients. *J Allergy Clin Immunol* 2006; **118**: 368–375.

Lu NZ, Cidlowski JA. The origin and functions of multiple human glucocorticoid receptor isoforms. *Ann N Y Acad Sci* 2004; **1024**: 102–123.

Matthews JG, Ito K, Barnes PJ, Adcock IM. Defective glucocorticoid receptor nuclear translocation and altered histone acetylation patterns in glucocorticoid-resistant patients. *J Allergy Clin Immunol* 2004; **113**: 1100–1108.

Montuschi P, Corradi M, Ciabattoni G et al. Increased 8-isoprostane, a marker of oxidative stress, in exhaled condensate of asthma patients. *Am J Respir Crit Care Med* 1999; **160**: 216–220.

Oakley RH, Jewell CM, Yudt MR et al. The dominant negative activity of the human glucocorticoid receptor beta isoform. Specificity and mechanisms of action. *J Biol Chem* 1999; **274**: 27857–27866.

Rogatsky I, Logan SK, Garabedian MJ. Antagonism of glucocorticoid receptor transcriptional activation by the c-Jun N-terminal kinase. *Proc Natl Acad Sci USA* 1998; **95**: 2050–2055.

Shaulian E, Karin M. AP-1 as a regulator of cell life and death. *Nat-Cell Biol* 2002; **4**: E131–136.

Sher ER, Leung DY, Surs W et al. Steroid-resistant asthma. Cellular mechanisms contributing to inadequate response to glucocorticoid therapy. *J Clin Invest* 1994; **93**: 33–39.

Silverman RA, Boudreaux ED, Woodruff PG et al. Cigarette smoking among asthmatic adults presenting to 64 emergency departments. *Chest* 2003; **123**: 1472–1479.

Siroux V, Pin I, Oryszczyn MP, et al. Relationships of active smoking to asthma and asthma severity in the EGEA study. Epidemiological study on the Genetics and Environment of Asthma. *Eur Respir J* 2000; **15**: 470–477.

Sousa AR, Lane SJ, Atkinson BA et al. The effects of prednisolone on the cutaneous tuberculin response in patients with corticosteroid-resistant bronchial asthma. *J Allergy Clin Immunol* 1996; **97**: 698–706.

Sousa AR, Lane SJ, Soh C, Lee TH. In vivo resistance to corticosteroids in bronchial asthma is associated with enhanced phosyphorylation of JUN N-terminal kinase and failure of prednisolone to inhibit JUN N-terminal kinase phosphorylation. *J Allergy Clin Immunol* 1999; **104**: 565–574.

Strickland I, Kisich K, Hauk PJ et al. High constitutive glucocorticoid receptor beta in human neutrophils enables them to reduce their spontaneous rate of cell death in response to corticosteroids. *J Exp Med* 2001; **193**: 585–593.

Swantek, JL, Cobb, MH, Geppert TD. Jun N-terminal kinase/stress-activated protein kinase (JNK/SAPK) is required for lipopolysaccharide stimulation of tumor necrosis factor alpha (TNF-alpha) translation: glucocorticoids inhibit TNF-alpha translation by blocking JNK/SAPK. *Mol Cell Biol* 1997; **17**: 6274–6282.

Thomson NC, Spears M. The influence of smoking on the treatment response in patients with asthma. *Curr Opin Allergy Clin Immunol* 2005; **5**: 57–63.

Thomson NC, Shepherd M, Spears M, Chaudhuri R. Corticosteroid insensitivity in smokers with asthma : clinical evidence, mechanisms, and management. *Treat Respir Med* 2006; **5**: 467–481.

Tsitoura DC, Rothman PB. Enhancement of MEK/ERK signalling promotes glucocorticoid resistance in CD4+ T-cells. *J Clin Invest* 2004; **113**: 619–627.

Turner MO, Noertjojo K, Vedal S et al. Risk factors for near-fatal asthma. A case-control study in hospitalized patients with asthma. *Am J Respir Crit Care Med* 1998; **157**: 1804–1809.

Tyler JK, Kadonaga JT. The "dark side" of chromatin remodeling: repressive effects on transcription. *Cell* 1999; **99**: 443–446.

Wang Z, Frederick J, Garabedian MJ. Deciphering the phosphorylation "code" of the glucocorticoid receptor in vivo. *J Biol Chem* 2002; **277**: 26573–26580.

Wenzel SE, Busse WW. Severe asthma: lessons from the Severe Asthma Research Program. *J Allergy Clin Immunol* 2007; **119**: 14–23.

8

Cigarette Smoke, Oxidative Stress and Corticosteroid Responsiveness

Irfan Rahman and David Adenuga

8.1 Oxidative Stress

Cigarette smoke is a complex admixture of debilitating gases, molecules, tar aggregates and particles. The smoke is also a repertoire of various free radicals that can initiate and propagate a continuous chain of reactive oxygen species (ROS) generation. Such events lead to cell damage via oxidation of proteins, DNA and lipids.

Reactive oxygen species – inhaled and endogenous oxidants

Endogenous oxidants

A free radical is any extremely short-lived chemical entity capable of independent existence and contains one or more unpaired electrons (Halliwell, 1991). The most important ROS of physiological significance are the superoxide anion ($O_2^{\bullet-}$), hydroxyl radical ($OH^{\bullet}$) and nitric oxide ($NO^{\bullet}$). Although hydrogen peroxide (H_2O_2) is not a free radical *per se*, it is however, capable of exhibiting effects akin to those of ROS. The primary ROS formed *in vivo* are $O_2^{\bullet-}$ and H_2O_2 (Halliwell and Gutteridge, 1989). H_2O_2 is generated through non-enzymatic or enzymatic dismutation of superoxide (Halliwell and Gutteridge, 1989). However, the most reactive and harmful ROS is $OH^{\bullet}$, which can be formed not only from H_2O_2 and $O_2^{\bullet-}$ but also via the reaction of $O_2^{\bullet-}$ with NO to produce peroxynitrite ($OONO^-$), which decomposes

Overcoming Steroid Insensitivity in Respiratory Disease   Edited by Ian M. Adcock and Kian Fan Chung
© 2008 John Wiley & Sons, Ltd.

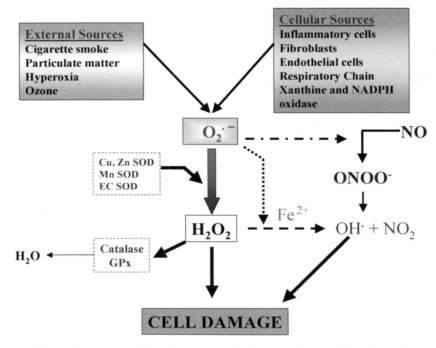

Figure 8.1 Inflammatory cells such as neutrophils, macrophages and eosinophils are the most important cells involved in endogenous generation of reactive oxygen species (ROS), intra- and extracellular generation of ROS and the antioxidant defence system. ($0_2^{\bullet-}$ = superoxide anion, NO = nitric oxide, H_2O_2= hydrogen peroxide, $OH^{\bullet}$ = hydroxyl radical, NO_2 = nitrogen dioxide, $ONOO^-$ = peroxynitrite, Fe^{2+} = ferrous ion, GPx = glutathione peroxidase)

to form NO_2 and $OH^{\bullet}$ (Figure 8.1) (Halliwell, 1991). Neutrophils, eosinophils and alveolar macrophages are the major lung sources of ROS (Kinnula et al., 1995). In addition, alveolar epithelial cells, bronchial epithelial cells and endothelial cells are also important generators of ROS in the lungs (Kinnula et al., 1992).

Inhaled oxidants: cigarette smoke and oxidative stress

Cigarette smoke is a repertoire for a number of potent oxidants, carcinogens/mutagens and chemicals and is therefore considered to be a prime suspect responsible for the development of chronic obstructive pulmonary disease (COPD), lung cancer and other cardiovascular diseases (Rahman and MacNee 1996, 1999). Each puff of cigarette is estimated to contain about 10^{17} oxidants/free radicals and the main stream smoke itself is a complex admixture of over 5000 different chemical compounds (Church and Pryor 1985; Pryor and Stone 1993). Side stream cigarette smoke contains more than 10^{15} reactive organic compounds per puff, and is mostly comprised of carbon monoxide, ammonia, formaldehyde, N-nitrosamines, benzo[a]pyrene, benzene, isoprene, ethane, pentane, nicotine, acrolein, acetaldehyde and other geno-toxic and carcinogeneic organic compounds. The gas phase of cigarette smoke con-tains short-lived oxidants, of which superoxide anion ($O_2^{\cdot-}$) and nitric oxide (NO) are predominant. NO and $O_2^{\cdot-}$ may rapidly interact to form the highly reactive and toxic peroxynitrite ($ONOO^-$) anion having a very high diffusion coefficient. The semiquinone radicals in the tar phase of cigarette can reduce oxygen to produce ROS, such as $O_2^{\cdot-}$, $^{\cdot}OH$ and H_2O_2 (Pryor and Stone, 1993).

Reactive oxygen species – lipid peroxidation products

Activated immune and inflammatory cells generate highly reactive and cytotoxic $O_2^{\cdot-}$ and $^{\cdot}OH$ species. When generated in close proximity to a cell, these free radi-cals can oxidize membrane phospholipids (lipid peroxidation), which may set up a chain of cell damaging reactions. Such peroxidative modifications of polyunsatu-rated fatty acids (PUFAs) may in turn trigger impairment of membrane functions, membrane-bound receptors, enzymes and receptor translocation. Furthermore, the loss of membrane fluidity may lead to increased tissue permeability, a process im-plicated in the aetiopathogenesis of diverse lung injuries (Morrison et al., 1999). A direct consequence of lipid peroxidation is the downstream generation of toxic products such as malondialdehyde (MDA), 4-hydroxy-2-nonenal (4-HNE), acrolein and F_2-isoprostanes (F_2IP). Some of these products such as 4-HNE and F_2IP have also been implicated in cellular signalling processes (Uchida et al., 1999). Oxidative stress-based pathophysiological events have been associated with the generation of aldehydes due to lipid peroxidation. Lipid peroxidation may also have a role in the signalling events in the molecular mechanisms involved in lung inflammation, as observed in COPD (Rahman et al., 1996, 2002).

8.2 Cigarette Smoke/Oxidative Stress-Induced NF-κB-mediated Pro-inflammatory Gene Expression

Nuclear factor kappa B (NF-κB) is an important cytosol to nucleus translocating transcription factor, pivotal to the inflammatory signalling process. During inacti-vated states, NF-κB is complexed with the inhibitor IκBα subunit, which prevents NF-κB binding to DNA. However, since both NF-κB and IκBα can rapidly shuttle between cytoplasm and the nucleus, the apparent cytoplasmic retention of NF-κB may simply represent an equilibrium state of a highly dynamic process. There are two pathways that can trigger NF-κB activation, one that occurs in the cytoplasm and one that traverses the nucleus. In the first case, NF-κB activators such as Tumor necrosis factor (TNF-α), Interleukin 1β (IL-1β), cigarette smoke and oxidants engage cell-surface receptors and transmit signals through the cytoplasm to the

IκB (IKK) complex. Activation of the IKK complex results in post-translational modification and proteasome-dependent degradation of IκBα; as a result, NF-κB is then free
to activate transcription of responsive genes. In the second case, activation of NF-κB is
triggered in response to DNA damage. The activation signal for IKK complex originates
in the nucleus and is transmitted to the cytoplasm. The critical events during NF-κB
activation, leading to inflammatory response, are generally redox sensitive (Figure 8.2).

It is now generally accepted that NF-κB regulates the expression of various
inflammatory genes, such as those for the cytokines Interleukin 8 (IL-8), TNFα
and inducible nitric oxide synthase (iNOS). Di Stefano and colleagues demonstrated
an increased expression of RelA/p65 subunit of NF-κB in bronchial epithelium of
smokers and patients with COPD (Di Stefano et al., 2002), which was negatively
correlated with the degree of airflow limitation in patients with COPD. Similarly,
Caramori and co-workers have reported increased levels of RelA/p65 subunit of
NF-κB in sputum macrophages but not in sputum neutrophils during exacerbations
of COPD. This suggests that inflammatory responses may vary with the cell type
(Caramori et al., 2003). The activation of NF-κB in monocytes/macrophages may
then, via release of pro-inflammatory mediators in lung epithelial fluid, trigger an

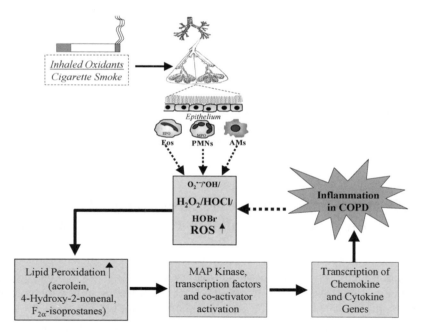

Figure 8.2   Mechanism of ROS-mediated lung inflammation. Inflammatory response is mediated by oxidants either inhaled and/or released by the activated neutrophils, alveolar macrophages, eosinophils and epithelial cells, leading to production of ROS and membrane lipid
peroxidation. Activation of transcription of the pro-inflammatory cytokine and chemokine
genes, upregulation of adhesion molecules and increased release of pro-inflammatory mediators are involved in the inflammatory responses in patients with COPD

amplified inflammatory cascade by activation of epithelial cells and recruitment of neutrophils in the airways (Rahman and Adcock, 2006).

8.3 Histone Acetylation and Deacetylation

In eukaryotic cells, transcriptional regulation of genes is strongly influenced by the way genetic information is packaged within the nucleus of the cell. Many factors, including specific DNA sequences, histones, non-histone chromosomal proteins, transcriptional activators/repressors and the transcription machinery, are all necessary for the assembly of an active transcriptional complex. Condensation of eukaryotic DNA as a tightly coiled structure in chromatin suppresses gene expression due to denied accessibility to the transcriptional apparatus. The nucleosome – the basic unit of chromatin – comprises H2A/H2B dimers and a tetramer of two H3/H4 dimers around which approximately 146 bp of DNA is wound.

The nucleosome cores are responsible for decreasing the accessibility of transcription factors such as NF-κB and activator protein 1 (AP-1) to the transcriptional complex. The binding and dissociation of histones from DNA depend on their acetylation status. When acetylated, histones dissociate leading to uncoiling of the DNA and thus exposing the DNA sequences, which may bind to the transcription factors. The acetylation of histone takes place on the lysine (K) residues at the N-terminal tails of the core histone proteins. Acetylation of K residues on histone 4 (K5, K8, K12, K16) is thought to regulate gene transcription. Histone acetylation is reversible and is regulated by a group of histone acetyltransferases (HATs) that promote acetylation. The nuclear receptor coactivators – steroid receptor coactivator 1 (SRC-1), cyclic AMP response element (CRE)-binding protein (CBP)/adenoviral protein E1A (p300) protein, CBP/p300 associated factor (P/CAF) and activator transcription factor-2 (ATF-2) – all possess intrinsic HAT activity. Of these, CBP/p300 and ATF-2, are vital for the coactivation of several transcription factors, including NF-κB and AP-1, and are regulated by the p38 MAPK pathway (Rahman et al., 2004). These activation complexes act in consonance with RNA polymerase II to initiate transcription. When deacetylated by histone deacetylases (HDACs), the histones bind back to the DNA, promote DNA rewinding and consequently block gene expression. Thus, in quiescent cells, levels of histone acetylation and or transcriptional activity are likely to be maintained by a balance between acetylation by HATs and deacetylation by HDACs (De Ruijter et al., 2003).

8.4 Corticosteroids

Corticosteroids/glucocorticoids or endogenous cortisol are potent anti-inflammatory 21-carbon hormones that mediate a vast array of tissue- and cell-specific biological pathways in humans. Differential responses of cells and tissues to corticosteroids and its effect on different signalling pathways may be due to the interaction of the glucocorticoid receptor (GR) with different tissue-specific coactivators or corepressors (Yudt and Cidlowski, 2002).

Glucocorticoid receptor (GR)

GR, a ligand-activated transcription factor of the hormone receptor family, is encoded from a single gene but several isoforms have been identified as splice variants. hGRα, the classical GR, is a single polypeptide chain with 777 amino acids. Glucocorticoid function is based on its binding to GRα, ubiquitously expressed in cells and localized to the cytoplasm (Yudt and Cidlowski, 2002). GRα has two isoforms A and B that are derived from differing translation start sites: GRα-A, a 94-kDa protein, utilizes Met-1 as its translation start site whereas the B isoform, a 91-kDa protein, utilizes Met-27 (Yudt and Cidlowski, 2002). The B isoform has a transactivation efficiency that is double that of the A isoform and differences in the ratio of the A and B isoforms may modulate differences in cell responses to glucocorticoid (Ito et al., 2006a). The GRβ isoform is a smaller protein that differs from GRα depending on splice variation in exon 9 of the GR gene. While GRα is primarily localized to the cytosol, GRβ is localized in the nucleus and is known also to bind glucocorticoid response elements (GREs) but has a non-functional ligand binding domain and is thus unable to activate gene transcription. The ability of GRβ to function as a dominant negative to GRα via formation of GRα/β heterodimers in *in vitro* experiments has led to its being touted as playing a possible role in glucocorticoid resistance. (Yudt and Cidlowski, 2002). However, *in vivo* analysis has shown that GRβ may not play a significant role in glucocorticoid resistance, as has been shown in overexpression studies where a fivefold excess of GRβ is required for it to function as a relevant dominant negative receptor. It is possible, however, that variability in the GRα/GRβ ratio may be a determining factor in the differential response of tissues to glucocorticoids. GRβ also does not bind antagonists and this may increase the GRα/GRβ ratio in certain cells, which may predispose them to increased glucocorticoid resistance (Yudt and Cidlowski, 2002; Rhen and Cidlowski, 2005).

GR interactions

Endogenous cortisol and synthetic corticosteroids are primarily known to act in two distinct ways:

Transactivation of gene expression by corticosteroids

Corticosteroids diffuse across the cell membrane where they bind to cytosolic GR bound to hsp90 and immunophilins such as FKBP51 and FKBP52. Ligand binding causes dissociation of hsp90 to expose the nuclear localization signal (NLS), which allows the active GR–ligand complex to translocate to the nucleus. In the nucleus, GR forms a homodimer with another GR where it binds to a GRE (GGTACAnnnT-GTTCT) of anti-inflammatory genes such as Annexin-1. Corticosteroids also induce IκBα (an inhibitor of NF-κB) and thus decrease the cellular inflammatory response, which is known to be primarily through the NF-κB pathway.

GR binding to DNA causes recruitment of coactivator complex containing transcription factors such as GRIP-1, SRC-1, CBP, RNA pol II and histone modifiers such as the SWI/SNF complex that have intrinsic histone acetylase properties. This increases histone acetylation, especially at histones H3 and H4 via CBP/P300, and increases accessibility of transcription factors such as NF-κB and AP-1, coactivators and RNA pol II to the transcription complex. However, physiological doses of corticosteroids have not been shown to cause a dramatic increase in Annexin-1 in bronchoalveolar lavage (BAL) fluid or an increase in IκBα in various cell types (Ito et al., 2006a). Corticosteroids at these concentrations are efficient at suppressing the release of inflammatory mediators from peripheral blood mononuclear cells in non-severe asthmatics (Ito et al., 2006a) and suppress the expression of NF-κB in cells of tracheo-bronchial lavage fluid in premature neonates (Aghai et al., 2006). This might be further proof that anti-inflammatory effects of corticosteroids may not be primarily through GR–GR homodimer induction of anti-inflammatory genes and that corticosteroids display anti-inflammatory properties via another pathway. The presence of negative GREs (nGREs) has also been argued as a mechanism by which corticosteroids might induce its systemic side effects. GR–GR homodimers are thought to bind to nGREs, recruit corepressors and promote gene silencing.

Transrepression of gene expression by corticosteroids

The primary mechanism by which corticosteroids exhibit potent anti-inflammatory properties is via repression of pro-inflammatory genes because most genes that are repressed in the presence of corticosteroids are not known to possess nGREs in their promoter regions. Mice deficient in the ability of GR to dimerize in the nucleus show that GR does bind to transcription factors such as AP-1 and NF-κB (Reichardt et al., 1998, 2001). It is thought that GR binding to transcription factors is followed by recruitment of corepressors (HDACs) that possess intrinsic histone deacetylase activity leading to gene silencing (Figure 8.3). HDACs, especially HDAC2, has been shown to be crucial in corticosteroid-mediated anti-inflammatory activity (Ito et al., 2005).

GR acetylation

Non-histone proteins are also acetylated by HATs and deacetylated by HDACs and this may be another important mechanism for the regulation of protein function (Glozak et al., 2005). Several nuclear receptors, including the oestrogen and

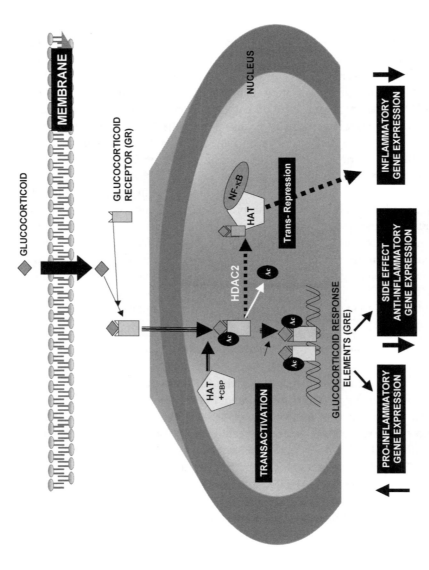

Figure 8.3 Binding of corticosteroid to glucocorticoid receptor (GR) results in acetylation of GR. Acetylation is effected by histone acetylase (HAT) and CRE-binding protein (CBP). The acetylated GR dimer then binds to glucocorticoid response elements and this leads to increased transcription of pro-inflammatory genes and suppression of anti-inflammatory gene expression. Deacetylation of GR by histone deacetylase (HDAC2) leads to inhibition of NF-κB, which thus switches off the expression of inflammatory genes

androgen receptors, may be acetylated and this affects the receptor–ligand interaction (Fu et al., 2004). It has been demonstrated recently that GR is acetylated after ligand binding and that this acetylated GR translocates to the nucleus to bind to GRE sites and activate genes such as secretory leukocyte protease inhibitor (SLPI) (Ito et al., 2006b). Acetylated GR is deacetylated by HDAC2 and this deacetylation is necessary before GR is able to inhibit NF-κB activation of inflammatory genes. The site of acetylation of GR is the lysine-rich region 492–495 with the sequence KTKK, which is analogous to the acetylation sites identified on other nuclear hormone receptors. Site-directed mutagenesis of the lysine residues K494 and K495 prevents GR acetylation and reduces activation of the SLPI gene by corticosteroids, whereas repression of NF-κB is unaffected (Ito et al., 2006b).

8.5   Histone Deacetylases

Four classes of proteins with histone deacetylase activity have been identified so far (de Ruijter et al., 2003):

(1) *Class I* includes HDAC 1, 2, 3 and 8 and they reside almost exclusively in the nucleus. HDAC1 and HDAC2 must be exclusively localized to the nucleus because they do not possess a nuclear export signal (NES). HDAC3, however, possesses both an NLS and an NES and therefore may also be able to localize to the cytoplasm. HDAC1 and HDAC2 are active only as parts of complexes that contain proteins involved in forming complexes with them on gene promoters. They may also be associated with proteins that modulate their deacetylase activity, as recombinant proteins have been found to be inactive.

(2) *Class II* includes HDACs 4–7, 9 and 10. Class II HDACs, although similar to class I molecules, are thought to possess the ability to shuttle between the nucleus and cytoplasm, even though HDAC6 seems to be predominantly located in the cytoplasm. Unlike class I HDACs, which that are thought to be expressed in most cell types, class II HDACs are thought to be expressed in a cell-specific manner, suggesting that they may be involved in more specific cell functions. They are thought to be required for cell differentiation.

(3) *Class III* comprises the "silent information regulator" (SIR2) family (sirtuins 1–7) of NAD^+-dependent proteins with intrinsic deacetylase activity. They are thought to be involved in aging, inflammation and cell senescence and have non-histone proteins (RelA/p65 and p53) as substrates.

(4) *Class IV* – The only known member of this class is HDAC11.

Cigarette smoke and corticosteroid resistance

Corticosteroids have been a mainstay as a major line of therapy for various inflammatory conditions such as asthma and other immune diseases. To the chagrin of physicians, a small proportion of asthmatics who are smokers still exhibit unresponsiveness towards even higher doses of oral corticosteroids. Such resistance to corticosteroid therapy has also been observed in other inflammatory and immune diseases such as rheumatoid arthritis and inflammatory bowel disease. The much widespread COPD is also highly unresponsive to corticosteroids and exhibits a largely steroid-resistant pattern of inflammation (Barnes, 2000; Barnes et al., 2005).

Corticosteroids suppress inflammation by inhibiting NF-κB-dependent gene expression, possibly by regulating HDAC and HAT activity (Figure 8.4). It has been shown that GR recruits HDAC2 specifically to acetylated histone H4 associated with the GM-CSF promoter (Ito et al., 2000). This observation is supported by another observation that HDAC2 knockdown using siRNA in epithelial cells could increase the induction of GM-CSF and decrease sensitivity to corticosteroids

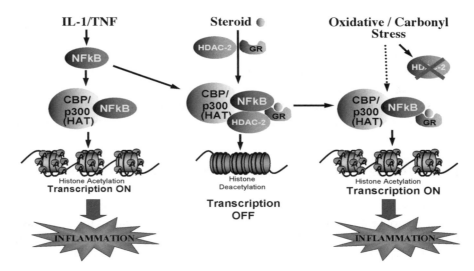

Figure 8.4 Diagram illustrating the process of histone acetylation leading to chromatin remodelling. Oxidative stress and cytokines activate the NF-κB pathway, leading to acetylation of chromatin on pro-inflammatory genes and increasing the accessibility of transcription factors. This leads to an increase in gene expression. Deacetylation results in DNA rewinding around histone proteins, decreasing gene transcription. The CRE-binding protein (CBP) and p300 function as intrinsic histone acetyltransferases (HATs). Activated corticosteroid receptors recruit histone deacetylase (HDAC) into the transcriptome complex, promoting histone deactylation, chromatin condensation and expulsion of DNA polymerases, shutting off gene expression. Oxidative stress inhibits HDAC2 activity as well as activating NF-κB, facilitating histone acetylation by the transcriptome complex even in the presence of activated glucocorticoid receptor

(Ito et al., 2006b). Current hypothesis suggests that in smokers with severe asthma, and in COPD patients, cigarette smoke-induced oxidative stress not only activates the NF-κB pathway but also alters the HDAC/HAT balance via post-translational modification of HDACs (Ito et al., 2001; Marwick et al. 2004; Yang et al., 2006). NF-κB nuclear translocation is increased in lungs of smokers, indicating that cigarette smoke does induce NF-κB activation leading to increased transcription of inflammatory genes (Szulakowski et al., 2006).

Role of HDAC2

The inability of corticosteroids to recruit HDAC2 or the presence of a defective or altered HDAC2 might explain the abnormal inflammatory response and the ineffectiveness of corticosteroid therapy seen in patients with COPD. In smoking subjects, increased acetylation of histones H3 and H4 also suggests an increased accessibility of transcription factors to gene promoters. The increase in acetylated H3, however, seems to persist in ex-smokers with COPD, suggesting that their abnormal inflammatory response could be due to increased H3 acetylation when compared to healthy smokers and smokers with COPD, as chronic inflammation seems to persist even after cessation of smoking (Szulakowski et al., 2006). In rat lungs, an elevation in H3 phosphorylation is also observed that correlates with p38-MAPK phosphorylation in response to cigarette smoke (Marwick et al., 2004). HDAC2 is recruited by the GR monomer on ligand binding and is crucial to corticosteroid function at physiological doses. HDAC2 expression and activity are decreased in peripheral blood mononuclear cells (PBMCs) and alveolar macrophages of COPD patients and chronic asthmatic patients who smoke (Cosio et al., 2004; Culpitt et al., 2002). The same decrease is also found in bronchial biopsies of COPD patients and correlates with disease severity, increased cytokine production and corticosteroid insensitivity (Di Stefano et al., 2002; Ito et al., 2005).

Cigarette smoke induces oxidative stress in cells and is a major source of exogenous oxygen radicals. Increased markers of oxidative stress, such as 8-isoprostane and 4-hydroxy-2-nonenal (4-HNE), have been found in the lungs of smokers and COPD patients, suggesting increased oxidant burden (Rahman and Adcock, 2006; Rahman et al., 2002). Immunoprecipitated HDAC2 in rat lungs shows increased staining for tyrosine nitration when incubated with cigarette smoke extract, which correlates with decreased activity (Marwick et al., 2004). Interestingly, the use of a synthetic NO/peroxynitrite donor also leads to increased tyrosine nitration of HDAC2 and subsequent decrease in HDAC2 activity (Marwick et al., 2004), suggesting that iNOS inhibitors might be good candidates for reversing HDAC2 modifications. Antioxidants also have the capacity to reduce these effects (Moodie et al., 2004), suggesting that cigarette smoke might not only induce NF-κB activation but may also affect HDAC/HAT balance, resulting in sustained increase in the inflammatory response of the lungs.

Role of HDAC1

While little is known about the role of HDAC1 in corticosteroid resistance, recent studies have shown that HDAC1 is crucial in suppressing NF-κB-dependent gene expression in unstimulated cells (Zhong et al., 2002). Immunoprecipitation studies in cells show that in unstimulated cells HDAC1 associates with p50 homodimers that bind to DNA and repress gene expression. On stimulation, NF-κB with RelA/p65 phosphorylated possibly by PKA recruits CBP with intrinsic HAT activity and translocates to the nucleus where it displaces the HDAC1/p50 complex to increase gene transcription (Zhong et al., 2002). Results also show that nuclear RelA/p65 associates with HDAC1 in unstimulated cells, and on stimulation RelA/p65 is phosphorylated, dissociates from HDAC1 and can then associate with CBP/p300 (Zhong et al., 2002). The role of HDAC1 in silencing the pro-inflammatory cytokine (IL-8) has also been shown (Ashburner et al., 2001). It is possible that post-translational modification of HDAC1 may occur, preventing it from efficiently binding unstimulated RelA/p65 and possibly predisposing the cell to a higher NF-κB activation than would normally be possible.

HDAC1 has been predominantly viewed as part of a corepressor complex whereas its deacetylase property has been identified as a possible coactivator for the corticosteroid receptor. On repressed chromatin, HDAC1 is predominantly acetylated and thus has very low activity. Transcriptionally active chromatin, however, possesses HDAC1, which is less acetylated and thus has a higher deacetylase activity. Studies show that mutation of key acetylation sites on HDAC1 completely abolishes its deacetylase activity. During induction of the MMTV promoter by GR, ligand-bound GR homodimers recruit HDAC1 to the MMTV promoter and rapidly induce gene expression. This increase in expression peaks at around 15–20 min, after which activity drops, correlating with rapid acetylation of HDAC1 by CBP recruited by GR (Qiu et al., 2006). This mechanism is likely a transactivation mechanism and may not have a direct effect on corticosteroid insensitivity towards inflammatory mediator expression. Another mechanism that has yet to be fully explored in terms of corticosteroid insensitivity is whether the GR itself becomes defective in response to cigarette smoke-induced oxidative stress. Nitrosylation of the GR may prevent ligand binding and disrupt its ability to translocate to the nucleus. Although no study has yet reported a defect in the GRs of patients with steroid-resistant asthma and COPD, reports of defects in ligand binding are available. While some studies have shown a reduced affinity for the GR by ligands that are reversible (Sher et al., 1994), reduced GR density may also present a similar problem. Increased expression of GRβ, a dominant negative isoform of GR, has been shown in BAL fluid macrophages of severe steroid-insensitive asthma (Goleva et al., 2006). Neutrophils that are also resistant to steroids also show an increased production of the isoform (Strickland et al., 2001). However, despite the presence of several isoforms and mutations of the GR protein, such mutants and isoforms do not appear to play a major role in glucocorticoid resistance (Ito et al., 2006a).

Role of HDAC3

The role of HDAC3 is proposed for deacetylation of RelA/p65 by Chen et al. (2001). NF-κB activity is dependent on its binding to IκBα, which by itself is an NF-κB-driven gene and serves as a negative feedback mechanism by which the cell regulates NF-κB activity. RelA/p65 itself is acetylated on lysine K310 by CBP/p300; it has been proposed that this acetylation reduces the ability of NF-κB to bind IκBα and increases the duration of NF-κB binding to promoter pro-inflammatory genes. HDAC3 removes the K63 acetyl group of NF-κB, thus allowing it to associate with IκBα and reduce the duration of DNA binding. Thus, it is possible that HDAC3 may possibly be linked to acetylation of GR or RelA/p65, and hence to steroid resistance.

Another mechanism by which GR may be altered is through phosphorylation by p38-MAPKs. In stimulated cells, p38 MAPK is known to phosphorylate GR and alter its ability to bind ligands, while the p38 inhibitor SB203580 has been shown to reverse corticosteroid resistance (Irusen et al., 2002).

Post-translational modifications of HDACs in response to cigarette smoke-derived NO and reactive aldehydes

4-Hydoxy-2-nonenal (4-HNE) has a high affinity towards cysteine, histidine and lysine residues, alters protein function and forms direct protein adducts. The role of 4-HNE in disease pathology has been suggested by the observation of increased levels of 4-HNE-modified proteins in airway and alveolar epithelial cells, endothelial cells and neutrophils of subjects afflicted with airway obstruction. The inverse co-relationship of 4-HNE with FEV_1 has further suggested a role for 4-HNE in the pathogenesis of COPD (Rahman et al., 2002).

Corticosteroids bound to GR recruit HDAC2 to NF-κB-dependent gene promoters, causing chromatin remodelling via deacetylation of core histones and subsequently suppressing pro-inflammatory gene transcription (Ito et al., 2000, 2001). HDAC1 and HDAC3 are also known to interact with RelA/p65 to exert pro-inflammatory gene repressor function (Ashburner et al., 2001; Zhong et al., 2002). Post-translational modifications to HDACs via oxidative stress and cigarette smoke have been implicated in steroid resistance, as observed in COPD patients (Rahman et al., 2004). *In vitro* experiments using monocytic cell lines have implicated cigarette smoke in decreasing HDAC activity and HDAC1, 2 and 3 protein levels after treatment with cigarette smoke extract (Yang et al., 2006). This decline in HDAC protein was however restored by pre-treating with GSH monoethyl ester, suggesting a role for oxidative stress in reduced HDAC activity. Immunoblot analysis also reveals significant increase in 4-HNE and nitrotyrosine post-translational modification of HDAC1, 2 and 3 proteins (Yang et al., 2006).

Alveolar macrophages and peripheral lung tissue from healthy smokers and COPD patients show a marked decrease in HDAC2 activity and expression compared to healthy non-smokers (Ito et al., 2001), which correlates with increased release of pro-inflammatory cytokines and reduced effectiveness of the corticosteroid dexamethasone (Ito et al., 2001). Alveolar macrophages of COPD patients also show a marked increase in nitrotyrosine formation (Di Stefano et al., 2002). It remains to be seen if other HDAC proteins are also modified post-translationally by 4-HNE and NO products *in vivo* in lung cells/macrophages of patients with COPD.

8.6   Reversing Glucocorticoids / Corticosteroid Resistance

Polyphenols and glucocorticoids / corticosteroid signalling

Oxidative stress is now known to play an insidious role in rendering corticosteroids less effective for the treatment of COPD and severe asthma. It has been reported recently that ROS-dependent abnormal expression of inflammatory genes may involve acetylation and deacetylation of histones (Kirkham and Rahman, 2006; Rahman and Adcock, 2006). Bronchial biopsies and alveolar macrophages from COPD patients and smoking controls demonstrated a significant decrease in both HDAC activity and HDAC protein levels, the magnitude of which increased with severity of disease (Ito et al., 2005). Since glucocorticoids act via recruitment of HDACs, it may therefore not be premature to consider that finding ways to increase HDAC2 expression would render the steroids more effective for the treatment of inflammatory diseases such as COPD. This notion is supported by the finding that theophylline increases HDAC2 activity and expression in lung macrophages and also increases the sensitivity of the cells to steroid treatment (Cosio et al., 2004; Ito et al., 2002a, b). However, it is unknown whether theophylline is effective under the conditions of oxidative stress.

Among the entire gamut of polyphenols, theophylline is the first drug that has been shown to activate HDAC2, resulting in marked potentiation of the anti-inflammatory effects of corticosteroids (Cosio et al., 2004; Ito et al., 2002a, b; Rahman et al., 2006). Dietary polyphenols such as curcumin (diferuloylmethane derived from tumeric powder) and resveratrol have been shown to exert their antioxidant/anti-inflammatory effects by virtue of their ability to control NF-κB activation and possibly by chromatin remodelling via modulation of HDAC2 activity (Culpitt et al., 2003; Donnelly et al., 2004; Rahman et al., 2006) (Figure 8.5). Such modulation of HDACs, in particular HDAC2, may lead to control of inflammatory gene expression in macrophages and lung epithelial cells. The authors have recently shown that curcumin, at nanomolar concentrations, was able to restore glucocorticoid function by upregulating HDAC2 expression and activity in monocyte/macrophage MonoMac6 and U937 cells (independent of any antioxidant activity) exposed to oxidative stress by cigarette smoke or hydrogen peroxide (Rahman et al., 2005). Interestingly, in MonoMac6 cell lines this was also associated with restoration of HDAC1 and HDAC3

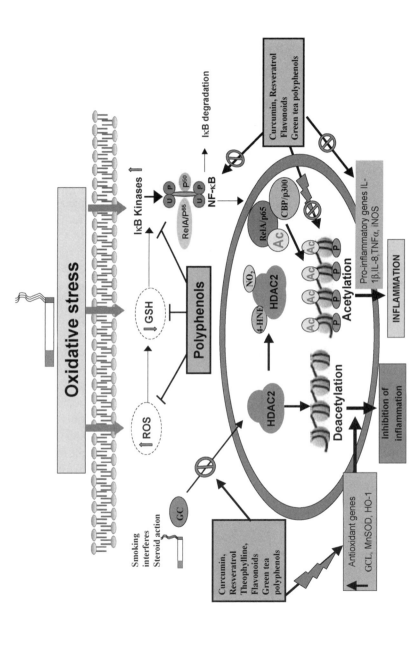

Figure 8.5 A schematic model for polyphenol- and theophylline-mediated modulation of cell signalling. Oxidative stress-induced inflammation is mediated by NF-κB activation and mitogen-activated protein kinases (MAPKs) and they affect a wide variety of cellular signalling processes leading to the generation of inflammatory mediators and chromatin remodelling. The latter allows expression of pro-inflammatory genes such as interleukin (IL)-1β, IL-8, tumour necrosis factor alpha (TNFα) and inducible nitric oxide synthase (iNOS). On the other hand, to counter the effects of oxidative stress, the cells also concomitantly express protective antioxidant genes such as glutamate cysteine ligase (GCL), manganese superoxide dismutase (MnSOD) and haem oxygenase (HO)-1. Polyphenols and theophylline inhibit pro-inflammatory gene expression via inhibition of IκBα, thus inhibiting NF-κB transactivation as well as restoring transrepressive pathways through the activation of histone deacetylases. A full-colour version of this figure can be found in the colour plate section of this book.

levels by thiol antioxidants (Yang et al., 2006). Clearly, oxidant-induced HAT–HDAC imbalance can thus be restored by dietary polyphenols. Such a mechanism would facilitate steroid-mediated HDAC2 recruitment, leading to attenuation of NF-κB-mediated chromatin/histone acetylation and therefore suppression of pro-inflammatory gene expression. The concept that HAT–HDAC imbalance regulates inflammatory gene expression and that this could be modulated by dietary polyphenols is corroborated by the findings that curcumin (100 μM) could inhibit HAT activity, preventing NF-κB-mediated chromatin acetylation (Kang et al., 2005). However, other possible mechanisms, such as stalling or reversing post-translational protein modifications induced by oxidants by which polyphenols inhibit inflammatory response, should not be overlooked. It is possible that dietary polyphenols may also assist in increasing the efficacy of corticosteroids by restoring HDAC2 activity. This might be achieved through the induction of enzymes such as tyrosine denitrase, carbonyl reductase or aldo–keto reductases. It is interesting to speculate that these dietary polyphenols and flavonols may not only act as antioxidant/anti-inflammatory agents but it may also increase the efficacy of glucocorticosteroids in COPD. However, this requires further examination *in vivo* using HDAC2 siRNA and knockout animal models.

A search for polyphenols or other compounds that would be more selective HDAC2 inducers is urgently needed. Novel HDAC2 activators might be discovered by high-throughput screening using HDAC2 activation, particularly under conditions of oxidative stress. Kinases or phosphatases that regulate HDAC2 activity in a similar manner to polyphenols/theophylline may also prove to be effective add-on therapies to corticosteroids. Many of the anti-inflammatory effects of corticosteroids appear to be mediated via inhibition of the transcriptional effects of NF-κB. Currently, small-molecule inhibitors of IKK2 that activate NF-κB are being developed. However, since corticosteroids have additional effects, it is not certain whether IKK2 inhibitors will parallel the clinical effectiveness of corticosteroids, and they may have side effects such as increased susceptibility to infections.

It may be likely that various p38-MAPK inhibitors might reduce steroid resistance both in *in vitro* and *in vivo* models of cigarette-smoke-mediated lung inflammation. Although these inhibitors act as anti-inflammatory treatments in patients with some forms of steroid-resistant asthma, they are not expected to benefit patients with the form of steroid resistance associated with a defect in acetylation of lysine 5 on histone H4. Studies involving a protein motif sequence scanning program (SCANPROSITE within Expasy, http://www.expasy.ch) have suggested that there are consensus phosphorylation sites within HDAC1, HDAC2 and HDAC3 where p38 MAPK can dock on the enzymes. Whereas a definite p38-MAPK docking site was detected only within HDAC3, a potential docking site was located only within HDAC1. Within HDAC2 no such docking sites were detected. The three HDACs also differed with respect to the presence of tyrosine phosphorylation sites. More *in vivo* studies are needed to determine the involvement of kinases, particularly p38 MAPKs and PI3K, in the regulation of HDACs under conditions of oxidative stress.

The above studies suggest that there is a potential to develop novel therapeutic agents that increase HDAC2 activity resulting in improved anti-inflammatory actions. These agents would act as steroid add-on therapies, enhancing the transrepression/transactivation ratio of steroids possessing a reduced side-effect profile.

8.7 Conclusion

There is now clear evidence for increased cigarette-smoke-derived ROS/free radicals being important in the pathogenesis of COPD. Oxidative stress causes imbalance in histone acetylation and deacetylation, leading to pro-inflammatory gene transcription. Oxidative stress also decreases HDAC2 by post-translational modifications by reactive aldehydes and NO products. HDAC, in particular HDAC2, is recruited with glucocorticoids in the corepressor complex to block the transcription of pro-inflammatory genes. The mechanism of glucocorticoid resistance in COPD and asthmatics is due to sustained oxidant generation, which may affect HDAC2 levels and/or glucocorticoid receptor interactions due to phosphorylation, acetylation or post-translational modifications of HDACs. Antioxidant compounds, particularly dietary polyphenols, may enhance the efficacy of glucocorticoids by quenching oxidants and reactive aldehydes or inducing phase II antioxidant genes, altering the acetylation state of histones or inducing HDACs in COPD patients. Dietary polyphenols such as resveratrol and curcumin have been shown to inhibit cigarette smoke/oxidant-induced NF-κB activation, histone acetylation and pro-inflammatory cytokine release and to restore glucocorticoid functions via a mechanism involving upregulation of HDAC2 activity. Dietary polyphenols regulate inflammatory response at the molecular level and this might be a way to restore glucocorticoid efficacy in the treatment of smoking-induced chronic inflammatory diseases. Considering the effects of curcumin and other polyphenols, it may thus be possible to discover other drugs in this class that could form the basis of a new class of anti-inflammatory drugs without the side effects that limit the use of theophylline in the treatment of COPD and steroid-resistant asthma.

References

Aghai ZH, Kumar S, Farhath S, Kumar MA et al. Dexamethasone suppresses expression of Nuclear Factor-kappaB in the cells of tracheobronchial lavage fluid in premature neonates with respiratory distress. *Pediatr Res* 2006; **59**: 811–815.

Ashburner BP, Westerheide SD, Baldwin Jr AS. The p65 (RelA) subunit of NF-kappaB interacts with the histone deacetylase (HDAC) corepressors HDAC1 and HDAC2 to negatively regulate gene expression. *Mol Cell Biol* 2001; **21**: 7065–7077.

Barnes PJ. Inhaled corticosteroids are not helpful in chronic obstructive pulmonary disease. *Am J Respir Crit Care Med* 2000; **161**: 342–344.

Barnes PJ, Adcock IM, Ito K. Histone acetylation and deacetylation: importance in inflammatory lung diseases. *Eur Respir J* 2005; **25**: 552–563.

Caramori G, Romagnoli M, Casolari P, Bellettato C et al. Nuclear localization of p65 in sputum macrophages but not in sputum neutrophils during COPD exacerbations. *Thorax* 2003; **58**: 348–351.

Chen L, Fischle W, Verdin E, Greene WC. Duration of nuclear NF-kappaB action regulated by reversible acetylation. *Science* 2001; **293**: 1653–1657.

Church T, Pryor WA. Free radical chemistry of cigarette smoke and its toxicological implications. *Environ Health Perspect* 1985; **64**: 111–126.

Cosio BG, Tsaprouni L, Ito K, Jazrawi E, Adcock IM, Barnes PJ. Theophylline restores histone deacetylase activity and steroid responses in COPD macrophages. *J Exp Med* 2004; **200**: 689–695.

Culpitt SV, Rogers DF, Fenwick PS, Shah P, De Matos C, Russell RE, Barnes PJ, Donnelly LE. Inhibition by red wine extract, resveratrol, of cytokine release by alveolar macrophages in COPD. *Thorax* 2003; **58**: 942–946.

Culpitt SV, Rogers DF, Shah P, De Matos C, Russel RE, Donnelly LE, Barnes PJ. Impaired inhibition by dexamethasone of cytokine release by alveolar macrophages from COPD patients. *Am J Respir Crit Care Med* 2002; **167**: 24–31.

Donnelly LE, Newton R, Kennedy GE, Fenwick PS, Leung RH, Ito K, Russell RE, Barnes PJ. Anti-Inflammatory Effects of Resveratrol in Lung Epithelial Cells: Molecular Mechanisms. *Am J Physiol Lung Cell Mol Physiol* 2004; **287**: L774–783.

De Ruijter AJ, Van Gennip AH, Caron HN, Kemp S, Van Kuilenburg AB. Histone deacetylases (HDACs): characterization of the classical HDAC *family. Biochem J* 2003; **370**: 737–749.

Di Stefano A, Caramori G, Oates T, Capelli A et al. Increased expression of nuclear factor-be in bronchial biopsies from smokers and patients with COPD. *Eur Respir J* 2002; **20**: 556–563.

Fu M, Wang C, Zhang X, Pestell RG. Acetylation of nuclear receptors in cellular growth and apoptosis. *Biochem Pharmacol* 2004; **68**: 1199–1208.

Glozak MA, Sengupta N, Zhang X, Seto E. Acetylation and deacetylation of non-histone proteins. *Gene* 2005; **363**: 15–23.

Goleva E, Li LB, Eves PT, Strand MJ, Martin RJ, Leung DY. Increased glucocorticoid receptor beta alters steroid response in glucocorticoid-insensitive asthma. *Am J Respir Crit Care Med* 2006; **173**: 607–616.

Halliwell B. Reactive oxygen species in living systems: source, biochemistry, and role in human disease. *Am J Med* 1991; **91**: 14S–22S.

Halliwell B, Gutteridge JMC. Free Radicals in Biology and Medicine. (2nd edn.), Oxford: Clarendon Press, 1989, pp. 1–20.

Irusen E, Matthews JG, Takahashi A, Barnes PJ, Chung KF, Adcock IM. p38 Mitogen-activated protein kinase-induced glucocorticoid receptor phosphorylation reduces its activity: role in steroid-insensitive asthma. *J Allergy Clin Immunol* 2002; **109**, 649–657.

Ito K, Barnes PJ, Adcock IM. Glucocorticoid receptor recruitment of histone deacetylase 2 inhibits IL-1β induced histone H4 acetylation on lysines 8 and 12. *Mol Cell Biol* 2000; **20**: 6891–6903.

Ito K, Chung KF, Adcock IM. Update on glucocorticoid action and resistance. *J Allergy Clin Immunol* 2006a; **117**: 522–543.

Ito K, Ito M, Elliott WM, Cosio B et al. Decreased Histone Deacetylase Activity in Chronic Obstructive Pulmonary Disease. *N Engl J Med* 2005; **352**: 1967–1976.

Ito K, Lim G, Caramori G, Chung KF, Barnes PJ, Adcock IM. Cigarette smoking reduces histone deacetylase 2 expression, enhances cytokine expression, and inhibits glucocorticoid actions in alveolar macrophages. *FASEB J* 2001; **15**: 1110–1112.

Ito K, Lim S, Caramori G, Cosio B, Chung KF, Adcock IM, Barnes PJ. A molecular mechanism of action of theophylline: induction of histone deacetylase activity to decrease inflammatory gene expression. *Proc Natl Acad Sci USA* 2002a; **99**: 8921–8926.

Ito K, Lim S, Chung KF, Barnes PJ, Adcock IM. Theophylline enhances histone deacetylase activity and restores glucocorticoid function during oxidative stress. *Am J Respir Crit Care Med* 2002b; **65**: A625.

Ito K, Yamamura S, Essilfie-Quaye S, Cosio B, Ito M, Barnes PJ, Adcock IM. Histone deacetylase 2-mediated deacetylation of the glucocorticoid receptor enables NF-κB suppression. *J Exp Med* 2006b; **203**: 7–13.

Kang J, Chen J, Shi Y, Jia J, Zhang Y. Curcumin-induced histone hypoacetylation: the role of reactive oxygen species. *Biochem Pharmacol* 2005; **69**: 1205–1213.

Kinnula VL, Chang L, Everitt JI, Crapo JD. Oxidants and antioxidants in alveolar epithelial type II cells: in situ, freshly isolated, and cultured cells. *Am J Physiol* 1992; **262**: L69–77.

Kinnula VL, Crapo JD, Raivio KO. Biology of disease: generation and disposal of reactive oxygen metabolites in the lung. *Lab Invest* 1995; **73**: 3–19.

Kirkham P, Rahman I. Oxidative stress in asthma and COPD: Antioxidants as a therapeutic strategy. *Pharm Ther* 2006; **111**: 476–494.

Marwick JA, Kirkham PA, Stevenson CS, Danahay H, Giddings J, Butler K, Donaldson K, MacNee W, Rahman I. Cigarette smoke alters chromatin remodeling and induces proinflammatory genes in rat lungs. *Am J Respir Cell Mol Biol* 2004; **31**: 633–642.

Moodie FM, Marwick JA, Anderson CS, Szulakowski P, Biswas SK, Bauter MR, Kilty I, Rahman I. Oxidative stress and cigarette smoke alter chromatin remodeling but differentially regulate NF-κB activation and proinflammatory cytokine release in alveolar epithelial cells. *FASEB J* 2004; **18**: 1897–1899.

Morrison D, Rahman I, Lannan S, MacNee W. Epithelial permeability, inflammation and oxidant stress in the airspaces of smokers. *Am J Respir Crit Care Med* 1999; **159**: 473–479.

Pryor WA, Stone K. Oxidants in cigarette smoke: radicals, hydrogen peroxides, peroxynitrate, and peroxynitrite. *Ann NY Acad Sci* 1993; **686**: 12–28.

Qiu Y, Zhao Y, Becker M, John S et al. HDAC1 acetylation is linked to progressive modulation of steroid receptor-induced gene transcription. *Mol Cell* 2006; **22**: 669–679.

Rahman I, Adcock IM. Oxidative stress and redox regulation of lung inflammation in COPD. *Eur Respir J* 2006; **28**: 219–242.

Rahman I, MacNee W. Role of oxidants/antioxidants in smoking-induced airways diseases. *Free Rad Biol Med* 1996; **21**: 669–681.

Rahman I, MacNee W. Lung glutathione and oxidative stress: Implications in cigarette smoke-induced airways disease. *Am J Physiol* 1999; **277**: L1067–L1088.

Rahman I, Bauter MR, Meja K, Kirkham P. Curcumin restores glucocorticoid function and inhibits cigarette smoke-mediated IL-8 release in oxidant stressed monocytic U937 cells. *ATS Abstract* 2005; A395.

Rahman I, Biswas SK, Kirkham PA. Regulation of inflammation and redox signaling by dietary polyphenols. *Biochem Pharmacol* 2006; **72**: 1439–1452.

Rahman I, Marwick J, Kirkham P. Redox modulation of chromatin remodeling: impact on histone acetylation and deacetylation, NF-κB and pro-inflammatory gene expression. *Biochem Pharmacol* 2004; **68**: 1255–1267.

Rahman I, Morrison D, Donaldson K, MacNee W. Systemic oxidative stress in asthma, COPD, and smokers. *Am J Respir Crit Care Med* 1996; **154**: 1055–1060.

Rahman I, Van Schadewijk AA, Crowther AJ, Hiemstra PS, Stolk J, Macnee W, De Boer WI. 4-Hydroxy-2-nonenal, a specific lipid peroxidation product, is elevated in lungs of patients with chronic obstructive pulmonary disease. *Am J Respir Crit Care Med* 2002; **166**: 490–495.

Reichardt HM, Kaestner KH, Tuckermann J, Kretz O et al. DNA binding of the glucocorticoid receptor is not essential for survival. *Cell* 1998; **93**: 531–541.

Reichardt HM, Tuckermann JP, Gottlicher M, Vujic M, Weih F, Angel P, Herrlich P, Schutz G. Repression of inflammatory responses in the absence of DNA binding by the glucocorticoid receptor. *EMBO J* 2001; **20**: 7168–7173.

Rhen T, Cidlowski JA. Anti-inflammatory action of glucocorticoids – new mechanisms for old drugs. *N Engl J Med* 2005; **353**: 1711–1723.

Sher ER, Leung DY, Surs W, Kam JC, Zieg G, Kamada AK, Szefler SJ. Steroid-resistant asthma. Cellular mechanisms contributing to inadequate response to glucocorticoid therapy. *J Clin Invest* 1994; **93**: 33–39.

Strickland I, Kisich K, Hauk PJ, Vottero A, Chrousos GP, Klemm DJ, Leung DY. High constitutive glucocorticoid receptor beta in human neutrophils enables them to reduce their spontaneous rate of cell death in response to corticosteroids. *J Exp Med* 2001; **193**: 585–593.

Szulakowski P, Crowther AJ, Jimenez LA, Donaldson K, Mayer R, Leonard TB, Macnee W, Drost EM. The effect of smoking on the transcriptional regulation of lung inflammation in patients with chronic obstructive pulmonary disease. *Am J Respir Crit Care Med* 2006; **174**: 41–50.

Uchida K, Shiraishi M, Naito Y, Torii N, Nakamura Y, Osawa T. Activation of stress signaling pathways by the end product of lipid peroxidation. *J Biol Chem* 1999; **274**: 2234–2242.

Yang SR, Chida AS, Bauter M, Shafiq N, Seweryniak K, Maggirwar SB, Kilty I, Rahman I. Cigarette smoke induces pro-inflammatory cytokine release by activation of NF-κB and post-translational modifications of histone deacetylase in macrophages. *Am J Physiol Lung Cell Mol Physiol* 2006; **29**: L46–L57.

Yudt MR, Cidlowski JA. The glucocorticoid receptor: coding a diversity of proteins and responses through a single gene. *Mol Endocrinol* 2002; **16**: 1719–1726.

Zhong H, May MJ, Jimi E, Ghosh S. The phosphorylation status of nuclear NF-kappa B determines its association with CBP/p300 or HDAC-1. *Mol Cell* 2002; **9**: 625–636.

9

Regulation of Glucocorticoid Sensitivity by Macrophage Migration Inhibitory Factor

Eric F. Morand

9.1 Introduction

Glucocorticoids (GC) have been used in the treatment of inflammatory diseases for over five decades. Despite their effectiveness, toxicity is common and generally dose dependent. Moreover, many diseases are characterized by GC resistance, which may be relative (in which higher doses are required in some individuals) or absolute (in which a given disease manifestation is not treatable with GC alone, e.g. proliferative lupus nephritis). Physicians treating inflammatory diseases universally seek to use lower doses of GC in every context, therefore the definition of factors regulating GC sensitivity is a major area of research.

As will be outlined, the twin observations that macrophage migration inhibitory factor (MIF) is glucocorticoid induced and yet antagonizes the effects of GC on the immune system suggest that MIF is such a regulatory factor. This further suggests that MIF could be targeted therapeutically in order to increase GC sensitivity.

9.2 MIF as a Pro-inflammatory Factor

MIF and inflammatory disease

Considerable evidence now supports the contention that MIF is an important pro-inflammatory factor. The range of diseases in which MIF has been implicated,

Overcoming Steroid Insensitivity in Respiratory Disease   Edited by Ian M. Adcock and Kian Fan Chung
© 2008 John Wiley & Sons, Ltd.

Table 9.1 Human chronic inflammatory diseases in which MIF is implicated

Human disease	References
Rheumatoid arthritis	Gregory et al., 2004; Ichiyama et al., 2004; Lacey et al., 2003; Leech et al., 1998, 1999, 2000, 2003; Mikulowska et al., 1997; Morand et al., 2002; Onodera et al., 2004; Sampey et al., 2001; Santos et al., 2001
Asthma and allergy	Kobayashi et al., 2006; Mizue et al., 2005; Rossi et al., 1998; Yamaguchi et al., 2000
Systemic lupus erythematosus	Foote et al., 2004; Hoi et al., 2006; Lan et al., 2000; Mizue et al., 2000; Sanchez et al., 2006
Atherosclerosis	Burger-Kentischer et al., 2002; Chen et al., 2004; Kong et al., 2005a, b; Lin et al., 2000; Pan et al., 2004; Schober et al., 2004
Inflammatory bowel disease	De Jong et al., 2001; Murakami et al., 2001, 2002; Nohara et al., 2004; Ohkawara et al., 2002, 2005; Ren et al., 2005
Glomerulonephritis	Lan et al., 1997; Yang et al., 1998
Psoriasis	Donn et al., 2004; Shimizu et al., 2001, 2002; Steinhoff et al., 1999
Multiple sclerosis	Denkinger et al., 2003; Niino et al., 2000; Powell et al., 2005
Diabetes	Yabunaka et al., 2000

through studies of MIF overexpression in humans and through studies of MIF neutralization or depletion in animal models, is large (Table 9.1). The significance of MIF in inflammatory disease in general can best be appreciated, however, by concentrating on a smaller number of diseases.

Rheumatoid arthritis (RA) is one of the most common chronic inflammatory diseases, affecting approximately 1% of adults. Evidence from recruitment patterns in clinical trials indicate that over 50% of RA patients receive chronic GC therapy, and recent studies suggest clear benefits on disease activity and damage from GC use (Svensson et al., 2005; Wassenberg et al., 2005). RA is a systemic connective tissue disease, characterized by a loss of immune tolerance and by extra-articular effects in the lungs, eyes, skin, subcutaneous tissues and vasculature, but it is most specifically characterized by chronic inflammation of synovial joints. The normally hypocellular synovial tissue undergoes dramatic expansion through recruitment of leukocytes (predominantly macrophages and CD4$^+$ T cells) and through dysregulated proliferation and apoptosis of resident cells known as fibroblast-like synoviocytes (FLS).

RA is among the best-studied diseases in terms of the pathogenic role of MIF. Human studies have demonstrated overexpression of MIF in cells and tissues from RA patients compared to controls, i.e. in RA patients with active disease compared to those with inactive disease (Leech et al., 1999; Morand et al., 2002). As recently reviewed, MIF has pro-inflammatory effects on almost all the pathways known to be implicated in the pathogenesis of synovitis in RA (Morand et al., 2003). These include induction of FLS expression of cytoplasmic phospholipase A_2 ($cPLA_2$) and cycolooxygenase-2 (COX-2), involved in prostaglandin synthesis (Sampey et al., 2001), upregulation of FLS proliferation and downregulation of apoptosis (Leech et al., 2003), upregulation of matrix metalloproteinases involved in cartilage and bone injury (Onodera et al., 2000, 2001; Pakozdi et al., 2006) and upregulation of a host of other cytokines known to be involved in RA pathogenesis, including TNF, IL-6 and IL-8 (Leech et al., 1999; Pakozdi et al., 2006; Santos et al., 2004). Effects on TNF are of particular interest given the clinical efficacy in RA of therapeutic agents that target this key cytokine. An effect of MIF on leukocyte recruitment to the joint has also been confirmed, with reduced leukocyte endothelial interactions in synovial and other tissues in MIF-deficient mice (Gregory et al., 2004). More recently, MIF has been shown to induce the selective recruitment of macrophages, partially via influencing the production of monocyte chemotactic protein-1 (MCP-1, also known as CCL-2) (Gregory et al., 2006). Finally, in patients with single nucleotide polymorphisms (SNP) of the *Mif* gene promoter, MIF overexpression is associated with negative long-term outcomes in disease-related joint damage (Baugh et al., 2002; Radstake et al., 2005). Together, these data have suggested MIF as a therapeutic target in RA.

Asthma is another disease almost universally treated with GC, and the potential for overexpression of MIF in asthma patients to contribute to GC resistance in this disease has been canvassed (Yamaguchi et al., 2000). In support of the theoretical role of MIF in GC resistance in asthma is the overlap between the observations that MIF induces activator protein-1 (AP-1) activation in human cells (Onodera et al., 2000, 2001), and that overactivation of AP-1 is implicated in GC resistance in asthma (Adcock et al., 1995; Lane et al., 1998). Significantly increased levels of MIF have been reported in the serum and induced sputum of asthmatics compared to healthy control subjects (Yamaguchi et al., 2000). Human eosinophils express MIF in response to stimuli such as IL-5, C5a or PMA and increased bronchoalveolar lavage (BAL) fluid MIF was reported in stable asthma patients (Rossi et al., 1998). Two recent studies examined rodent models of ovalbumin (OVA)-induced allergic airway inflammation. MIF was increased in the airway mucosa of OVA-challenged Brown Norway rats and was markedly increased in BAL fluid of OVA-challenged rats. Anti-MIF mAb treatment significantly reduced total cell counts, neutrophils and eosinophils in the BAL fluid of OVA-challenged rats (Kobayashi et al., 2006). Significantly, anti-MIF mAb also attenuated OVA-induced airway hyper-responsiveness to OVA and methacholine. However, anti-MIF mAb did not affect the level of serum OVA-specific IgE, suggesting a lack of effect on the Th2 immune response *per se*. Mizue et al reported similar findings in MIF-deficient mice (Mizue et al., 2005). MIF deficiency was associated with reduced leukocyte infiltration in the lungs, lowered BAL fluid eosinophils, eotaxin and IL-15, and lower lung tissue eotaxin, IL-5 and IL-13. This was accompanied by a reduction in airway hyperresponsiveness, but in contrast to the findings in the rat study using anti-MIF mAb the MIF deficiency was associated with reduced OVA-specific T-cell responses and Th2 cytokine expression. In support of these findings, Nakamaru et al. (2005) reported on MIF-deficient mice in a model of OVA-induced allergic rhinitis. Antigen-induced nasal clinical features were significantly reduced in MIF KO mice compared to WT mice, along with reduced infiltrating eosinophils and mucosal TNFα in MIF KO mice.

Similar issues relating to glucocorticoid use and resistance apply in chronic obstructive pulmonary disease (COPD), and the recently revealed effects of MIF on neutrophil and macrophage migration are of potential relevance. There are no published clinical studies of MIF in human COPD. In a model of acute lung injury in the rat, administration of lipopolysaccharide (LPS) resulted in accumulation of neutrophils in alveolar spaces, and MIF immunostaining was detected in bronchial epithelial cells and alveolar macrophages (Makita et al., 1998). Pre-treatment with anti-MIF antibody significantly attenuated neutrophil accumulation, which may relate to the observed reduction in levels of the chemokine macrophage inflammatory protein-1α (MIP-1α). The findings of this study were recently extended and confirmed by Lai et al. (2003) in a study of endotoxin-induced pulmonary inflammation. These findings have not been supported by all studies, however (Korsgren et al., 2000).

One other disease is of special note in relation to the theme of MIF and GC use. Systemic lupus erythematosus (SLE) is a less common autoimmune disease for which there has been no new therapy approved in over 30 years. Most SLE patients are treated with GC and non-selective immunosuppressants, and GC toxicity such as osteoporosis is a major issue in the management of such patients. We recently reported a highly protected phenotype in MIF-deficient MRL/*lpr* lupus-prone mice, with a 50% prolongation of life and a near-total protection from severe crescentic glomerulonephritis (Hoi et al., 2006). The latter was associated with reductions in macrophage recruitment to the glomerulus and reduced MCP-1 expression. We had previously reported elevations in serum MIF concentrations in patients with SLE, associated with increased accumulation of disease-related damage over time (Foote et al., 2004), and the *Mif* over-expression SNP noted earlier in relation to RA has also been reported in association with SLE (Sanchez et al., 2006). Specific GC-sparing through MIF antagonism would be of particular value in SLE.

Finally, both inflammatory diseases *per se* and GC therapy of these diseases are associated with increased risk of atherosclerotic vascular disease and premature death. Indeed, in SLE, premature vascular death is now the leading cause of death. A strong evidence base supports the role of MIF in the pathogenesis of atherosclerosis, and it can be hypothesized that increased MIF expression in inflammatory disease, further increased by GC therapy, may contribute to accelerated atherosclerosis in such individuals, as recently reviewed (Morand et al., 2006).

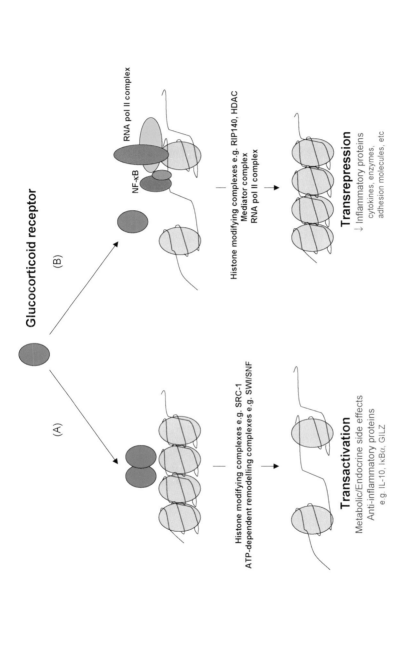

Figure 4.1 Mechanisms of transcriptional control by glucocorticoids. (A) Gene induction (transactivation) by the dimerized glucocorticoid receptor (GR) is mediated through a variety of interacting proteins, including the ATP-dependent chromatin remodelling enzymes that alter the packing of the nucleosomes and cofactors that either have histone-modifying activity or can recruit histone-modifying enzymes. Histone tails can be both methylated and acetylated, and the degree of modification of the histones regulates transcription rates. (B) Some of these processes are also targeted during GR-mediated transrepression of NF-κB activity. Thus, GR can engage with the transcriptional machinery through the mediator complex, which seems to function to integrate signals from the promoter and communicate with RNA polymerase II. In addition, differential recruitment of corepressor molecules by GR can reverse NF-κB-associated changes in histone modifications. Different genes in different cells are influenced by these activities to varying degrees, thus allowing considerable scope for pharmacological modulation

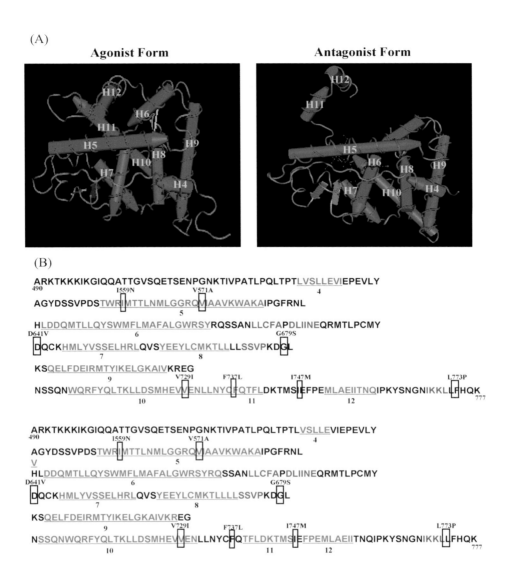

Figure 5.4 Crystal structure of the ligand-binding domain (LBD) of the human glucocorticoid receptor (hGR). (A) Stereotactic conformation of the agonist (*left*) and antagonist (*right*) form of the LBD of hGRα. The α-helices (H4–H12) are depicted as cylinders, whereas broad arrows represent the β-turn. (B) Location of the known mutations of hGR in the agonist (*upper panel*) and antagonist (*lower panel*) form of the LBD of hGRα. Helices are indicated in red and are underlined, while β-sheets are indicated in green. Two mutations (I559 and V571A) are located within H5, while four mutations (V729I, F737L, I747M and L773P) are located within or close to helices 11 and 12. The ligand-binding pocket is formed by helices 3, 5, 11 and 12. Upon ligand binding, the receptor undergoes major conformational changes, which alter the position of H11 and H12 and generate an interaction surface that allows coactivators to bind to the LBD through their LXXLL motifs. Helix 12 plays a critical role in the formation of both the ligand-binding pocket and the AF-2 surface that facilitates interaction with coactivators. The fact that most hGR mutations are clustered around H5, H11 and H12 indicates that these helices play an important role in glucocorticoid signal transduction

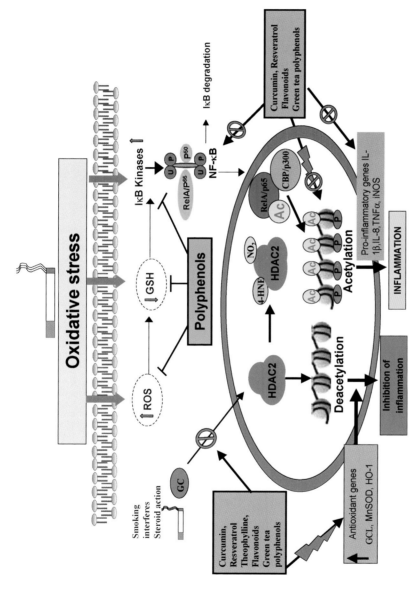

Figure 8.5 A schematic model for polyphenol- and theophylline-mediated modulation of cell signalling. Oxidative stress-induced inflammation is mediated by NF-κB activation and mitogen-activated protein kinases (MAPKs) and they affect a wide variety of cellular signalling processes leading to the generation of inflammatory mediators and chromatin remodelling. The latter allows expression of pro-inflammatory genes such as interleukin (IL)-1β, IL-8, tumour necrosis factor alpha (TNFα) and inducible nitric oxide synthase (iNOS). On the other hand, to counter the effects of oxidative stress, the cells also concomitantly express protective antioxidant genes such as glutamate cysteine ligase (GCL), manganese superoxide dismutase (MnSOD) and haem oxygenase (HO)-1. Polyphenols and theophylline inhibit pro-inflammatory gene expression via inhibition of IκBα, thus inhibiting NF-κB transactivation as well as restoring transrepressive pathways through the activation of histone deacetylases

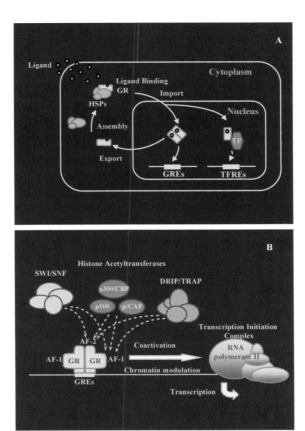

Figure 5.2 (A) Nucleocytoplasmic shuttling of the glucocorticoid receptor. Upon binding to the ligand, the activated hGRα dissociates from HSPs and translocates into the nucleus, where it homodimerizes and binds to GREs in the promoter region of target genes. (B) Schematic representation of the interaction of AF-1 and AF-2 of hGRα with coactivators. AF: activation function; DRIP/TRAP: vitamin D receptor-interacting protein/thyroid hormone receptor-associated protein; GR, glucocorticoid receptor; GREs, glucocorticoid response elements; HSP: heat shock protein; SWI/SNF: switching/sucrose non-fermenting; TF: transcription factor; TFRE: transcription factor response element

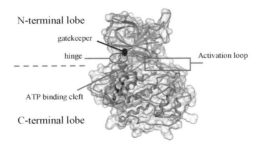

Figure 12.1 Molecular model of GSKb-3 as a template to indicate standard kinase nomenclature. A ribbon diagram (green) showing secondary structure elements (helices in red, strands in cyan). The molecular surface is represented in grey

Mechanisms of action of MIF

Activation of MAP kinases but not NF-κB by MIF

It is fair to say that the mechanisms of action of MIF remain incompletely under-stood. The first evidence for a specific cell surface receptor for MIF was published in 2003 (Leng et al., 2003). This work demonstrated the binding of MIF to the extracellular domain of the MHC Class II invariant chain, CD74 (also known as Ii). It is of note that the extracellular domain of CD74 has a predicted structure that is trimeric in form (Kukol et al., 2002). Recently it has been reported that CD74 and CD44 cooperate in transducing extracellular signals by MIF (Shi et al., 2006). Cells required the expression of both CD74 and CD44 in order to respond to MIF in the form of SRC kinase activation, a pathway recently separately demonstrated as highly significant to MIF-induced cell signalling (Lue et al., 2006). A separate re-port also documented binding of MIF with CD44 (Meyer-Siegler and Vera, 2005).

MIF induces a uniquely sustained phosphorylation of the mitogen-activated protein (MAPK) extracellular signal-regulated kinase (ERK)-1/2 (Mitchell et al., 1999). The activation by MIF of ERK and also of p38 MAPK has been shown in RA FLS (Lacey et al., 2003; Santos et al., 2004). We have also recently reported a significant deficiency in IL-1 and TNF-induced MAPK activation in MIF-deficient cells (Toh et al., 2006). Consistent with the activation of MAPKs by MIF, several studies have documented activation of the *c*-jun element of the AP-1 transcription factor by MIF (Onodera et al., 2000, 2001). MIF has also been shown to interact with the intracellular protein JAB-1, a coactivator of AP-1 transcription, but the effect reported was to diminish AP-1-dependent gene transcription (Bucala, 2000; Kleemann et al., 2000). More recently, it was reported that the MIF–JAP-1 interac-tion was permissive for MIF-induced ERK MAPK activation, despite being inhibi-tory of sustained ERK MAPK activation (Lue et al., 2006).

In contrast to the evidence for the activation by MIF of MAPKs little evidence for a direct activating effect of MIF on NF-κB has been adduced. For example, in RA FLS, despite inducing cell activation as outlined, recombinant MIF did not induce nuclear translocation of NF-κB subunits, and anti-MIF mAb concentrations that prevented IL-1-induced cell activation had no effect on IL-1-induced NF-κB (Lacey et al., 2003). In more recent studies, no effect of MIF deficiency on NF-κB activa-tion by IL-1 was observed, despite clear effects on activation of MAPKs (Toh et al., 2006). Reductions in NF-κB activation have been reported in MIF −/− mice cells in response to LPS (Roger et al., 2001), but this may reflect the reduction in TLR-4 expression by these cells and does not demonstrate direct activation of NF-κB by MIF. MIF does not directly affect I-κB kinase activity, as measured by Western blotting of I-κB protein (Daun and Cannon, 2000), and TNF induction of NF-κB reporter gene expression was identical in cells transfected with MIF antisense and control transfected cells (Kleemann et al., 2000). Onodera et al reported upregula-tion of NF-κB DNA binding by recombinant MIF in cultured human RA FLS, but only at extreme supraphysiological concentrations (1000 ng/ml); induction of AP-1 DNA binding (which would be consistent with MAPK activation) was observed at a more physiological concentration (Onodera et al., 2004).

MIF and p53

The potential mechanisms of action of MIF in disease pathogenesis and in the regulation of GC sensitivity have been recently broadened by evidence that MIF is the only pro-inflammatory cytokine capable of functionally inactivating the tumour suppressor protein p53 (Hudson et al., 1999). Relevant data come from a study in which macrophage viability in the setting of endotoxaemia was maintained via an inhibitory effect of endogenous MIF on p53 (Mitchell et al., 2002). In this study, macrophage apoptosis in response to LPS was potentiated in MIF$-/-$ mice, and rMIF suppressed macrophage apoptosis. MIF induces COX-2 in RA FLS (Sampey et al., 2001), and downstream PGE_2 production may be required for MIF inhibition of p53 activity (Mitchell et al., 2002). The survival of primary murine embryonic fibroblasts that overexpress MIF is also extended, and this has been shown to be p53 dependent (Hudson et al., 1999). Leech et al. (2003) reported that MIF directly inhibits p53 expression and apoptosis in human RA FLS while stimulating pro-liferation, supporting the hypothesis proposed above. These studies also demon-strated upregulation of p53 and downregulation of apoptosis in MIF $-/-$ cells and inflamed synovial tissues.

Indirect effects of MIF

Considerable evidence favours an indirect as well as a direct role of MIF in cellular activation. For example, IL-1 and TNF induce an activation of RA FLS that is more intense than that maximally inducible by MIF, yet the effects of IL-1 and TNF are completely prevented by anti-MIF mAb. This situation is also the case for cytokine-induced $cPLA_2$ and COX-2 expression and cellular proliferation (Lacey et al., 2003; Sampey et al., 2001). Similarly, although MIF is not a T-cell mitogen, anti-MIF mAb is a powerful inhibitor of *in vitro* T-cell proliferation and of *in vivo* delayed-type hypersensitivity (DTH) reactions (Bacher et al., 1996; Bernhagen et al., 1996), and MIF $-/-$ T-cells exhibit markedly reduced antigen-specific proliferation (L.L. Santos and E.F. Morand, unpublished observations). The effects of directly added exogenous MIF on a given system are often of lesser magnitude than the effects of preventing the contribution of MIF via neutralizing mAb or MIF gene deletion. These findings suggest that, in addition to direct effects on cell activation, MIF ex-erts a significant facilitatory effect on events entrained by other stimuli. The endog-enous expression of pre-formed MIF in resting cells, its autocrine/paracrine release early in immune responses, its physical relationship with signalling molecules such as JAB-1 and observations of attenuated MAPK activation in MIF-deficient cells are all consistent with this hypothesis. Recent studies even suggest that cells obtained from MIF $-/-$ mice diminished expression of receptors for IL-1 and TNF (Toh et al., 2006).

9.3   Relationship between MIF and Glucocorticoids

Regulation of MIF by GC

It is now widely appreciated that physiological GCs exert a powerful inhibitory influence on the immune system (Chrousos, 1995). Inflammation activates the hypothalamic-pituitary adrenal (HPA) axis via the action of circulating cytokines such as IL-6, leading to increased production of GC and subsequent attenuation of the inflammatory response. The production of endogenous GC during inflammation therefore constitutes an anti-inflammatory regulatory or feedback control loop. It is essential for normal function of the immune system to proceed despite the inhibitory effects of endogenous GC, and indeed all normal immune responses in mammals occur in the context of physiological GC concentrations. Whereas metabolic effects of physiological GC released during stress are desirable, maintaining activation of the immune system despite increased GC requires the existence of GC counter-regulatory systems. In addition to its direct role in inflammation, MIF has emerged as a GC-induced GC-counter-regulatory factor of considerable significance.

Although first described over 30 years ago, resurgent interest in MIF in the last 10 years was largely stimulated by the observation of its regulation by GC (Calandra et al., 1995). Consistent across most *in vitro* studies is a biphasic pattern of MIF regulation by GC. Although MIF concentrations in cell culture supernatants are suppressible by a high concentration of GC, MIF release is increased by low physiological concentrations, for example around 10^{-10} M hydrocortisone (Calandra et al., 1995). Within the immune system, MIF is secreted in response to GC stimulation in both monocytes and T cells (Bacher et al., 1996; Calandra et al., 1995). This has been confirmed in a variety of other cell types, including pancreatic islet cells (Waeber et al., 1997) and neuronal cells (Vedder et al., 2000). Leech et al. (1999) confirmed a concentration-dependent biphasic regulation of MIF by GC in human RA FLS *in vitro*. Evidence for endogenous GC upregulation of MIF *in vivo* has been obtained in experimental arthritis (Leech et al., 2000), in that tissue MIF was reduced in adrenalectomized rats. Others have methodically investigated the regulation of MIF expression by exogenous glucocorticoids *in vivo* in the rat (Fingerle-Rowson et al., 2003). Administration of dexamethasone was found to increase MIF protein expression in immune and endocrine tissues, skin and muscle. This increase was reported to be due to a post-transcriptional regulatory effect because tissue MIF mRNA levels were not influenced. In vivo regulation of serum MIF by exogenous GC in humans has been demonstrated in patients with SLE (Foote et al., 2004), but no evidence for endogenous changes in cortisol level altering MIF has been produced (Petrovsky and Bucala, 2002).

Functional antagonistic effects of MIF and GC and the regulation of GC sensitivity

Central to the role of MIF as a GC counter-regulatory factor is the observation that, despite being induced by GC, MIF is able to directly antagonize the effects of GC. This has been shown to be the case for macrophage TNF, IL-1β, IL-6 and IL-8 secretion (Calandra et al., 1995; Donnelly et al., 1997), for T-cell proliferation and IL-2 release (Bacher et al., 1996), and in cells from inflamed human lung tissue (Donnelly et al., 1997). In these experiments, GC-induced suppression of a given pro-inflammatory event was attenuated by the addition of MIF. MIF is present in healthy human serum at concentrations (3–5 ng/ml) that, *in vitro* exert GC-counter-regulatory activity. MIF also exhibits a GC-antagonist effect *in vivo* in models involving both innate and adaptive immune responses, such as endotoxic shock and antigen-induced arthritis (Calandra et al., 1995; Santos et al., 2001). In both of these models, inhibition of disease by GC was attenuated by administration of exogenous MIF.

While other pro-inflammatory stimuli, such as other cytokines, can also oppose the actions of GC, these are generally suppressed by GC and are therefore not present in the relevant locations. MIF, on the other hand, being inducible by GC, has the unique opportunity to act in opposition to GC. The proposal arising from these observations, that MIF acts in balance with GC to affect the "set-point" and hence the outcome of an inflammatory response (Bucala, 1996), has now been confirmed. New data from two groups demonstrate that MIF does indeed regulate GC sensitivity. Aeberli et al demonstrated that the sensitivity to suppression by dexamethasone of LPS-induced TNF in peritoneal macrophages was three-fold greater in MIF $-/-$ cells compared to wild-type controls (Aeberli et al., 2006). This work was independently demonstrated in the lab of Calandra et al. in almost identical experiments (Roger et al., 2005). These studies demonstrated that for a given concentration of GC a greater suppressive effect was observed in the absence of MIF than in its presence. The effect of MIF on GC sensitivity is depicted in Figure 9.1.

It can be hypothesized on the basis of these observations that therapeutic antagonism of MIF would inhibit the natural GC antagonist role of MIF, thereby allowing GC, either endogenous or exogenous, to prevail (Aeberli et al., 2006). This would be the first direct example of a so-called "steroid-sparing" therapy. The practical effect would be the opportunity to use lower (or zero) doses of exogenous GC when combined with MIF antagonism, thus reducing dose-dependent GC toxicity. In support of this, anti-MIF mAb administration has been shown to replace endogenous GC in a model of arthritis, in which the lethal effect of adrenalectomy in rats developing adjuvant arthritis was completely prevented by MIF neutralization (Leech et al., 2000).

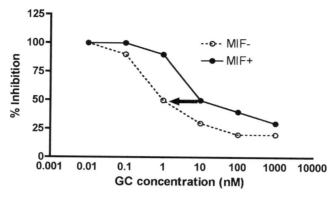

Figure 9.1   Left-shift of GC responsiveness in the absence of MIF. In this figure, the effect of MIF on GC sensitivity is illustrated. Suppression of a given inflammatory process by GC is indicated as % inhibition, where 100% represents the degree of activation in the absence of GC. MIF-deficient cells have been shown in two studies (Aeberli et al., 2006; Roger et al., 2005) to left-shift the dose–response curve to GC, increasing the suppressive effect of a given GC concentration. To obtain a desired degree of suppression, therefore, a lower concentration of GC is required

Mechanisms of MIF–GC antagonism

MIF and NF-κB

The mechanisms through which MIF antagonizes the effects of GC have not been fully elucidated. Cell activation via NF-κB is highly GC sensitive, such that inhibition of NF-κB represents a major means by which GCs inhibit the inflammatory response (Barnes, 1998). Daun et al reported that while MIF did not directly induce NF-κB activation, it impaired effects of GC on the NF-κB inhibitory molecule I-κB (Daun et al., 2000). In contrast, we and others (as noted above) have found no evidence that MIF acts through NF-κB signal transduction (Kleemann et al., 2000; Lacey et al., 2003; Toh et al., 2006). Moreover, recent studies by the author using MIF-deficient cells have not confirmed an effect of MIF on the expression of I-κB (Aeberli et al., 2006). The possibility that effects of MIF on NF-κB explain its effects on GC sensitivity therefore remains uncertain at best.

MIF and MAP kinases

Antagonism of GC-mediated suppression of inflammatory cell activation could instead depend on the preferential utilization by MIF of MAPK signalling pathways. MAPK pathways are activated by a wide variety of pro-inflammatory and growth factor stimuli, and are involved in a wide range of pathologies such that direct MAPK antagonists are under development by multiple pharmaceutical companies.

There are no direct effects of the GC–receptor complex on MAPKs. GCs, do, however, induce the expression of MAPK phosphatase (MKP)-1, an endogenous negative regulator of MAPK activation that dephosphorylates activated MAPKs (Lasa et al., 2002; Toh et al., 2004). Several recent studies have underlined the significance of the inhibitory effect of MKP-1 on the activation of innate immune responses (Chi et al., 2006; Salojin et al., 2006; Zhao et al., 2006). As noted above, two groups have recently reported that MIF is a negative regulator of GC sensitivity *in vitro* (Aeberli et al., 2006; Roger et al., 2005). Both studies also demonstrated that MIF is a negative regulator of GC-induced MKP-1 expression. The absence of MIF resulted in greater sensitivity to induction of MKP-1 by dexamethasone, and exogenous MIF directly inhibited dexamethasone-induced MKP-1 expression. This is consistent with the idea that, in disease, MIF permits overactivation of MAPKs and that MIF attenuation of GC-induced MKP-1 is the mechanism of MIF's role in controlling GC sensitivity. This model is presented in Figure 9.2.

Other effects of MIF

The effects of MIF on p53 may also be relevant to the functional interaction of MIF and GC. p53 interacts directly with the GR and with the GR–DNA complex,

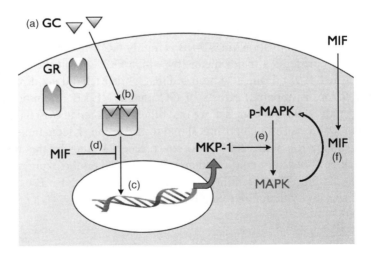

Figure 9.2 Antagonism of GC effects on MKP-1 by MIF. Extracellular GC molecules enter the cell (a) and bind to cytoplasmic GC receptors (GR) (b). The ligand-bound GR activates transcription and eventual expression of MKP-1 (c). MIF inhibits GC-induced MKP-1 expression through, as yet, uncertain mechanisms. The dephosphorylation of phosphorylated MAPKs (p-MAPK) by MKP-1 (e) is therefore suppressed, leading to persistence of activated MAPKs. In addition, MIF directly stimulates the phosphorylation of MAPKs, adding further to a net pro-inflammatory result

resulting in inhibition of GR-mediated transactivation events (Maiyar et al., 1997) as well as inhibition of the actions of p53. Other aspects of GC action, in contrast, require the expression of p53 and are attenuated in its absence (Urban et al., 2003). Moreover, expression of MKP-1 is dependent at least in part on p53 (Li et al., 2003; Yang and Wu, 2004), suggesting the as-yet untested hypothesis that MIF-dependent inhibition of p53 could underlie MIF-dependent inhibition of GC-induced MKP-1 (Aeberli et al., 2006).

Potential alternative mechanisms for the negative regulatory effects of MIF on the anti-inflammatory effects of GC include MAPK-dependent phosphorylation of GR. The MAPK JNK has been reported to directly phosphorylate and hence in-activate the GR (Rogatsky et al., 1998). There is no evidence to date that MIF is implicated in this pathway but reduced JNK activation in the absence of MIF has been reported (Toh et al., 2006). One recent study demonstrated inhibitory effects of MIF on the expression of heat shock protein (hsp) 40 and hsp70, wherein MIF de-ficiency resulted in increased hsp expression (Ohkawara et al., 2006). The potential for effects on other systems known to be involved in the regulation of GC sensitivity such as HDAC is speculative.

9.4 Conclusions

MIF is a broad-spectrum pro-inflammatory molecule implicated in the pathogenesis of a wide range of chronic diseases commonly treated with GC. MIF not only atten-uates the anti-inflammatory effects of GC, but its expression is induced by GC and it is therefore in a unique position to antagonize GC effects in the context of inflamma-tion. The effect of MIF on GC sensitivity has recently been demonstrated, confirm-ing the long-held hypothesis that MIF acts as a physiological counter-regulator of the effects of GC. Although the definitive mechanisms of action of MIF remain under investigation, clear effects on MAPKs and on GC-induced expression of the MAPK inhibitory phosphatase MKP-1 appear likely to explain the recently observed effect of MIF on GC sensitivity. The potential for therapeutic MIF antagonism increasing GC sensitivity *in vivo*, resulting in a clinical "steroid-sparing" effect, is supported by the existing data. Demonstration of such effects *in vivo* and confirmation of the mechanisms of these effects are likely to coincide with the clinical development of MIF antagonist approaches under development at several pharmaceutical companies worldwide.

References

Adcock IM, Lane SJ, Brown CR, Lee TH, Barnes PJ. Abnormal glucocorticoid receptor-activator protein 1 interaction in steroid-resistant asthma. *J Exp Med* 1995; **182**: 1951–1958.

Aeberli D, Leech M, Morand EF. Macrophage migration inhibitory factor and glucocorticoid sensitivity. *Rheumatology (Oxf)* 2006; **45**: 937–943.

Aeberli D, Yang YH, Mansell A, Santos L, Leech M, Morand EF. Macrophage migration inhibitory factor modulates glucocorticoid sensitivity in macrophages via effects on map kinase phosphatase-1 and p38 map kinase. *FEBS Lett* 2006; **580**: 974–981.

Bacher M, Metz CN, Calandra T, Mayer K et al. An essential regulatory role for macrophage migration inhibitory factor in T-cell activation. *Proc Natl Acad Sci USA* 1996; **93**: 7849–7854.

Barnes PJ. Anti-inflammatory actions of glucocorticoids–molecular mechanisms. *Clin Sci* 1998; **94**: 557–572.

Baugh JA, Chitnis S, Donnelly SC, Baugh JA et al. A functional promoter polymorphism in the macrophage migration inhibitory factor (MIF) gene associated with disease severity in rheumatoid arthritis. *Genes Immun* 2002; **3**: 170–176.

Bernhagen J, Bacher M, Calandra T, Metz CN, Doty SB, Donnelly T, Bucala R. An essential role for macrophage migration inhibitory factor in the tuberculin delayed-type hypersensitivity reaction. *J Exp Med* 1996; **183**: 277–282.

Bucala R. Mif rediscovered: Cytokine, pituitary hormone, and glucocorticoid-induced regulator of the immune response. *FASEB J* 1996; **10**: 1607–1613.

Bucala R. Signal transduction. A most interesting factor. *Nature* 2000; **408**: 146–147.

Burger-Kentischer A, Goebel H, Seiler R, Fraedrich G et al. Expression of macrophage migration inhibitory factor in different stages of human atherosclerosis. *Circulation* 2002; **105**: 1561–1566.

Calandra T, Bernhagen J, Metz CN, Spiegel LA et al. MIF as a glucocorticoid-induced modulator of cytokine production. *Nature* 1995; **377**: 68–71.

Chen Z, Sakuma M, Zago AC, Zhang X et al. Evidence for a role of macrophage migration inhibitory factor in vascular disease. *Arterioscler Thromb Vasc Biol* 2004; **24**: 709–714.

Chi H, Barry SP, Roth RJ, Wu JJ, Jones EA, Bennett AM, Flavell RA. Dynamic regulation of pro- and anti-inflammatory cytokines by MAPK phosphatase 1 (MKP-1) in innate immune responses. *Proc Natl Acad Sci USA* 2006; **103**: 2274–2279.

Chrousos GP. The hypothalamic-pituitary-adrenal axis and immune-mediated inflammation. *New Engl J Med* 1995; **332**: 1351–1362.

Daun JM, Cannon JG. Macrophage migration inhibitory factor antagonizes hydrocortisone-induced increases in cytosolic IκBα. *Am J Physiol* 2000; **279**: R1043–R1049.

de Jong YP, Abadia-Molina AC, Satoskar AR, Clarke K et al. Development of chronic colitis is dependent on the cytokine MIF. *Nat Immunol* 2001; **2**: 1061–1066.

Denkinger CM, Denkinger M, Kort JJ, Metz C, Forsthuber TG. In vivo blockade of macrophage migration inhibitory factor ameliorates acute experimental autoimmune encephalomyelitis by impairing the homing of encephalitogenic T cells to the central nervous system. *J Immunol* 2003; **170**: 1274–1282.

Donn RP, Plant D, Jury F, Richards HL, Worthington J, Ray DW, Griffiths CE. Macrophage migration inhibitory factor gene polymorphism is associated with psoriasis. *J Invest Dermatol* 2004; **123**: 484–487.

Donnelly SC, Haslett C, Reid PT, Grant IS et al. Regulatory role for macrophage migration inhibitory factor in acute respiratory distress syndrome. *Nature Med* 1997; **3**: 320–323.

Fingerle-Rowson G, Koch P, Bikoff R, Lin X et al. Regulation of macrophage migration inhibitory factor expression by glucocorticoids in vivo. *Am J Pathol* 2003; **162**: 47–56.

Foote A, Briganti EM, Kipen Y, Santos L, Leech M, Morand EF. Macrophage migration inhibitory factor in systemic lupus erythematosus. *J Rheumatol* 2004; **31**: 268–273.

Gregory JL, Leech MT, David JR, Yang YH, Dacumos A, Hickey MJ. Reduced leukocyte–endothelial cell interactions in the inflamed microcirculation of macrophage migration inhibitory factor-deficient mice. *Arthritis Rheum* 2004; **50**: 3023–3034.

Gregory JL, Morand EF, McKeown SJ, Ralph JA et al. Macrophage migration inhibitory factor induces macrophage recruitment via CC chemokine ligand 2. *J Immunol* 2006; **177**: 8072–8079.

Hoi A, Hickey MJ, Hall P, Yamana J et al. Mif deficiency attenuates macrophage recruitment, glomerulonephritis and lethality in *mrl/lpr* mice. *J Immunol* 2006; **177**: 5687–5696.

Hudson JD, Shoaibi MA, Maestro R, Carnero A, Hannon GJ, Beach DH. A proinflammatory cytokine inhibits p53 tumor suppressor activity. *J Exp Med* 1999; **190**: 1375–1382.

Ichiyama H, Onodera S, Nishihira J, Ishibashi T et al. Inhibition of joint inflammation and destruction induced by anti-type II collagen antibody/lipopolysaccharide (LPS)-induced arthritis in mice due to deletion of macrophage migration inhibitory factor (MIF). *Cytokine* 2004; **26**: 187–194.

Kleemann R, Hausser A, Geiger G, Mischke R et al. Intracellular action of the cytokine MIF to modulate AP-1 activity and the cell cycle through JAB1. *Nature* 2000; **408**: 211–216.

Kobayashi M, Nasuhara Y, Kamachi A, Tanino Y et al. Role of macrophage migration inhibitory factor in ovalbumin-induced airway inflammation in rats. *Eur Respir J* 2006; **27**: 726–734.

Kong YZ, Huang XR, Ouyang X, Tan JJ et al. Evidence for vascular macrophage migration inhibitory factor in destabilization of human atherosclerotic plaques. *Cardiovasc Res* 2005a; **65**: 272–282.

Kong YZ, Yu X, Tang JJ, Ouyang X et al. Macrophage migration inhibitory factor induces mmp-9 expression: Implications for destabilization of human atherosclerotic plaques. *Atherosclerosis* 2005; **178**: 207–215.

Korsgren M, Kallstrom L, Uller L, Bjerke T, Sundler F, Persson CG, Korsgren O. Role of macrophage migration inhibitory factor (MIF) in allergic and endotoxin-induced airway inflammation in mice. *Mediat Inflamm* 2000; **9**: 15–23.

Kukol A, Torres J, Arkin IT. A structure for the trimeric MHC Class II-associated invariant chain transmembrane domain. *J Mol Biol* 2002; **320**: 1109–1117.

Lacey D, Sampey A, Mitchell R, Bucala R, Santos L, Leech M, Morand E. Control of fibroblast-like synoviocyte proliferation by macrophage migration inhibitory factor. *Arthritis Rheum* 2003; **48**: 103–109.

Lai KN, Leung JC, Metz CN, Lai FM, Bucala R, Lan HY. Role for macrophage migration inhibitory factor in acute respiratory distress syndrome. *J Pathol* 2003; **199**: 496–508.

Lan HY, Bacher M, Yang N, Mu W et al. The pathogenic role of macrophage migration inhibitory factor in immunologically induced kidney disease in the rat. *J Exp Med* 1997; **185**: 1455–1465.

Lan HY, Yang N, Nikolic-Paterson DJ, Yu XQ et al. Expression of macrophage migration inhibitory factor in human glomerulonephritis. *Kidney Int* 2000; **57**: 499–509.

Lane SJ, Adcock IM, Richards D, Hawrylowicz C, Barnes PJ, Lee TH. Corticosteroid-resistant bronchial asthma is associated with increased *c-fos* expression in monocytes and T lymphocytes. *J Clin Invest* 1998; **102**: 2156–2164.

Lasa M, Abraham SM, Boucheron C, Saklatvala J, Clark AR. Dexamethasone causes sustained expression of mitogen-activated protein kinase (MAPK) phosphatase 1 and phosphatase-mediated inhibition of MAPK p38. *Mol Cell Biol* 2002; **22**: 7802–7811.

Leech M, Lacey DC, Xue JR, Santos L et al. Macrophage migration inhibitory factor (MIF) regulates p53 in inflammatory arthritis. *Arthritis Rheum* 2003; **48**: 1881–1889.

Leech M, Metz C, Bucala R, Morand EF. Regulation of macrophage migration inhibitory factor by endogenous glucocorticoids in rat adjuvant-induced arthritis. Arthritis Rheum 2000; **43**:827–833.

Leech M, Metz C, Hall P, Hutchinson P et al. Macrophage migration inhibitory factor in rheumatoid arthritis: Evidence of proinflammatory function and regulation by glucocorticoids. *Arthritis Rheum* 1999; **42**: 1601–1608.

Leech M, Metz CN, Santos LL, Peng T, Holdsworth SR, Bucala R, Morand EF. Involvement of macrophage migration inhibitory factor in the evolution of rat adjuvant arthritis. *Arthritis Rheum* 1998; **41**: 910–917.

Leng L, Metz CN, Fang Y, Xu J et al. MIF signal transduction initiated by binding to CD74. *J Exp Med* 2003; **197**: 1467–1476.

Li M, Zhou JY, Ge Y, Matherly LH, Wu GS. The phosphatase MKP1 is a transcriptional target of p53 involved in cell cycle regulation. *J Biol Chem* 2003; **278**: 41059–41068.

Lin SG, Yu XY, Chen YX, Huang XR et al. De novo expression of macrophage migration inhibitory factor in atherogenesis in rabbits. *Circ Res* 2000; **87**: 1202–1208.

Lue H, Kapurniotu A, Fingerle-Rowson G, Roger T et al. Rapid and transient activation of the ERK MAPK signalling pathway by macrophage migration inhibitory factor (MIF) and dependence on JAB1/CSN5 and SRC kinase activity. *Cell Signal* 2006; **18**: 688–703.

Maiyar AC, Phu PT, Huang AJ, Firestone GL. Repression of glucocorticoid receptor transactivation and DNA binding of a glucocorticoid response element within the serum/glucocorticoid-inducible protein kinase (SGK) gene promoter by the p53 tumor suppressor protein. *Mol Endocrinol* 1997; **11**: 312–329.

Makita H, Nishimura M, Miyamoto K, Nakano T et al. Effect of anti-macrophage migration inhibitory factor antibody on lipopolysaccharide-induced pulmonary neutrophil accumulation. *Am J Respir Crit Care Med* 1998; **158**: 573–579.

Meyer-Siegler KL, Vera PL. Substance P induced changes in CD74 and CD44 in the rat bladder. *J Urol* 2005; **173**: 615–620.

Mikulowska A, Metz CN, Bucala R, Holmdahl R. Macrophage migration inhibitory factor is involved in the pathogenesis of collagen type II-induced arthritis in mice. *J Immunol* 1997; **158**: 5514–5517.

Mitchell RA, Liao H, Chesney J, Fingerle-Rowson G, Baugh J, David J, Bucala R. Macrophage migration inhibitory factor (MIF) sustains macrophage proinflammatory function by inhibiting p53: Regulatory role in the innate immune response. *Proc Natl Acad Sci USA* 2002; **99**: 345–350.

Mitchell RA, Metz CN, Peng T, Bucala R. Sustained mitogen-activated protein kinase (MAPK) and cytoplasmic phospholipase A2 activation by macrophage migration inhibitory factor (MIF). Regulatory role in cell proliferation and glucocorticoid action. *J Biol Chem* 1999; **274**: 18100–18106.

Mizue Y, Ghani S, Leng L, McDonald C et al. Role for macrophage migration inhibitory factor in asthma. *Proc Natl Acad Sci USA* 2005; **102**: 14410–14415.

Mizue Y, Nishihira J, Miyazaki T, Fujiwara S et al. Quantitation of macrophage migration inhibitory factor (MIF) using the one-step sandwich enzyme immunosorbent assay: Elevated serum MIF concentrations in patients with autoimmune diseases and identification of MIF in erythrocytes. *Int J Mol Med* 2000; **5**: 397–403.

Morand EF, Bucala R, Leech M. Macrophage migration inhibitory factor: An emerging therapeutic target in rheumatoid arthritis. *Arthritis Rheum* 2003; **48**: 291–299.

Morand EF, Leech M, Bernhagen J. MIF: A new cytokine link between rheumatoid arthritis and atherosclerosis. *Nat Rev Drug Discov* 2006; **5**: 399–410.

Morand EF, Leech M, Weedon H, Metz C, Bucala R, Smith MD. Macrophage migration inhibitory factor in rheumatoid arthritis: Clinical correlations. *Rheumatology (Oxf)* 2002; **41**: 558–562.

Murakami H, Akbar SM, Matsui H, Horiike N, Onji M. Macrophage migration inhibitory factor activates antigen-presenting dendritic cells and induces inflammatory cytokines in ulcerative colitis. Clin Exp Immunol 2002; **128**:504–510.

Murakami H, Akbar SM, Matsui H, Onji M. Macrophage migration inhibitory factor in the sera and at the colonic mucosa in patients with ulcerative colitis: Clinical implications and pathogenic significance. Eur J Clin Invest 2001; **31**:337–343.

Nakamaru Y, Oridate N, Nishihira J, Takagi D, Furuta Y, Fukuda S. Macrophage migration inhibitory factor (MIF) contributes to the development of allergic rhinitis. *Cytokine* 2005; **31**: 103–108.

Niino M, Ogata A, Kikuchi S, Tashiro K, Nishihira J. Macrophage migration inhibitory factor in the cerebrospinal fluid of patients with conventional and optic-spinal forms of multiple sclerosis and neuro-behcet's disease. *J Neurol Sci* 2000; **179**: 127–131.

Nohara H, Okayama N, Inoue N, Koike Y et al. Association of the −173 G/C polymorphism of the macrophage migration inhibitory factor gene with ulcerative colitis. *J Gastroenterol* 2004; **39**: 242–246.

Ohkawara T, Miyashita K, Nishihira J, Mitsuyama K et al. Transgenic over-expression of macrophage migration inhibitory factor renders mice markedly more susceptible to experimental colitis. *Clin Exp Immunol* 2005; **140**: 241–248.

Ohkawara T, Nishihira J, Ishiguro Y, Otsubo E et al. Resistance to experimental colitis depends on cytoprotective heat shock proteins in macrophage migration inhibitory factor null mice. *Immunol Lett* 2006; **107**: 148–154.

Ohkawara T, Nishihira J, Takeda H, Hige S et al. Amelioration of dextran sulfate sodium-induced colitis by anti-macrophage migration inhibitory factor antibody in mice. *Gastroenterology* 2002; **123**: 256–270.

Onodera S, Kaneda K, Mizue Y, Koyama Y, Fujinaga M, Nishihira J. Macrophage migration inhibitory factor up-regulates expression of matrix metalloproteinases in synovial fibroblasts of rheumatoid arthritis. *J Biol Chem* 2000; **275**: 444–450.

Onodera S, Nishihira J, Iwabuchi K, Koyama Y, Yoshida K, Tanaka S, Minami A. Macrophage migration inhibitory factor up-regulates matrix metalloproteinase-9 and -13 in rat osteoblasts. Relevance to intracellular signaling pathways. *J Biol Chem* 2001; **20**: 20.

Onodera S, Nishihira J, Koyama Y, Majima T et al. Macrophage migration inhibitory factor up-regulates the expression of interleukin-8 messenger RNA in synovial fibroblasts of rheumatoid arthritis patients: Common transcriptional regulatory mechanism between interleukin-8 and interleukin-1beta. *Arthritis Rheum* 2004; **50**: 1437–1447.

Pakozdi A, Amin MA, Haas CS, Martinez RJ et al. Macrophage migration inhibitory factor: A mediator of matrix metalloproteinase-2 production in rheumatoid arthritis. *Arthritis Res Ther* 2006; **8**: R132.

Pan JH, Sukhova GK, Yang JT, Wang B et al. Macrophage migration inhibitory factor deficiency impairs atherosclerosis in low-density lipoprotein receptor-deficient mice. *Circulation* 2004; **109**: 3149–3153.

Petrovsky N, Bucala R. Macrophage migration inhibitory factor: A critical neurohumoral mediator. *Front Horm Res* 2002; **29**: 83–90.

Powell ND, Papenfuss TL, McClain MA, Gienapp IE, Shawler TM, Satoskar AR, Whitacre CC. Cutting edge: Macrophage migration inhibitory factor is necessary for progression of experimental autoimmune encephalomyelitis. *J Immunol* 2005; **175**: 5611–5614.

Radstake TR, Sweep FC, Welsing P, Franke B et al. Correlation of rheumatoid arthritis severity with the genetic functional variants and circulating levels of macrophage migration inhibitory factor. *Arthritis Rheum* 2005; **52**: 3020–3029.

Ren Y, Lin CL, Li Z, Chen XY et al. Up-regulation of macrophage migration inhibitory factor in infants with acute neonatal necrotizing enterocolitis. *Histopathology* 2005; **46**: 659–667.

Rogatsky I, Logan SK, Garabedian MJ. Antagonism of glucocorticoid receptor transcriptional activation by the C-jun N-terminal kinase. *Proc Natl Acad Sci USA* 1998; **95**: 2050–2055.

Roger T, Chanson AL, Knaup-Reymond M, Calandra T. Macrophage migration inhibitory factor promotes innate immune responses by suppressing glucocorticoid-induced expression of mitogen-activated protein kinase phosphatase-1. *Eur J Immunol* 2005; **35**: 3405–3413.

Roger T, David J, Glauser MP, Calandra T. MIF regulates innate immune responses through modulation of toll-like receptor 4. *Nature* 2001; **414**: 920–924.

Rossi AG, Haslett C, Hirani N, Greening AP et al. Human circulating eosinophils secrete macrophage migration inhibitory factor (MIF). Potential role in asthma. *J Clin Invest* 1998; **101**: 2869–2874.

Salojin KV, Owusu IB, Millerchip KA, Potter M, Platt KA, Oravecz T. Essential role of MAPK phosphatase-1 in the negative control of innate immune responses. *J Immunol* 2006; **176**: 1899–1907.

Sampey AV, Hall PH, Mitchell RA, Metz CN, Morand EF. Regulation of synoviocyte phospholipase A2 and cyclooxygenase 2 by macrophage migration inhibitory factor. *Arthritis Rheum* 2001; **44**: 1273–1280.

Sanchez E, Gomez LM, Lopez-Nevot MA, Gonzalez-Gay MA et al. Evidence of association of macrophage migration inhibitory factor gene polymorphisms with systemic lupus erythematosus. *Genes Immun* 2006; **7**: 433–436.

Santos LL, Hall P, Metz CN, Bucala R, Morand EF. Role of macrophage migration inhibitory factor (MIF) in murine antigen-induced arthritis: Interaction with glucocorticoids. Clin Exp Immunol 2001; **123**: 309–314.

Santos LL, Lacey D, Yang Y, Leech M, Morand EF. Activation of synovial cell p38 MAP kinase by macrophage migration inhibitory factor. *J Rheumatol* 2004; 31: 1038–1043.

Schober A, Bernhagen J, Thiele M Zeiffer U et al. Stabilization of atherosclerotic plaques by blockade of macrophage migration inhibitory factor after vascular injury in apolipoprotein E-deficient mice. *Circulation* 2004; **109**: 380–385.

Shi X, Leng L, Wang T, Wang W et al. CD44 is the signaling component of the macrophage migration inhibitory factor–CD74 receptor complex. *Immunity* 2006; 25: 595–606.

Shimizu T, Nishihira J, Mizue Y, Nakamura H et al. Histochemical analysis of macrophage migration inhibitory factor in psoriasis vulgaris. *Histochem Cell Biol* 2002; **118**: 251–257.

Shimizu T, Nishihira J, Mizue Y, Nakamura H et al. High macrophage migration inhibitory factor (MIF) serum levels associated with extended psoriasis. *J Invest Dermatol* 2001; **116**: 989–990.

Steinhoff M, Meinhardt A, Steinhoff A, Gemsa D, Bucala R, Bacher M. Evidence for a role of macrophage migration inhibitory factor in psoriatic skin disease. *Br J Dermatol* 1999; **141**: 1061–1066.

Svensson B, Boonen A, Albertsson K, van der Heijde D, Keller C, Hafstrom I. Low-dose prednisolone in addition to the initial disease-modifying antirheumatic drug in patients with early active rheumatoid arthritis reduces joint destruction and increases the remission rate: A two-year randomized trial. *Arthritis Rheum* 2005; 52: 3360–3370.

Toh M-L, Aeberli D, Lacey D, Yang Y et al. Regulation of Il-1 and TNF receptor expression and function by endogenous MIF. *J Immunol* 2006; **177**: 4818–4825.

Toh M-L, Yang Y, Leech M, Morand EF. Expression of MAP kinase phosphatase-1, a negative regulator of MAP kinases, in rheumatoid arthritis: Upregulation by Il-1 and glucocorticoids. *Arthritis Rheum* 2004; 50: 3118–3128.

Urban G, Golden T, Aragon IV, Cowsert L, Cooper SR, Dean NM, Honkanen RE. Identification of a functional link for the p53 tumor suppressor protein in dexamethasone-induced growth suppression. *J Biol Chem* 2003; **278**: 9747–9753.

Vedder H, Krieg J, Gerlach B, Gemsa D, Bacher M. Expression and glucocorticoid regulation of macrophage migration inhibitory factor (MIF) in hippocampal and neocortical rat brain cells in culture. *Brain Res* 2000; **869**: 25–30.

Waeber G, Calandra T, Roduit R, Haefliger JA et al. Insulin secretion is regulated by the glucose-dependent production of Islet beta cell macrophage migration inhibitory factor. *Proc Natl Acad Sci USA* 1997; **94**: 4782–4787.

Wassenberg S, Rau R, Steinfeld P, Zeidler H. Very low-dose prednisolone in early rheumatoid arthritis retards radiographic progression over two years: A multicenter, double-blind, placebo-controlled trial. *Arthritis Rheum* 2005; **52**: 3371–3380.

Yabunaka N, Nishihira J, Mizue Y, Tsuji M et al. Elevated serum content of macrophage migration inhibitory factor in patients with type 2 diabetes. *Diabetes Care* 2000; **23**: 256–258.

Yamaguchi E, Nishihira J, Shimizu T, Takahashi T et al. Macrophage migration inhibitory factor (MIF) in bronchial asthma. *Clin Exp Allergy* 2000; **30**: 1244–1249.

Yang H, Wu GS. p53 transactivates the phosphatase MKP1 through both intronic and exonic p53 responsive elements. *Cancer Biol Ther* 2004; **3**: 1277–1282.

Yang NS, Nikolic-Paterson DJ, Ng YY, Mu W et al. Reversal of established rat crescentic glomerulonephritis by blockade of macrophage migration inhibitory factor (MIF)–potential role of MIF in regulating glucocorticoid production. *Mol Med* 1998; **4**: 413–424.

Zhao Q, Wang X, Nelin LD, Yao Y et al. Map kinase phosphatase 1 controls innate immune responses and suppresses endotoxic shock. *J Exp Med* 2006; **203**: 131–140.

10

Steroid-sparing Strategies: Long-acting Inhaled β_2-Agonists

Anna Miller-Larsson and **Olof Selroos**

10.1   Introduction

The combination of inhaled corticosteroids (ICS) and long-acting inhaled β_2-agonists (LABA) is widely used in the treatment of patients with asthma and chronic obstructive pulmonary disease (COPD). In COPD fixed daily doses of ICS are recommended and approved, e.g. budesonide (BUD) 800 µg and fluticasone propionate (FP) 1000 µg per day. ICS/LABA combinations such as budesonide/formoterol (BUD/FORM) and salmeterol/fluticasone (SALM/FP) are highly effective in COPD for reducing severe exacerbations and improving patients' health-related quality of life (Calverley et al., 2003; Szafranski et al., 2003) but the rationale for adding LABA to ICS in COPD patients was not with the intention of reducing the ICS dose.

10.2   Why and When is a Steroid-sparing Effect of LABA Important in Asthma?

ICS represent the first-line treatment of all patients with persistent asthma (Global Initiative for Asthma (GINA), 2002). The majority of asthmatics have a mild disease that usually responds well to ICS alone and with rapid-acting β_2-agonists used as needed (GINA, 2002). Patients with moderate to severe asthma are rarely totally steroid resistant but they may require higher ICS doses that can potentially result in signs of systemic corticosteroid activity. Therefore, in general terms, patients requiring doses of BUD above 1000 µg/day or FP above 500 µg/day are candidates

Overcoming Steroid Insensitivity in Respiratory Disease   Edited by Ian M. Adcock and Kian Fan Chung
© 2008 John Wiley & Sons, Ltd.

for steroid-sparing regimens as these higher doses have been shown to suppress the hypothalamic-pituitary-adrenal (HPA) axis and to exhibit other signs of systemic glucocorticoid (GC) activity (Barnes et al., 1998; Lipworth and Jackson, 2000; Wales et al., 1999). An ICS/LABA combination can result in improved asthma control without the need to increase ICS doses to a range that can cause systemic GC activity.

A recent meta-analysis including 10 studies in adult patients with asthma showed no difference in severe asthma exacerbations requiring oral steroids when comparing reduced ICS doses (mean reduction 60%) in ICS/LABA combinations to a fixed moderate to high dose of ICS alone (Gibson et al., 2005).

10.3 Effects of Lower Dose ICS/LABA versus a Higher Dose ICS on Lung Function, Symptoms and Use of Reliever Medication

The first study to look at the effects of treating patients with a lower dose of ICS/ LABA compared with a higher dose of ICS was a 6-month trial evaluating the efficacy of adding SALM 50 μg twice daily (b.i.d.) to a standard dose of beclomethasone dipropionate (BDP) 200 μg b.i.d. compared with BDP 500 μg b.i.d. alone (Greening et al., 1994). Significantly better airway function, fewer asthma symptoms and a reduced need for reliever medication were seen in patients treated with the SALM/BDP combination therapy compared with the higher dose BDP alone. No differences in safety profile were reported. The study was not powered for detection of differences in exacerbation rates. A similar study in patients with more severe asthma compared BDP 500 μg in combination with SALM 50 or 100 μg b.i.d. against BDP 1000 μg b.i.d. (Woolcock et al., 1996). As in the previous study, combination therapy was significantly more effective than higher dose BDP in improving lung function and asthma symptoms, and in reducing the use of reliever medication. No difference in efficacy was found between the two doses of SALM as its dose–response curve for doses above 50 μg is rather flat (Palmqvist et al., 1999), but the prevalence of tremor was threefold and significantly higher in the higher dose SALM group.

Improved lung function, reductions in asthma symptoms and need for reliever medication have also been described in studies where FORM was added to low-dose BUD compared with a higher dose of BUD alone (Lalloo et al., 2003) and in studies where BUD 160 μg (delivered dose corresponding to 200 μg metered dose) plus FORM 4.5 μg b.i.d. was compared with FP 250 μg b.i.d. (Bateman et al., 2003). In addition, further studies have confirmed that adding SALM 50 μg b.i.d. to FP 100 μg b.i.d. in a single inhaler was superior to FP 250 μg b.i.d. (Bloom et al., 2003; Busse et al., 2003) and that SALM/FP 50/250 μg b.i.d. was better than FP 500 μg b.i.d. (Ind et al., 2003). Comparisons of SALM/FP 50/100 μg versus BUD 400 μg b.i.d. (Johansson et al., 2001), SALM/FP 50/250 μg versus BUD 800 μg b.i.d. (Jenkins et al., 2000) and SALM/FP 50/100 μg versus triamcinolone 600 μg b.i.d. (Baraniuk et al., 1999) all showed the ICS/LABA combinations to be better than the higher ICS dose alone. These findings have been summarized in a recent review (Gibson et al., 2005).

All the aforementioned studies have used lung function measurements, asthma symptoms and use of as-needed reliever medication as study variables. It is not surprising that adding a potent and long-acting bronchodilator to the therapeutic regimen results in improvements in these variables compared to treatment without LABA. These studies were not designed or powered for detection of differences in exacerbation rates, which may increase in the absence of adequate doses of ICS.

10.4 Effects of Lower Dose ICS/LABA versus Higher Dose ICS on Exacerbations

Variables measuring asthma control are required to address the importance of the ICS/LABA combinations. The FACET (Formoterol And Corticosteroids Establishing Therapy) study was the first asthma study to use the exacerbation rate as the primary efficacy variable (Pauwels et al., 1997). Severe and mild exacerbations were evaluated separately. Patients with moderately severe asthma were treated for 1 year with either a low (100 μg b.i.d.) or moderate (400 μg b.i.d.) dose of BUD plus FORM 9 μg b.i.d. or placebo (instead of FORM). The addition of FORM to both doses of BUD and increasing the BUD dose fourfold significantly reduced the rate of both severe and mild exacerbations. The fourfold increase in BUD dose alone reduced the rate of severe exacerbations significantly more than the low-dose BUD/FORM, but no difference in mild exacerbations were found between low-dose BUD/FORM and the higher dose BUD groups (P = 0.76). A separate analysis showed no difference in the profile of symptoms and lung function changes before, during and after the exacerbations between the four treatment groups (Tattersfield et al., 1999). Thus, it was confirmed that the use of the LABA in combination with ICS helped to reduce exacerbations of all types and did not mask deteriorations in asthma control before, during or after these events. The study also confirmed that in moderate to severe asthma the 200 μg/day dose of BUD was not optimal in preventing severe exacerbations in patients using ICS alone or in combination with LABA.

In patients with mild persistent asthma not well controlled on ICS alone, the addition of FORM 4.5 μg b.i.d. to BUD 100 μg b.i.d. resulted in a significantly reduced rate of severe exacerbations compared with a twofold higher dose of BUD (group B in the OPTIMA study, i.e. patients not well controlled in their asthma on ICS alone O'Byrne et al., 2001). In agreement with the OPTIMA results, other studies have shown that doubling the dose of ICS is largely ineffective in preventing asthma exacerbations (FitzGerald et al., 2004a; Harrison et al., 2004). Thus, a permanent (Pauwels et al., 1997) or temporary (Foresi et al., 2000) fourfold increase in ICS dose is normally required to achieve a reduction in severe exacerbations. Systematic reviews have now confirmed that a lower dose of ICS in combination with a LABA is more effective than a double dose of ICS alone in preventing severe exacerbations in mild to severe persistent asthma (Sin et al., 2004).

10.5   Protocols with Tapering ICS Doses With and Without LABA while Maintaining Asthma Control

Studies with a steroid tapering design, which by necessity include well-controlled patients before allowing downward dose titration of ICS, normally have the disadvantage of insufficient time at each dose step to assess control before allowing further dose reduction. However, a well-designed double-blind, crossover study was reported by Wilding et al., (1997). Patients with mild or moderate asthma taking at least 200 μg of BDP or BUD received 50 μg of SALM or placebo b.i.d. for 6 months each, with a 1-month washout. The ICS dose was adjusted according to guidelines. Compared with placebo, a modest 17% reduction in ICS dose was observed with SALM (95% CI 12–22%). Lung function and symptom control improved with SALM.

Self et al., (1998) reported the results of a small 12-month study ($n = 24$) in patients with moderate to severe asthma requiring daily doses of at least 1000 μg of ICS. Patients were randomized to receive 50 μg of SALM or placebo b.i.d. and the ICS dose was then reduced by at least 10% every 4 weeks as long as airway function and need for reliever medication remained constant. There was no significant difference in ICS mean doses at the end of the trial but a trend was seen and patients in the SALM group were 2.3 times more likely to have some ICS dosage reduction compared to patients in the placebo group (95% CI 0.8–6.9).

Nielsen et al., (1999) investigated the steroid-sparing effects of LABA in 34 patients using 800–1600 μg/day of ICS. Firstly, the dose of BDP was reduced by 200 μg per week until asthma deteriorated. The minimal acceptable dose (MAD) was thus defined as the dose step above deterioration. The patients then received three times the MAD for 2 weeks before being randomized to receive, in addition, 50 μg of SALM or placebo b.i.d. and the MAD was again determined. The MAD BDP was significantly lower in the SALM group compared with placebo ($P < 0.01$), and a 50% reduction of the MAD was achieved by more patients treated with SALM than with placebo ($P = 0.001$). Asthma symptoms and use of as-needed medication were also significantly lower in the SALM group.

The largest ICS tapering study included 175 patients not well controlled in their asthma during a 6-week run-in period on triamcinolone 400 μg b.i.d. (Lemanske et al., 2001). Patients were then randomized to additional treatment with SALM 50 μg b.i.d. ($n = 154$) or placebo ($n = 21$) for 2 weeks. The placebo group and half of the SALM group were subsequently randomly assigned to have their ICS therapy reduced by 50% for 8 weeks, which was then discontinued for 8 weeks. The other half of the SALM group continued the ICS/LABA treatment for 16 weeks. The results showed that the ICS dose could be reduced by 50% without a statistically significant deterioration in asthma control, although a threefold numerical increase in exacerbations was seen in this period. Discontinuation of all ICS after 8 weeks resulted in significant deterioration in both symptom and exacerbation control. As 8 weeks may be an inadequate period to assess stability, it remains uncertain if a 50% dose reduction was achieved successfully in this study. What is clear is that monotherapy with LABA alone cannot be recommended. This finding was confirmed in a study that showed that SALM could mask an increase in inflammation following the complete withdrawal of ICS (McIvor et al., 1998).

10.6 Reducing ICS Doses Using an Adjustable ICS/LABA Dosing Regimen

Of the ICS/LABA combinations available, the BUD/FORM combination exhibits dose–response relationships for both of its components in the treatment of asthma (Busse et al., 1998; Ringdal et al., 1998). Thus, the doses of BUD/FORM can be adjusted depending on asthma severity without changing the inhaler device. This cannot be done with SALM/FP as the dose–response curve of SALM is flat for doses above 50 μg (Palmqvist et al., 1999; Ullman and Svedmyr, 1988; Woolcock et al., 1996). The principles of adjustable maintenance dosing of BUD/FORM have been reviewed by Buhl (2003) and Ankerst (2005). In brief, patients with moderately severe asthma are given two doses of BUD/FORM b.i.d. to gain control. Those patients achieving good asthma control can reduce their maintenance dose to one inhalation b.i.d.. However, in case of predefined worsening, the dose should be increased for 1–2 weeks to four doses b.i.d.. After achieving good asthma control, the dose can then be reduced to one inhalation b.i.d.. All patients use a rapid- and short-acting β_2-agonist for temporary relief of symptoms. In the clinical studies the results of the adjustable treatment regimens with BUD/FORM were compared with a fixed maintenance dose.

Several studies utilizing the adjustable maintenance dosing of BUD/FORM have been published (Aalbers et al., 2004; Buhl et al., 2004; Canonica et al., 2004; FitzGerald et al., 2003; Ind et al., 2004; Leuppi et al., 2003; Ställberg et al., 2003). A recent review (FitzGerald et al., 2004b) summarized the results of the seven first mentioned studies plus data from one further study presented in abstract form (Michils et al., 2003).

In the first 6-month study by Ställberg et al., 2003 ($n = 1034$) the patients were equally well controlled in terms of their asthma symptoms in the higher dose BUD/FORM fixed or lower dose regimen using adjustable maintenance treatment. However, there were significantly fewer exacerbations in the adjustable maintenance treatment group – 6.2% versus 9.5% (odds ratio 0.63, 95% CI 0.40–1.00, P = 0.049) despite a significant 40% reduction in ICS dose (P < 0.001) (Figure 10.1). In a 5-month Canadian study (FitzGerald et al., 2003) ($n = 995$) asthma symptom severity was again equally maintained with both treatment regimens but exacerbations were significantly fewer in the adjustable treatment group – 4.0% versus 8.9%

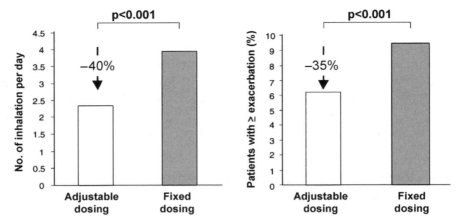

Figure 10.1 Mean number of BUD/FORM inhalations in asthma patients treated with an adjustable dosing regimen or fixed dosing (*left*), and the per cent of patients with ≥ 1 severe asthma exacerbation (*right*). Adapted from Ställberg et al. (2003)

in the fixed treatment group (P = 0.002), with a 36% reduction in the average BUD maintenance dose in the adjustable treatment group (P < 0.001).

Overall, the seven cited studies show that there were no clinically relevant differences in lung function, asthma symptoms or night-time awakenings but there were fewer exacerbations (FitzGerald et al., 2004b). However, the use of BUD/FORM was consistently lowered by 13–40% compared with fixed dosing, thus demonstrating a steroid-sparing effect. In these studies patients required an action plan to achieve the clinical benefits obtained with the adjustable maintenance treatment approach and this could be considered a potential drawback of this treatment approach. An alternative treatment approach that involves automatic adjustments in BUD/FORM dose at the first sign of symptoms, i.e. when patients require a reliever, may have greater potential in everyday clinical practice.

10.7 Reducing ICS Doses Using the Symbicort® Maintenance and Reliever Therapy

Due to the rapid onset of action, FORM can be used as a reliever medication in asthma (Seberová and Andersson, 2000). Bronchodilatation after inhalation of BUD is also detectable within hours after administration (Ellul-Micallef and Johansson, 1983). Therefore, patients with moderate to severe asthma can be treated by using only one inhaler, the BUD/FORM combination inhaler, for both maintenance and as-needed use, without requiring an additional short-acting β_2-agonist bronchodilator for as-needed use. This concept has been coined SMART (Symbicort® Maintenance And Reliever Therapy) (Gibson, 2005).

Three large clinical studies comparing BUD/FORM SMART with fixed ICS/LABA or higher ICS dosing have been published (O'Byrne et al., 2005; Rabe et al., 2006; Scicchitano et al., 2004).

In a 12-month study ($n = 1890$) of the SMART concept two inhalations of BUD/FORM 160/4.5 μg once daily with additional doses as needed were compared with a higher dose of BUD (two inhalations 160 μg b.i.d.) with terbutaline as needed in patients with moderate to severe asthma (Scicchitano et al., 2004). The mean doses of BUD used in the study were 466 and 640 μg per day in the SMART group and the higher BUD dose group, respectively. Nevertheless, compared with the higher ICS dose, in the SMART group the time to the first asthma exacerbation was significantly prolonged ($P < 0.001$) and the risk of having a severe asthma exacerbation was reduced by 39% ($P < 0.001$).

Similarly, in a 6-month study in patients with mild to moderate asthma ($n = 697$) an increased efficacy (larger improvements in airway function, reduced risk of exacerbations and hospitalizations) and a steroid-sparing effect were found with the SMART concept. The mean BUD doses were 240 and 320 μg per day in the SMART group and the higher BUD dose group, respectively, with 77% fewer oral steroid treatment days in the SMART group (Rabe et al., 2006).

A third double-blind 12-month study in adults and children with moderately severe asthma compared the SMART concept (BUD/FORM 80/4.5 μg b.i.d. plus additional doses as needed) with BUD/FORM in a fixed dose of 80/4.5 μg b.i.d. with terbutaline as needed and with a four times higher dose of BUD (320 μg b.i.d.) with terbutaline as needed ($n = 2760$) (O'Byrne et al., 2005). Children 4–11 years old inhaled the medication once daily in the evening. BUD/FORM SMART improved airway function significantly more than the two other treatments. It prolonged the time to the first asthma exacerbation ($P < 0.001$), resulting in a 45–47% lower exacerbation risk versus BUD/FORM in fixed dosing (hazard ratio 0.55, 95% CI 0.44–0.67) or the four times higher BUD dose (hazard ratio 0.53, 95% CI 0.43–0.65). Table 10.1 shows

Table 10.1   Total mean ICS doses and the number of days when patients had to use oral steroids in three asthma studies investigating the SMART (Symbicort® Maintenance And Reliever Therapy) concept. Data from Scicchitano et al. (2004), O'Byrne et al. (2005) and Rabe et al. (2006)

	Rabe et al. (2006)		O'Byrne et al. (adults) (2005)			Scicchitano et al. (2004)	
	BUD 160 μg 2×1	SMART 80/4.5 μg 2×1 + p.r.n.	BUD 160 μg 2×2	BUD/FORM 80/4.5 μg 1×2	SMART 80/4.5 μg 1×2 + p.r.n.	BUD 160 μg 2×2	SMART 160/4.5 μg 2×1 + p.r.n.
Total BUD dose (μg/day)	320	242	640	160	240	640	466
Systemic steroids (no. of days)	498	114	2577	2918	1255	3177	1776

Table 10.2 Total mean ICS doses and the number of days when children with asthma had to use oral steroids in three studies investigating the SMART (Symbicort® Maintenance And Reliever Therapy) concept. Data from Bisgaard et al. (2006)

	SMART	BUD/FORM	BUD
BUD fixed dose/day (µg)	80	80	320
BUD as needed/day (µg)	46	–	–
Total BUD dose/day (µg)	126	80	320
Systemic GCs (no. of days)[a]	32	230	141

[a] Due to asthma exacerbations.

the steroid-sparing capacity of the SMART concept. The adult patients used mean doses of BUD of 240, 160 and 640 µg in the BUD/FORM SMART, BUD/FORM fixed dosing and higher dose BUD groups, respectively, and in addition oral steroids on 1255, 2918 and 2577 days during the entire study period. The overall steroid use in the three cited studies and the corresponding steroid-sparing capacity of the SMART concept are shown in Table 10.1. In children ($n = 341$) the BUD doses were 126, 80 and 320 µg per day and the number of days with oral steroids were 32, 230 and 141, respectively. Thus, in children, a significant steroid-sparing effect was demonstrable with the BUD/FORM SMART concept (Table 10.2).

In a study comparing BUD/FORM SMART with SALM/FP in adjustable doses (by changing the inhaler used, based on actual asthma control) and salbutamol used as needed, the SMART concept, as in the above-mentioned studies, resulted in significantly fewer exacerbations and a clear steroid-sparing effect (Figure 10.2) (Vogelmeier et al., 2005).

10.8   Does Enhanced Anti-inflammatory Efficacy Explain Steroid-sparing Effects in ICS/LABA Therapy?

It is conceivable that superior asthma control by ICS/LABA therapy, and especially the reduction of disease exacerbations at lower ICS doses than with ICS monotherapy, is at least partly achieved by enhanced control over airway inflammation and possibly over airway remodelling. Indeed, enhanced anti-inflammatory and some anti-remodelling effects of ICS/LABA were shown in airway and lung structure cells and inflammatory cells. In many studies, the greatest potentiation of steroid anti-inflammatory activity by the addition of LABA was obtained at low steroid concentrations. This suggests that there is a link between an enhanced anti-inflammatory efficacy and steroid-sparing effects in ICS/LABA therapy.

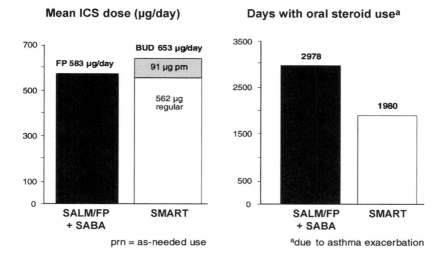

Figure 10.2 Mean doses of ICS when used as BUD/FORM according to the SMART (Symbicort® Maintenance And Reliever Therapy) concept and as SALM/FP with salbutamol as reliever therapy (*left*), and the number of days when oral steroids had to be used due to asthma exacerbations (*right*). The SMART concept resulted in an overall steroid-sparing effect. Adapted from Vogelmeier et al. (2005)

Airway and lung structure cells

Complementary, additive or even synergistic anti-inflammatory effects of GCs and LABA were shown in *in vitro* studies in structural airway and lung cells, which are probably the main source of inflammatory mediators, recruiting inflammatory cells into the asthmatic airways. For example, the production of granulocyte macrophage-colony stimulating factor (GM-CSF), a cytokine which activates and enhances survival of eosinophils, was additively decreased by the combination of BUD and FORM in cultured bronchial epithelial cells and lung fibroblasts exposed to pro-inflammatory cytokines (Korn et al., 2001; Spoelstra et al., 2002). Similarly, in cultured human airway smooth-muscle cells, FP and SALM additively decreased the levels of the TNFα-induced eosinophil chemokine eotaxin (Nie et al., 2005; Pang and Knox, 2001), and synergistically decreased the neutrophil chemokine interleukin-8 (IL-8) (Pang and Knox, 2000). In the same cells, SALM rendered a low concentration of dexamethasone more effective in the inhibition of TNFα-induced eosinophil chemokine RANTES (regulated on activation normal T-cell expressed and secreted) (Ammit et al., 2002). Similarly, in induced sputum cells isolated from asthmatics, FORM or salbutamol potentiated the inhibitory effects of BDP on the release of GM-CSF, RANTES and IL-8 (Profita et al., 2005). The BUD/FORM and SALM/FP combinations also additively decreased expression of the adhesion molecules, intercellular adhesion molecule-1 (ICAM-1) and vascular adhesion molecule-1 (VCAM-1) in cultured human lung fibroblasts (Silvestri et al., 2001; Spoelstra et al., 2002). These molecules are important for infiltration of inflammatory cells into the airway and lung tissue, and ICAM-1 is also the receptor for 90% of rhinovirus. Rhinovirus infections are the main trigger of asthma exacerbations, and bronchial epithelial cells from asthmatic patients seem to have a deficient innate immune response to these infections (Contoli et al., 2006; Wark et al., 2005). Importantly, FP and SALM were recently shown to additively or synergistically suppress lymphocyte and neutrophil chemokines (Edwards et al., 2006) as well as angiogenic and pro-fibrotic factors (Volonaki et al., 2006) induced by rhinovirus in cultured human bronchial epithelial cells.

In asthma, airway and lung structural cells are involved in airway remodelling, which is probably driven by chronic inflammatory processes and boosted by disease exacerbations. Airway remodelling includes enhanced proliferation of airway smooth-muscle cells, goblet cell hyperplasia and airway wall fibrosis characterized by increased synthesis of specific collagens, fibronectin and proteoglycans by myofibroblasts. These alterations may lead to increased airway wall thickness, reduced airway calibre and altered function of airway smooth-muscles cells and may all contribute to increased airway hyper-responsiveness, which is a constant feature of asthma. It seems that airway remodelling may be relatively insensitive to ICS monotherapy and the question of whether the addition of LABA leads to a better asthma control arises. *In vitro* data are quite supportive. BUD and FORM synergistically inhibited serum-stimulated proliferation of human cultured airway smooth-muscle cells (Roth et al., 2002) and proteoglycan production by serum- or TGFβ-stimulated cultured human lung fibroblasts (Todorova et al., 2006 and 2007). Either FP or SALM alone partially inhibited TGFβ-induced α-smooth-muscle actin (a marker of myofibroblasts) in cultured human lung fibroblasts, whereas FP plus SALM resulted in nearly complete inhibition (Baouz et al., 2005). *In vivo* data are more controversial. FP administered together with SALM counteracted goblet cell hyperplasia in the airways of allergic rats, however the amount of fibronectin and collagen in the airway wall was enhanced compared to FP alone (Vanacker et al., 2002). In patients with asthma on a low dose of ICS, an increase in the density of vascularity (number of vessels/mm^2) in the subepithelial lamina propria was reduced by 3 months' supplementary treatment with inhaled SALM (50 μg b.i.d.) but not with supplementary FP (100 μg b.i.d.) (Orsida et al., 2001). In asthma, during acute inflammation and exacerbations, an increased plasma leakage from subepithelial microvessels leads to airway oedema, which may contribute to airway narrowing. Acute, histamine-induced plasma leakage in human bronchial airways was rapidly and significantly reduced by FORM (two consecutive inhalations of 12 μg each) (Greiff et al., 1998), whereas topical BUD (studied in human nasal airways) exerted only slight inhibitory effects (Greiff et al., 1997).

Inflammatory cells

Compared to airway structural cells, data on the effects of addition of LABA to GCs on inflammatory cells seem to be more contentious. For example, SALM was shown to enhance the inhibitory effect of dexamethasone on human monocyte proliferation and cytokine release (Oddera et al., 1998), however it blocked the inhibition of superoxide generation induced by dexamethasone in human eosinophils (Nielson and Hadjokas, 1998), which are key inflammatory cells in asthma and are associated with asthma severity. In contrast, BUD and FORM additively or synergistically decreased superoxide generation in human eosinophils activated by conditioned medium from bronchial epithelial cells (Persdotter et al., 2007). Similarly, FP and SALM additively blocked eosinophil adhesion (Myo et al., 2004), and synergistically inhibited *in vitro* survival of peripheral blood T cells from asthmatic subjects (Pace et al., 2004). *In vivo,* inhaled FORM (24 μg b.i.d. for 2 months) reduced the number of mast cells and eosinophils in bronchial submucosa and epithelium in mild asthmatics (Wallin et al., 1999, 2002). The number of eosinophils in the bronchial lamina propria was also reduced by inhaled SALM (50 μg b.i.d. for 12 weeks) in asthmatic patients who were already using ICS (Li et al., 1999). Furthermore, addition of SALM (50 μg b.i.d.) to FP (200 μg b.i.d.) in 3-month inhalation therapy significantly decreased submucosal mast cells to the level obtained by monotherapy with a higher FP dose (500 μg b.i.d.), whereas monotherapy with FP at 200 μg b.i.d. was not effective (Wallin et al., 2003). In contrast to these results in bronchial biopsies, the number of sputum eosinophils in mild asthma was not decreased by addition of FORM (12 μg b.i.d.) to BUD (100 μg b.i.d.) after 1-month inhalation therapy (Green et al., 2006). Moreover, even in a 1-year study, the addition of SALM (50 μg b.i.d.) to FP (250 μg b.i.d.) had no effect on cell numbers and cytokine levels in sputum after allergen exposure (Koopmans et al., 2006). The difference between sputum and biopsy studies may suggest that LABA decrease eosinophil numbers in the airway wall at least partly by an increase of their clearance into the airway lumen.

While infiltration and activation of eosinophils are sensitive to ICS therapy, ICS seems to have little effect on airway neutrophilia, which is common in severe asthma exacerbations. ICS may even increase airway neutrophilia, as shown for FP (100 μg b.i.d. for 12 weeks) (Reid et al., 2003). Therefore, complementary effects of LABA may increase control over neutrophilic inflammation by ICS/LABA treatment. Indeed, FORM inhibited superoxide generation and elastase release by human neutrophils *in vitro* (Tintinger et al., 2000), and 4 weeks' treatment with inhaled FORM (24 μg b.i.d.) decreased neutrophil numbers and IL-8 levels in induced sputum in patients with mild asthma, while BUD (400 μg b.i.d. for 4 weeks) had less effect (Maneechotesuwan et al., 2005). SALM had no effects in the aforementioned Tintinger et al., study, but inhaled SALM (50 μg b.i.d. for 6 weeks) reduced neutrophil numbers in bronchial biopsies in mild stable asthma (Jeffery et al., 2002). The reduction of neutrophil chemoattractant IL-8 in the airways, as well as an induction of neutrophil apoptosis, may contribute to decreased airway neutrophilia by LABA (Jeffery et al., 2002; Maneechotesuwan et al., 2005; Reid et al., 2003). LABA are also known inhibitors of mast cell activation and these effects may complement or add to the effects of GCs, as shown with SALM and FP in immunologically activated human cultured mast cells (Akabane et al., 2006).

Dose and timing of ICS/LABA administration

A *sine qua non* for enhanced anti-inflammatory activity by ICS/LABA therapy is that inflammation is not fully controlled by ICS monotherapy so there is a potential for further improvement. The dose–response relationship for ICS is relatively flat because already low doses exert significant anti-inflammatory effects. This may explain why, in mild asthma, addition of inhaled FORM (12 µg b.i.d.) to BUD (100 or 400 µg b.i.d.) over an 8-week period did not further decrease eosinophil and mast cell immunostaining in bronchial biopsies, as the maximal effect was obtained already by BUD at 100 µg and was equal to that achieved by BUD at 400 µg (Overbeek et al., 2005). In a longer study by Kips et al., (2000), 1-month treatment with a high BUD dose (800 µg b.i.d.) significantly decreased the number of eosinophils in induced sputum and no further improvement was observed during the following year when patients were treated with moderate doses of BUD (400 µg b.i.d.) alone or low doses (100 µg b.i.d.) together with FORM (12 µg b.i.d.). Similarly, there were no significant differences on multiple indices of airway inflammation monitored in asthmatics treated for 24 weeks with FP 250 µg b.i.d. compared to combination therapy with a lower dose of FP (100 µg) inhaled twice daily in one inhaler with SALM (50 µg) (Jarjour et al., 2006). Importantly, these studies demonstrate that low doses of ICS administered together with a LABA effectively control airway inflammation and are as effective as higher ICS doses, thus twice daily treatment with ICS/LABA is ICS sparing without masking inflammation.

Besides dosing, the timing of ICS/LABA inhalation in relation to allergen exposure is also important for the anti-inflammatory efficacy of combination therapy. In the previously mentioned Koopmans et al., study (2006), the authors pointed out that the lack of anti-inflammatory effect of SALM added to FP might have been caused by the fact that 12 h had passed between the last drug treatment and allergen challenge exposure. This seems to apply to ICS as well. Accordingly, a single dose of FP (250 µg) given 30 min before allergen challenge decreased allergen-induced late response, hyper-responsiveness and sputum eosinophils, whereas 2 weeks' treatment with FP (250 µg b.i.d.) had no significant effects when the last FP dose was given 24 h before allergen challenge (Parameswaran et al., 2000). These results were recently confirmed and extended in a study by Subbarao et al., (2005) showing that the protective effects of inhaled FP or BUD (both 200 µg b.i.d. for 7 days) against allergen challenge-induced early and late allergic responses and sputum eosinophilia were partially lost when allergen exposure occurred 12 h after the last ICS dose, and protection against bronchial hyper-responsiveness was completely lost. In contrast,

BUD (800 μg) inhaled after allergen exposure and followed by two additional inhalations at 2-h intervals inhibited the late asthmatic response and airway responsiveness (Paggiaro et al., 1994). Similarly, other studies have shown that ICS treatment continued during and after allergen exposure results in up to 50% decrease of the early response and nearly complete abolition of the late response, airway eosinophilia and allergen-induced airway hyper-reactivity (for review see Subbarao et al., 2005). Collectively, these results suggest that both ICS and LABA exert relatively rapid effects in asthmatic patients, and that maximal protection against allergen-induced responses requires more frequent inhalations of ICS/LABA around allergen exposure and during exacerbation periods. These findings provide the rationale for the adjustable Symbicort® dosing regimen and SMART, where Symbicort® dosing frequency is adjusted in response to symptom worsening or improvement to achieve maximal asthma control at the lowest effective doses.

10.9 Possible Mechanisms of Steroid-sparing Effects by Addition of LABA to ICS

It seems that there is a spectrum of responsiveness to steroids in asthma and that it is related to disease severity (Barnes, 2004). Multiple mechanisms may be responsible and they may differ between patients. There are experimental data to suggest that LABA are able to interfere with some of these mechanisms in a way that may decrease steroid requirements for an effective control of severe asthma and asthma exacerbations, and thereby achieving steroid-sparing effects.

Glucocorticoid receptor translocation

A prerequisite of GC action is an effective translocation of glucocorticoid receptor (GR), in a complex with a bound GC, from cell cytoplasm into the nucleus. GR translocation was shown to be significantly decreased in peripheral blood mononuclear cells (PBMCs) isolated from patients with steroid-resistant asthma and exposed to a GC *in vitro* (Matthews et al., 2004). Unexpectedly, Eickelberg et al., (1999) demonstrated that β_2-agonists are able to translocate GR in a ligand-independent way. These *in vitro* findings in human lung fibroblasts and vascular smooth-muscle cells were later confirmed by others in PBMCs and monocyte/macrophage cell lines (Yanagawa et al., 2001) and airway smooth-muscle cells (Roth et al., 2002). This effect was also shown *in vivo* in patients with asthma – in blood leukocytes after FORM inhalation (Leufgen et al., 2002) and in epithelial cells and macrophages from induced sputum after inhalation of SALM (Usmani et al., 2005). where the combination of a low FP dose with SALM resulted in an augmented GR translocation, compared to FP alone. However, LABA-induced GR-translocation could not be shown in cultured human bronchial epithelial cell (Loven et al., 2007; Yanagawa et al., 2001). In sputum eosinophils and macrophages isolated from asthmatics, *ex vivo* incubation with FORM or salbutamol had no effect on GR nuclear localization, however both β_2-agonists significantly increased GR translocation induced by BDP (Profita et al., 2005). Importantly, To et al. (2005a) demonstrated that the impaired dexamethasone-induced GR translocation in PBMCs from patients with steroid-insensitive severe asthma was restored to normal levels by cell co-incubation with a clinically relevant concentration of FORM (10^{-9} M). The mechanisms responsible for increased nuclear localization of GR by β_2-agonists are not yet clear, and besides an increased translocation of GR from cell cytoplasm into the cell nucleus they may include a decrease of GR export from the nucleus (Haque et al., 2006).

Gene transcription

Restoration of GR nuclear localization by the addition of LABA potentially leads to the restoration of the anti-inflammatory effects of GCs. Indeed, the sensitivity of dexamethasone to inhibit TNFα-induced IL-8 production in PBMCs from steroid-insensitive asthmatics was restored by addition of FORM (10^{-9} M) (To et al., 2005a) or SALM (10^{-8} M) (To et al., 2005b). GCs suppress inflammatory genes (transrepression) by inhibition of pro-inflammatory transcription factors, such as nuclear factor-κB (NF-κB) and activator protein-1 (AP-1). The evidence is growing that LABA, besides promoting GR translocation, may also suppress activation of NF-κB and AP-1 and as a result add to the GC-induced transrepression (Baouz et al., 2005; Fragaki et al., 2006; Nie et al., 2005; Wilson et al., 2001).

Recent findings suggest that in a substantial percentage of patients with severe asthma there is no defect of GR translocation in PBMCs but there is a reduction of histone deacetylase (HDAC) activity, resulting in reduced transrepressive effects of GCs (Hew et al., 2006; Mercado et al., 2006). Marked reduction of HDAC activity was also shown in alveolar macrophages and lung parenchyma in COPD, where it is related to the degree of inflammation and disease severity, and probably also contributes to relative steroid resistance (Barnes et al., 2005). HDACs and histone acetylases are important GR coactivator proteins, and they are critical for gene transrepression and transactivation, respectively. Impaired deacetylation of GR in alveolar macrophages from COPD patients was recently shown to be critical for the inability of GCs to repress NF-κB-mediated gene expression (Ito et al., 2006). Interestingly, LABA were shown to have the ability, like GCs, to inhibit TNFα-induced histone acetylation and subsequent NF-κB binding to a pro-inflammatory gene promoter, resulting in supression of gene transcription (Nie et al., 2005).

Although transrepression seems to be the most important mechanism by which GCs exert anti-inflammatory effects, transactivation of anti-inflammatory genes by GCs may be essential for anti-inflammatory control of severe asthma (Matthews et al., 2004). LABA were shown to increase GR binding to its DNA binding sites, and as a consequence also increased transactivation of several anti-inflammatory genes such as interleukin-10 (IL-10) (Adcock et al., 2003), secretory leuko-proteinase inhibitor (SLPI) and mitogen-activated protein kinase phosphatase-1 (MKP-1) (Usmani et al., 2005; Jazrawi et al., 2005). The activation of MKP-1 might be important for the restoration of GC sensitivity via dephosphorylation and inhibition of p38 mitogen-activated protein kinase, which appears to play a crucial role in GR deactivation (Clark and Lasa, 2003). Importantly, most recently it was shown in human bronchial epithelial cell line and in primary human airway smooth muscle cells that GC-inducible gene expression was additively or synergistically inhanced by LABA to a level that could not be achieved by GCs alone (Kaur et al., 2007). Additionally, maximal responses exerted by GCs were achieved at approximately 10-fold lower GC concentrations in the presence of LABA. Gene transactivation seems to require higher concentrations of GCs than gene transrepression (Adcock et al., 1999). This may contribute to increased GC requirement for control of amplified inflammatory processes in severe asthma and asthma exacerbations. Therefore, enhanced transactivation of anti-inflammatory genes by addition of LABA to ICS may essentially contribute to the steroid-sparing effect of ICS/LABA therapy.

A coordinated control of transcription of various genes by GCs and LABA may also directly affect some aspects of airway remodelling in asthma (besides indirect effects via decrease of inflammation). For example, the enhanced anti-proliferative effect of BUD and FORM in primary cell cultures of human airway smooth muscle cells was, besides an increased GR translocation, the result of synergistically enhanced promoter activation of p21 (cip1/waf1) gene (a negative cell-cycle control protein inhibiting cell proliferation), induced by interaction between GR and β_2-agonist-activated CCAAT-enhancer binding protein-α (C/EBP-α) (Roth et al., 2002). Recently, a synergistic induction of another negative cell-cyle control protein gene, p57KIP2, was shown by GC/LABA treatment in primary human airway smooth muscle cells, suggesting synergistic inhibition of airway smooth muscle cell hyperplasia characteristic of asthma.

Dosing frequency of ICS/LABA

Allergen exposures and rhinoviral infections play a critical role in the induction of exacerbations in asthma. Allergen exposure requires more intensive ICS therapy in patients with allergic asthma, probably due to amplified airway inflammation and induction of a decrease in sensitivity to ICS via multiple mechanisms (Leung and Bloom, 2003). Likewise, virus-induced exacerbations are relatively resistant to ICS, and reduction of GR translocation by rhinovirus may be a contributing factor (Bellettato et al., 2003). As reviewed in this chapter, temporarily increased steroid requirements in asthma exacerbations may be kept down by addition of LABA, and mechanisms responsible include increased anti-inflammatory efficacy and enhanced steroid responsiveness. However, in addition, the previously mentioned findings of the relatively short-lived protective effects of ICS and LABA against allergen-challenge responses provide the rationale for adjustable ICS/LABA dosing frequency as a more effective and steroid-sparing therapy than fixed twice-daily dosing regimen.

An early study of Toogood et al., (1982) demonstrated that the same total dose of inhaled BUD divided into four-times-daily inhalation was more effective in severe unstable asthma than when delivered twice daily, indicating that an increase of ICS dosing frequency is more important than the total ICS dose delivered. As efficacy of ICS in the airways depends on ICS concentrations in airway tissue, it is likely that ICS local kinetics provides an explanation for the results of Toogood et al., (1982). ICS concentrations achieved in airway tissue after inhalation are high ($\sim10^{-7}$ M) but they decline rapidly over the next few hours, reaching a 10–100-fold lower but more stable level (Jendbro et al., 2001; Miller-Larsson et al., 1998). These lower concentrations are obviously sufficient to control low inflammatory activity during periods of good asthma control. However, they seem to be insufficient to inhibit amplified inflammation and to counteract induction of relative steroid insensitivity during asthma exacerbations. More frequent inhalations and high airway concentrations may also induce, and allow greater benefits from, rapid non-genomic effects of GCs (Norman et al., 2004), which may be especially important in acute asthma. From kinetics and modelling studies, the conclusion can be drawn that an increase of ICS dosing frequency from 2 to 3–4 per day increases ICS concentrations in the airway tissue more than when doubling the ICS dose delivered twice daily (Jendbro et al., 2001). This would explain why increasing the ICS dosing frequency is more effective than increasing the dose itself. It is likely that this is also valid for LABA as their airway efficacy is also determined by their airway kinetics.

Together these findings provide an explanation for effective and steroid-sparing therapy with adjustable dosing frequency of BUD/FORM (including SMART). Accordingly, increased BUD/FORM dosing frequency during approaching exacerbations increases BUD and FORM concentrations in airway and lung tissue and thus enables effective inhibition of rising inflammation and bronchoconstriction. Decreased BUD/FORM dosing frequency during well-controlled periods maintains sufficient drug concentrations in airway and lung tissue for maximal control and safety.

References

Aalbers R, Backer V, Kava TTK, Omenaas ER, Sandström T, Jorup C, Welte T. Adjustable maintenance dosing with budesonide/formoterol improves asthma control compared with fixed-dose salmeterol/fluticasone. *Curr Med Res Opin* 2004; **20**: 225–240.

Adcock IM, Nasuhara Y, Stevens DA, Barnes PJ. Ligand-induced differentiation of glucocorticoid receptor (GR) trans-repression and transactivation: preferential targetting of NF-κB and lack of I-κB involvement. *Br J Pharmacol* 1999; **127**: 1003–10011.

Adcock IM, Yanagawa H, Hewitt AH, Buck H. Effects of long-acting β-agonists and glucocorticoids on cytokine expression. *Am J Respir Crit Care Med* 2003; **167**: A356.

Akabane H, Murata M, Kufota M, Takashima E, Tanaka H, Inagaki N, Horifa M, Nagai H. Effects of salmeterol xinafoate and fluticasone propionate on immunological activation of human cultured mast cells. *Allergol Int* 2006; **55**: 387–393.

Ammit AJ, Lazaar AL, Irani C, O'Neill GM et al. Tumor necrosis factor-α-induced secretion of RANTES and interleukin-6 from human airway smooth muscle cells: modulation by glucocorticoids and beta-agonists. *Am J Respir Cell Mol Biol* 2002; **26**: 465–474.

Ankerst J. Combination inhalers containing inhaled corticosteroids and long-acting β_2-agonists: improved clinical efficacy and dosing options in patients with asthma. *J Asthma* 2005; **42**: 715–724.

Baouz S, Giron-Michel J, Azzarone B, Giuliani M et al. Lung myofibroblasts as targets of salmeterol and fluticasone propionate: inhibition of α-SMA and NF-κB. *Int Immunol* 2005; **17**: 1473–1481.

Baraniuk J, Murray JJ, Nathan RA, Berger WE et al. Fluticasone alone or in combination with salmeterol versus triamcinolone in asthma. *Chest* 1999; **116**: 625–632.

Barnes PJ. Corticosteroid resistance in airway disease *Proc Am Thorac Soc* 2004; **1**: 264–268.

Barnes PJ, Adcock IM, Ito K. Histone acetylation and deacetylation: importance in inflammatory lung diseases. *Eur Respir J* 2005; **25**: 552–563.

Barnes PJ, Pedersen S, Busse WW. Efficacy and safety of inhaled corticosteroids. New developments. *Am J Respir Crit Care Med* 1998; **157**: S1–S53.

Bateman ED, Bantje TA, Joao Gomes M, Toumbis M, Huber R, Naya I, Eliraz A. Combination therapy with single inhaler budesonide/formoterol compared with high dose of fluticasone propionate alone in patients with moderate persistent asthma. *Am J Respir Med* 2003; **2**: 275–281.

Bellettato C, Adcock IM, Ito K, Caramori G et al. Rhinovirus infection reduces glucocorticoid receptor nuclear translocation in airway epithelial cells. *Am J Respir Crit Care Med* 2003; **167**: A578.

Bisgaard H, LeRoux P, Bjåmer D, Dymek A, Vermeulen JH, Hultquist C. Budesonide/formoterol maintenance plus reliever therapy: a new strategy in pediatric asthma. *Chest* 2006; **130**: 1733–1743.

Bloom J, Calhoun W, Koenig S, Yancey S et al. Fluticasone propionate/salmeterol 100/50 mcg is inhaled steroid sparing in patients who require fluticasone propionate 250 mcg for asthma stability. *Am J Respir Crit Care Med* 2003; **167**: A891.

Buhl R. Budesonide/formoterol for the treatment of asthma. *Expert Opin Pharmacother* 2003; **4**: 1393–1406.

Buhl R, Kardos P, Richter K, Meyer-Sabellek W, Brüggenjürgen B, Willich SN, Vogelmeier C. The effect of adjustable dosing with budesonide/formoterol on health-related quality of life and asthma control compared with fixed dosing. *Curr Med Res Opin* 2004; **20**: 1209–1220.

Busse WW, Chervinsky P, Condemi J, Lumry WR, Petty TL, Rennard S, Townley RG. Budesonide delivered by Turbuhaler is effective in a dose-dependent fashion when used in the treatment of adults with chronic asthma. *J Allergy Clin Immunol* 1998; **101**: 457–463.

Busse W, Koenig SM, Oppenheimer J, Sahn SA et al. Steroid-sparing effects of fluticasone propionate 100 µg and salmeterol 50 µg administered twice daily in a single product in patients previously controlled with fluticasone propionate 250 µg administered twice daily. *J Allergy Clin Immunol* 2003; **111**: 57–65.

Calverley PM, Boonsawat W, Cseke Z, Zhong N, Peterson S, Olsson H. Maintenance therapy with budesonide and formoterol in chronic obstructive pulmonary disease. *Eur Respir J* 2003; **22**: 912–919.

Canonica GW, Castellani P, Cazzola M, Fabbri LM et al. Adjustable maintenance dosing with budesonide/formoterol in a single inhaler provides effective asthma symptom control at a lower dose than fixed maintenance dosing. *Pulm Pharmacol Ther* 2004; **17**: 239–247.

Clark AR, Lasa M. Crosstalk between glucocorticoids and mitogen-activated protein kinase signalling pathways. *Curr Opin Pharmacol* 2003; **3**: 404–411.

Contoli M, Message SD, Laza-Stanca V, Edwards MR et al. Role of deficient type III interferon-lambda production in asthma exacerbations. *Nat Med* 2006; **12**: 1023–1026.

Edwards MR, Johnson MW, Johnston SL. Combination therapy: Synergistic suppression of virus-induced chemokines in airway epithelial cells. *Am J Respir Cell Mol Biol* 2006; **34**: 616–624.

Eickelberg O, Roth M, Lörx R, Bruce V, Rüdiger J, Johnson M, Block LH. Ligand-independent activation of the glucocorticoid receptor by β_2-adrenergic receptor agonists in primary human lung fibroblasts and vascular smooth muscle cells. *J Biol Chem* 1999; **274**: 1005–1010.

Ellul-Micallef R, Johansson SÅ. Acute dose–response studies in bronchial asthma with a new corticosteroid, budesonide. *Brit J Clin Pharmacol* 1983; **15**: 419–422.

FitzGerald JM, Becker A, Sears MR, Mink S, Chung K, Lee J, Canadian Asthma Exacerbation Study Group. Doubling the dose of budesonide versus maintenance treatment in asthma exacerbations. *Thorax* 2004a; **59**: 550–556.

FitzGerald JM, Olsson P, Michils A. Adjustable maintenance dosing with budesonide/formoterol in a single inhaler – efficacy and safety. *Int J Clin Pract* 2004b; **58**: 18–25.

FitzGerald JM, Sears MR, Boulet L-P, Becker AB et al. Adjustable maintenance dosing with budesonide/formoterol reduces asthma exacerbations compared with traditional fixed dosing: a five-month multicentre Canadian study. *Can Respir J* 2003; **10**: 427–434.

Foresi A, Morelli MC, Catena E. Low-dose budesonide with the addition of an increased dose during exacerbations is effective in long-term asthma control. *Chest* 2000; **117**: 400–406.

Fragaki K, Kileztky C, Trentesaux C, Zahm JM, Bajolet O, Johnson M, Puchelle E. Downregulation by a long-acting β_2-adrenergic receptor agonist and corticosteroid of Staphylococcus aureus-induced airway epithelial inflammatory mediator production. *Am J Physiol Lung Cell Mol Physiol* 2006; **291**: L11–18.

Gibson PG. Teaching old drugs new tricks: asthma therapy adjusted by patient perception or noninvasive markers. *Eur Respir J* 2005; **25**: 397–399.

Gibson PG, Powell H, Ducharme F. Long-acting beta$_2$-agonists as an inhaled corticosteroid-sparing agent for chronic asthma in adults and children. *Cochrane Database Systematic Review* 2005; 4: CD005076.

Global Initiative for Asthma (GINA). Global Strategy for Asthma Management and Prevention. Publication no. NIH-NHLI 02-3569. Bethesda, MD: National Institutes of Health 2002.

Green RH, Brightling CE, McKenna S, Hargadon B et al. Comparison of asthma treatment given in addition to inhaled corticosteroids on airway inflammation and responsiveness. *Eur Respir J* 2006; **27**: 1144–1151.

Greening AP, Ind PW, Northfield M, Shaw G. Added salmeterol versus higher-dose corticosteroid in asthma patients with symptoms on existing inhaled steroid. *Lancet* 1994; **344**: 219–224.

Greiff L, Andersson M, Svensson C, Akerlund A, Alkner U, Persson CG. Effects of two weeks of topical budesonide treatment on microvascular exudative responsiveness in healthy human nasal airways. *Eur Respir J* 1997; **10**: 841–845.

Greiff L, Wollmer P, Andersson M, Svensson C, Persson CGA. Effects of formoterol on histamine induced plasma exudation in induced sputum from normal subjects. *Thorax* 1998; **53**, 1010–1013.

Harrison TW, Oborne J, Newton S, Tattersfield AE. Doubling the dose of inhaled corticosteroid to prevent asthma exacerbations: randomised controlled trial. *Lancet* 2004; **363**: 271–275.

Haque RA, Johnson M, Adcock IM, Barnes PJ. Addition of salmeterol to fluticasone prolongs retention of glucocorticoid receptors within the nucleus of BEAS-2B cells and enhances downstream glucocorticoid effects. *Proc Am Thorac Soc* 2006; **3**: A78.

Hew M, Bhavsar P, Torrego A, Meah S et al. Relative corticosteroid insensitivity of peripheral blood mononuclear cells in severe asthma. *Am J Respir Crit Care Med* 2006; **174**: 134–141.

Ind PW, Dal Negro R, Colman NC, Fletcher CP, Browning D, James MH. Addition of salmeterol to fluticasone propionate treatment in moderate-to-severe asthma. *Respir Med* 2003; **97**: 555–562.

Ind PW, Haughney J, Price D, Rosen J-P, Kennelly J. Adjustable and fixed dosing with budesonide/formoterol via a single inhaler in asthma patients: the ASSURE study. *Respir Med* 2004; **98**: 464–475.

Ito K, Yamamura S, Essilfie-Quaye S, Cosio B, Ito M, Barnes PJ, Adcock IM. Histone deacetylase 2-mediated deacetylation of the glucocorticoid receptor enables NF-κB suppression. *J Exp Med* 2006; **203**: 7–13.

Jarjour NN, Wilson SJ, Koenig SM, Laviolette M et al. Control of airway inflammation maintained at a lower steroid dose with 100/50 μg of fluticasone propionate/salmeterol. *J Allergy Clin Immunol* 2006; **118**: 44–52.

Jazrawi E, Ito K, Barnes PJ, Adcock IM. Effect of budesonide and formoterol on glucocorticoid receptor DNA binding and transactivation in BEAS-2B cells *Proc Am Thorac Soc* 2005; **2**: A108.

Jeffery PK, Venge P, Gizycki MJ, Egerod I, Dahl R, Faurschou P. Effects of salmeterol on mucosal inflammation in asthma: a placebo-controlled study. *Eur Respir J* 2002; **20**: 1378–1385.

Jendbro M, Johansson CJ, Strandberg P, Falk-Nilsson H, Edsbäcker S. Pharmacokinetics of budesonide and its major ester metabolite after inhalation and intravenous administration of budesonide in the rat. *Drug Metab Dispos* 2001; **29**: 769–776.

Jenkins C, Woolcock AJ, Saarelainen P, Lundbäck B, James MH. Salmeterol/fluticasone propionate combination therapy 50/250 μg bid is more effective than budesonide 800 μg bid in treating moderate-to-severe asthma. *Respir Med* 2000; **94**: 715–723.

Johansson G, McIvor RA, Purello D'Ambrosio F, Gratziou C, James MH. Comparison of salmeterol/fluticasone propionate combination with budesonide in patients with mild-to-moderate asthma. *Clin Drug Invest* 2001; **21**: 633–642.

Kaur M, Chivers JE, Giembycz MA, Newton R. Long-acting β$_2$-adrenoceptor agonists synergistically enhance glucocorticoid-dependent transcription in human airways epithelial and smooth muscle cells. *Mol Pharmacol* 2007; [Epub ahead of print].

Kips JC, O'Connor J, Inman MD, Svensson K, Pauwels RA, O'Byrne PM. A long-term study of the antiinflammatory effect of low-dose budesonide plus formoterol versus high-dose budesonide in asthma. *Am J Respir Crit Care Med* 2000; **161**: 996–1001.

Koopmans JG, Lutter R, Jansen HM, van der Zee JS. Adding salmeterol to an inhaled corticosteroid: long term effects on bronchial inflammation in asthma. *Thorax* 2006; **61**: 306–312.

Korn SH, Jerre A, Brattsand R. Effects of formoterol and budesonide on GM-CSF and IL-8 secretion by triggered human bronchial epithelial cells. *Eur Respir J* 2001; **17**: 1070–1077.

Lalloo UG, Malolepszy J, Kozma D, Krofta K, Ankerst J, Johansen B, Thomson NC. Budesonide and formoterol in a single inhaler improves asthma control compared with increasing the dose of corticosteroid in adults with mild-to-moderate asthma. *Chest* 2003; **123**: 1480–1487.

Lemanske RF, Sorkness CA, Mauger EA, Lazarus SC et al. Inhaled corticosteroid reduction and elimination in patients with persistent asthma receiving salmeterol. *J Amer Med Assoc* 2001; **285**: 2594–2603.

Leufgen H, Rüdiger JJ, Herrmann MJ, Meyer L et al. Glucocorticoid receptor activation by steroids and long-acting β$_2$-agonists *in vivo*: A double-blind crossover study. *Am J Respir Crit Care Med* 2002; **165**: A618.

Leung DY, Bloom JW. Update on glucocorticoid action and resistance. *J Allergy Clin Immunol* 2003; **111**: 3–22.

Leuppi JD, Salzberg M, Meyer L, Bucher SE, Nief M, Brutsche MH, Tamm M. An individualized, adjustable maintenance regimen of budesonide/formoterol provides effective asthma symptom control at a lower overall dose than fixed dosing. *Swiss Med Wkly* 2003; **133**: 302–309.

Li X, Ward C, Thien F, Bish R et al. An antiinflammatory effect of salmeterol, a long-acting β$_2$ agonist, assessed in airway biopsies and bronchoalveolar lavage in asthma. *Am J Respir Crit Care Med* 1999; **160**: 1493–1499.

Lipworth BJ, Jackson M. Safety of inhaled and intranasal corticosteroids. Lessons for the new millennium. *Drug Safety* 2000; **23**: 11–33.

Lovén J, Svitacheva N, Jerre A, Miller-Larsson A, Korn SH. Anti-inflammatory activity of β$_2$-agonists in primary lung epithelial cells is independent of glucocorticoid receptor. *Eur Respir J* 2007; **30**: 848–856.

Maneechotesuwan K, Essilfie-Quaye S, Meah S, Kelly C, Kharitonov SA, Adcock IM, Barnes PJ. Formoterol attenuates neutrophilic airway inflammation in asthma. *Chest* 2005; **128**: 1936–1942.

Matthews JG, Ito K, Barnes PJ, Adcock IM. Defective glucocorticoid receptor nuclear translocation and altered histone acetylation patterns in glucocorticoid-resistant patients. *J Allergy Clin Immunol* 2004; **113**: 1100–1108.

McIvor RA, Pizzichini E, Turner MO, Hussack P, Hargreave FE, Sears MR. Potential masking effects of salmeterol on airway inflammation in asthma. *Am J Respir Crit Care Med* 1998; **158**: 924–930.

Mercado N, To Y, Ito M, Adcock IM, Barnes PJ, Ito K. Two novel phenotypes in severe asthma may require distinct treatments. *Proc Am Thorac Soc* 2006; **3**: A16.

Michils A, Peché R, Verbraeken J, Vandenhoven G, Wollaert L, Duquenne V. SURF Study: real-life effectiveness of budesonide/formoterol (B/F) adjustable maintenance dosing. *Allergy Clin Immunol Int* 2003; **15**: 56, [Abstract P-2-39].

Miller-Larsson A, Mattsson H, Hjertberg E, Dahlbäck M, Tunek A, Brattsand R. Reversible fatty acid conjugation of budesonide. Novel mechanism for prolonged retention of topically applied steroid in airway tissue. *Drug Metab Dispos* 1998; **26**: 623–630.

Myo S, Zhu X, Myou S, Meliton AY et al. Additive blockade of β_2-integrin adhesion of eosinophils by salmeterol and fluticasone propionate. *Eur Respir J* 2004; **23**: 511–517.

Nie M, Knox AJ, Pang L. β_2-Adrenoceptor agonists, like glucocorticoids, repress eotaxin gene transcription by selective inhibition of histone H4 acetylation. *J Immunol* 2005; **175**: 478–86.

Nielsen LP, Pedersen B, Faurschou P, Madsen F, Wilcke JTR, Dahl R. Salmeterol reduces the need for inhaled corticosteroids in steroid-dependent asthmatics. *Respir Med* 1999; **93**: 863–868.

Nielson CP, Hadjokas NE. Beta-adrenoceptor agonists block corticosteroid inhibition in eosinophils. *Am J Respir Crit Care Med* 1998; **157**: 184–191.

Norman AW, Mizwicki MT, Norman DP. Steroid-hormone rapid actions, membrane receptors and a conformational ensemble model. *Nat Rev Drug Discov* 2004; **3**: 27–41.

O'Byrne PM, Barnes PJ, Rodriguez-Rousin R, Runnerstrom E, Sandstrom T, Svensson K, Tattersfield AE. Low dose inhaled budesonide and formoterol in mild persistent asthma. The OPTIMA randomized trial. *Am J Respir Crit Care Med* 2001; **164**: 1392–1397.

O'Byrne PM, Bisgaard H, Godard PP, Pistolesi M et al. Budesonide/formoterol combination therapy as both maintenance and reliever medication in asthma. *Am J Respir Crit Care Med* 2005; **171**: 129–136.

Oddera S, Silvestri M, Testi R, Rossi GA. Salmeterol enhances the inhibitory activity of dexamethasone on allergen-induced blood mononuclear cell activation. *Respiration* 1998; **65**: 199–204.

Orsida BE, Ward C, Li X, Bish R, Wilson JW, Thien F, Walters EH. Effect of a long-acting β_2-agonist over three months on airway wall vascular remodeling in asthma. *Am J Respir Crit Care Med* 2001; **164**: 117–121.

Overbeek SE, Mulder PG, Baelemans SM, Hoogsteden HC, Prins JB. Formoterol added to low-dose budesonide has no additional antiinflammatory effect in asthmatic patients. *Chest* 2005; **128**: 1121–1127.

Pace E, Gagliardo R, Melis M, La Grutta S et al. Synergistic effects of fluticasone propionate and salmeterol on *in vitro* T-cell activation and apoptosis in asthma. *J Allergy Clin Immunol* 2004; **114**: 1216–1223.

Paggiaro PL, Dente FL, Morelli MC, Bancalari L et al. Postallergen inhaled budesonide reduces late asthmatic response and inhibits the associated increase of airway responsiveness to methacholine in asthmatics. *Am J Respir Crit Care Med* 1994; **149**: 1447–1451.

Palmqvist M, Ibsen T, Mellén A, Lötvall J. Comparison of the relative efficacy of formoterol and salmeterol in asthmatic patients. *Am J Respir Crit Care Med* 1999; **160**: 244–249.

Pang L, Knox AJ. Synergistic inhibition by β_2-agonists and corticosteroids on tumor necrosis factor-α-induced interleukin-8 release from cultured human airway smooth-muscle cells. *Am J Respir Cell Mol Biol* 2000; **23**: 79–85.

Pang L, Knox AJ. Regulation of TNF-α-induced eotaxin release from cultured human airway smooth muscle cells by β_2-agonists and corticosteroids. *FASEB J* 2001; **15**: 261–269.

Parameswaran K, Inman MD, Watson RM, Morris MM et al. Protective effects of fluticasone on allergen-induced airway responses and sputum inflammatory markers. *Can Respir J* 2000; **7**: 313–319.

Pauwels RA, Löfdahl C-G, Postma DS, Tattersfield AE, O'Byrne PM, Barnes PJ, Ullman A. Effect of inhaled formoterol and budesonide on exacerbations of asthma. *N Engl J Med* 1997; **337**: 1405–1411.

Persdotter S, Lindahl M, Malm-Erjefält M, von Wachenfeldt, Korn SH, Stevens T, Miller-Larsson A. Cooperative effects of budesonide and formoterol on eosinophil superoxide production stimulated by bronchial epithelial cell conditioned medium. *Intern Arch Allergy Immunol* 2007; **143**: 201–210.

Profita M, Gagliardo R, Di Giorgi R, Pompeo F et al. Biochemical interaction between effects of beclomethasone dipropionate and salbutamol or formoterol in sputum cells from mild to moderate asthmatics. *Allergy* 2005; **60**: 323–329.

Rabe KF, Pizzichini E, Ställberg B, Romero S et al. Budesonide/formoterol in a single inhaler for maintenance and relief in mild-to-moderate asthma. A randomized, double-blind trial. *Chest* 2006; **129**: 246–256.

Reid DW, Ward C, Wang N, Zheng L, Bish R, Orsida B, Walters EH. Possible anti-inflammatory effect of salmeterol against interleukin-8 and neutrophil activation in asthma in vivo. *Eur Respir J* 2003; **21**: 994–999.

Ringdal N, Derom E, Wåhlin-Boll E, Pauwels R. Onset and duration of action of single doses of formoterol inhaled via Turbuhaler. *Respir Med* 1998; **92**: 1017–1021.

Roth M, Johnson PRA, Rüdiger JJ, King GG et al. Interaction between glucocorticoids and β_2 agonists on bronchial airway smooth muscle cells through synchronised cellular signalling. *Lancet* 2002; **360**: 1293–1299.

Scicchitano R, Aalbers R, Ukena D, Manjra A et al. Efficacy and safety of budesonide/formoterol single inhaler therapy versus a higher dose of budesonide in moderate to severe asthma. *Curr Med Res Opin* 2004; **20**: 1403–1418.

Seberová E, Andersson A. Oxis (formoterol given by Turbuhaler) showed as rapid an onset of action as salbutamol given by a pMDI. *Respir Med* 2000; **94**: 607–611.

Self T, Rumbak MJ, Kelso T, Eberle L et al. Does salmeterol facilitate "step-down" therapy in patients with asthma receiving moderate to high doses of inhaled corticosteroids? *Curr Ther Res* 1998; **59**: 803–811.

Silvestri M, Fregonese L, Sabatini F, Dasic G, Rossi GA. Fluticasone and salmeterol downregulate in vitro, fibroblast proliferation and ICAM-1 or H-CAM expression. *Eur Respir J* 2001; **18**: 139–145.

Sin DD, Man J, Sharpe H, Gan WQ, Man SFP. Pharmacological management to reduce exacerbations in adults with asthma: A systematic review and meta-analysis. *J Am Med Assoc* 2004; **292**: 367–376.

Spoelstra FM, Postma DS, Hovenga H, Noordhoek JA, Kauffman HF. Additive anti-inflammatory effect of formoterol and budesonide on human lung fibroblasts. *Thorax* 2002; **57**: 237–241.

Ställberg B, Olsson P, Jörgensen LA, Lindarck N, Ekström T. Budesonide/formoterol adjustable maintenance dosing reduces asthma exacerbations versus fixed dosing. *Int J Clin Pract* 2003; **57**: 656–661.

Subbarao P, Dorman SC, Rerecich T, Watson RM, Gauvreau GM, O'Byrne PM. Protection by budesonide and fluticasone on allergen-induced airway responses after discontinuation of therapy. *J Allergy Clin Immunol* 2005; **115**: 745–750.

Szafranski W, Cukier A, Ramirez A, Menga G et al. Efficacy and safety of budesonide/formoterol in the management of obstructive pulmonary disease. *Eur Respir J* 2003; **21**: 74–81.

Tattersfield AE, Postma DS, Barnes PJ, Svensson K et al. Exacerbations of asthma. A descriptive study of 425 severe exacerbations. *Am J Respir Crit Care Med* 1999; **160**: 594–599.

Tintinger GR, Anderson R, Theron AJ, Ramafi G, Ker JA. Comparison of the effects of selective and non-selective beta-adrenoreceptor agonists on the pro-inflammatory activities of human neutrophils *in vitro*. *Inflammation* 2000; **24**: 239–249.

To Y, Ito M, Adcock IM, Barnes PJ, Ito K. Formoterol restores corticosteroid responses in corticosteroid-insensitive asthma. *Eur Respir J* 2005a; **26**: 50s.

To Y, Adcock IM, Barnes PJ, Ito K. Salmeterol treatment improves corticosteroid responsiveness in patients with corticosteroid-insensitive severe asthma *Eur Respir J* 2005b; **26**: 465s.

Todorova L, Gürcan E, Miller-Larsson A, Westergren-Thorsson G. Lung fibroblast proteoglycan production induced by serum is inhibited by budesonide and formoterol. *Am J Respir Cell Mol Biol* 2006; **34**: 92–100.

Todorova L, Bjermer L, Miller-Larsson A, Westergren-Thorsson G. Inhibitory effects of fudesonide and formoterol in combination on TGFβ-induced proteoglycan production by bronchial biopsy fibroblasts from healthy and mild asthmatic subjects. *Eur Respir J* 2007; **30**: 352s

Toogood JH, Baskerville JC, Jennings B, Lefcoe NM, Johansson SA. Influence of dosing frequency and schedule on the response of chronic asthmatics to the aerosol steroid, budesonide. *J Allergy Clin Immunol* 1982; **70**: 288–298.

Ullman A, Svedmyr N. Salmeterol, a new long acting inhaled beta2adrenoceptor agonist: comparison with salbutamol in adult asthmatic patients. *Thorax* 1988; **43**: 674–678.

Usmani OS, Ito K, Maneechotesuwan K, Ito M, Johnson M, Barnes PJ, Adcock IM. Glucocorticoid receptor nuclear translocation in airway cells after inhaledcombination therapy. *Am J Respir Crit Care Med* 2005; **172**: 704–712.

Vanacker NJ, Palmans E, Pauwels RA, Kips JC. Effect of combining salmeterol and fluticasone on the progression of airway remodeling. *Am J Respir Crit Care Med* 2002; **166**: 1128–1134.

Vogelmeier C, D'Urzo A, Pauwels R, Merino JM et al. Budesonide/formoterol maintenance and reliever therapy: an effective asthma treatment option? *Eur Respir J* 2005; **26**: 819–828.

Volonaki E, Psarras S, Xepapadaki P, Psomali D, Gourgiotis D, Papadopoulos NG. Synergistic effects of fluticasone propionate and salmeterol on inhibiting rhinovirus-induced epithelial production of remodelling - associated growth factors. *Clin Exp Allergy* 2006; **36**: 1268–1273.

Wales D, Makker H, Kane J, McDowell P, O'Driscoll BR. Systemic bioavailability and potency of high-dose inhaled corticosteroids. A comparison of four inhaler devices and three drugs in healthy adult volunteers. *Chest* 1999; **115**: 1278–1284.

Wallin A, Sandström T, Cioppa GD, Holgate S, Wilson S. The effects of regular inhaled formoterol and budesonide on preformed Th-2 cytokines in mild asthmatics. *Respir Med* 2002; **96**: 1021–1025.

Wallin A, Sandström T, Söderberg M, Howarth P et al. The effects of regular inhaled formoterol, budesonide, and placebo on mucosal inflammation and clinical indices in mild asthma. *Am J Respir Crit Care Med* 1999; **159**: 79–86.

Wallin A, Sue-Chu M, Bjermer L, Ward J et al. Effect of inhaled fluticasone with and without salmeterol on airway inflammation in asthma. *J Allergy Clin Immunol* 2003; **112**: 72–78.

Wark PA, Johnston SL, Bucchieri F, Powell R et al. Asthmatic bronchial epithelial cells have a deficient innate immune response to infection with rhinovirus. *J Exp Med* 2005; **201**: 937–947.

Wilding P, Clark M, Thompson Coon J, Lewis S et al. Effect of long term treatment with salmeterol on asthma control: a double blind, randomised crossover study. *BMJ* 1997; **314**: 1441–1446.

Wilson SJ, Wallin A, Della-Cioppa G, Sandstrom T, Holgate ST. Effects of budesonide and formoterol on NF-κB, adhesion molecules, and cytokines in asthma. *Am J Respir Crit Care Med* 2001; **164**: 1047–1052.

Woolcock A, Lundback B, Ringdal, Jacques LA. Comparison of the addition of salmeterol to inhaled steroids with doubling the dose of inhaled steroids. *Am J Respir Crit Care Med* 1996; **153**: 1481–1488.

Yanagawa H, Ito K, Barnes PJ, Adcock IM. Formoterol-induced glucocorticoid receptor nuclear translocation in monocytes and U937 cells but not epithelial cell lines. *Am J Respir Crit Care Med* 2001; **163**: A734.

11

Steroid-sparing Strategies: Other Combinations

Gaetano Caramori, Kazuhiro Ito and Alberto Papi

11.1 Introduction

In this chapter we will analyse the scientific and clinical rationale of using other steroid-sparing strategies in the treatment of asthma and/or chronic obstructive pulmonary disease (COPD), excluding long-acting inhaled β_2-agonists and kinase inhibitors that are reviewed in other chapters of this book.

11.2 Theophylline as Steroid-sparing Treatment in Asthma and COPD

Despite the extensive use of theophylline in the treatment of asthma, the molecular mechanisms of action of this drug have not been completely clarified (Barnes, 2003a, 2005). Several mechanisms of action have been proposed. Theophylline is a non-selective phosphodiesterase (PDE) inhibitor and increases intracellular cyclic adenosine monophosphate (cAMP) and cyclic guanosine monophosphate (cGMP) levels, resulting in airway smooth-muscle relaxation and inhibition of inflammatory cell activation. Theophylline is a relatively weak inhibitor of PDEs, although there is evidence to suggest that PDE activity is elevated in the inflammatory cells of atopic subjects, and thus an altered responsiveness to PDE inhibitors may, in part, explain the mechanism of action of theophylline (Barnes, 2003a, 2005). Glucocorticoid suppression of inflammatory genes requires recruitment of histone deacetylases (HDACs) to the activation complex by the glucocorticoid receptor (GR)

Overcoming Steroid Insensitivity in Respiratory Disease   Edited by Ian M. Adcock and Kian Fan Chung
© 2008 John Wiley & Sons, Ltd.

(Barnes et al., 2005). HDACs are not effective in switching off inflammatory genes unless recruited to the active inflammatory site by activated GRs. Increased oxidative stress in COPD reduces HDAC2 expression and activity, thus potentially limiting glucocorticoid effectiveness in suppressing inflammation, as evidenced by *in vitro* studies and clinically in patients with COPD (Barnes, 2006). Theophylline, at concentrations that do not inhibit PDE4 activity, enhances HDAC2 activity and functionally this enhances glucocorticoid effects. Theophylline activates different subtypes of HDAC, under conditions of oxidative stress, with equal activation of HDAC1 and HDAC2. There appears to be a relatively selective effect on Class I HDACs, with less effect on Class II HDACs (Barnes, 2005). The mechanism whereby low concentrations of theophylline activate HDAC is not yet known, but it is not mediated by either PDE inhibition or adenosine receptor antagonism, because PDE inhibitors (non-selective and PDE3, PDE4 and PDE5 selective inhibitors) and adenosine A_1 and A_2 receptor antagonists do not mimic this action of theophylline (Barnes, 2005). Current studies are investigating nuclear signal transduction pathways that regulate HDAC2 activity and the effect of theophylline on these pathways (Figure 11.1). The

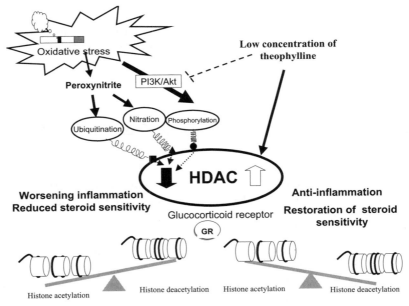

Figure 11.1 Increased oxidative stress in chronic obstructive pulmonary disease (COPD) reduces histone deacetylase (HDAC) expression and activity through its ubiquitination, nitration and phosphorylation [mediated by phosphoinositide 3-kinases (PI3K) and V-akt murine thymoma viral oncogene homolog (Akt) kinases] increasing the histone acetylation/deacetylation balance and thus potentially worsening inflammation and limiting glucocorticoid effectiveness in suppressing inflammation. Theophylline, at low concentrations that do not inhibit phosphodiesterase 4(PDE4) activity, enhances HDAC activity and inhibits the PI3K/Akt kinases. This functionally decreases the histone acetylation/deacetylation balance and thus potentially limits inflammation and enhances glucocorticoid effects

novel action of theophylline predicts that theophylline alone would have a relatively weak anti-inflammatory action, whereas theophylline should potentiate the anti-inflammatory actions of glucocorticoids (Barnes, 2005).

Asthma

Clinically, theophylline has been used in the treatment of asthma for many decades and it is still used worldwide for the treatment of asthma. However, theophylline has only recently been shown to have significant anti-inflammatory effects in asthma (Caramori and Adcock, 2003). Thus, theophylline has been shown to inhibit the activation of eosinophils, neutrophils, monocytes and T lymphocytes (Barnes, 2003a; Barnes et al., 2005). Low-dose theophylline reduces the increase in eosinophils in bronchial biopsies after allergen challenge and withdrawal of theophylline in patients with severe persistent asthma is associated with an increase in airway T lymphocytes (Caramori and Adcock, 2003).

Theophylline alone or in combination with inhaled glucocorticoids may maintain asthma control but in asthmatics regular treatment with sustained-release theophylline does not reduce the severity of bronchial hyper-responsiveness (Caramori and Adcock, 2003).

Long-term treatment with sustained-release theophylline alone is effective in controlling asthma symptoms and improving lung function in patients with mild persistent asthma (Global Initiative for Asthma (GINA) 2006). The use of theophylline, however, has declined owing to the widespread use of inhaled glucocorticoids, which remain the most effective treatment for asthma (Barnes, 2003a, 2005). One of the limitations of theophylline in the past has been the side effects observed in many patients at the traditional bronchodilator doses associated with plasma levels of theophylline between 10 and 20 mg/l. However, anti-inflammatory benefits appear to occur at lower plasma theophylline levels (<10 mg/l), and the incidence of any adverse effects is minimized (Barnes, 2003a, 2005). Many studies have demonstrated that low-dose theophylline added to inhaled glucocorticoids is equally efficacious when compared with increasing the dose of inhaled glucocorticoids in symptomatic patients established on inhaled glucocorticoid therapy (Evans et al., 1997; Ukena et al., 1997). However, in these patients, long-acting inhaled β_2-agonists are at least as effective as theophylline and with fewer adverse effects (GINA, 2006; Kankaanranta et al., 2004; Shah et al., 2003).

COPD

Despite most current COPD guidelines stating that theophylline is of limited value in the routine management of COPD, many controlled clinical trials support its utility in stable COPD patients and further larger studies are required for comparison with the other available bronchodilators. Airway biopsy studies are required to evaluate whether low-dose theophylline has, as demonstrated in bronchial asthma, a significant *in vivo* anti-inflammatory activity (Caramori and Adcock, 2003). Long-acting inhaled β2-agonists (LABA) seem to have additive effects when used in combination with anticholinergics or theophylline. Again, further controlled clinical trials are required to evaluate the long-term effects in stable COPD of LABA in combination with anticholinergics (in separate inhalers or in a single inhaler) and low-dose theophylline (Tennant et al., 2003).

11.3   Selective Inhibitors of PDE4

A class of promising novel anti-inflammatories for asthma and COPD are the selective inhibitors of PDE4. Phosphodiesterases hydrolyse intracellular cyclic nucleotides such as cAMP and cGMP into inactive 5′ monophosphates, and exist as 11 families. They are found in a variety of inflammatory and structural cells of the lung. Inhibitors of PDEs allow the elevation of cAMP and cGMPs, which leads to a variety of cellular effects, including airway smooth-muscle relaxation and inhibition of cellular inflammation or of immune responses (Chung, 2006a). PDE4 inhibitors specifically prevent the hydrolysis of cAMP. PDE4 is expressed in macrophages, eosinophils, neutrophils, T cells, bronchial epithelial and airway smooth-muscle cells (Figure 11.2). These

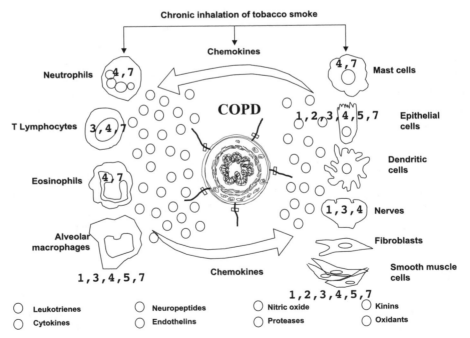

Figure 11.2 Expression of different isoforms of phosphodiesterase enzymes in the inflammatory and structural cells of lung with chronic obstructive pulmonary disease (COPD)

compounds inhibit the hydrolysis of intracellular cAMP, which may result in bron-chodilation and suppression of inflammation. Selective PDE4 inhibitors have broad spectrum anti-inflammatory effects such as inhibition of cell trafficking, and activation of many inflammatory cells such as neutrophils, eosinophils, macrophages and T cells (Caramori and Adcock, 2003; Chung, 2006a) (Figure 11.3).

There are many compounds in this new class of drugs in clinical development. The second generation PDE4 inhibitors, cilomilast and roflumilast, have reached clinical trial stage and have beneficial effects in asthma and COPD. The emerging results of clinical trials on PDE4 inhibitors in asthma and COPD should be interpreted with cautious optimism since much of the evidence has been published only in abstract form to date (Lipworth, 2005). The next few years should resolve important issues about the potential role of these drugs as oral non-steroidal anti-inflammatory therapy for asthma and COPD and their place in management guidelines (Lipworth, 2005).

Ultimately, clinicians will want to know whether PDE4 inhibitors are anything more than expensive "designer" theophylline, the archetypal non-selective PDE inhibitor (Lipworth, 2005). A potential problem with PDE4 inhibitors is their side-effect profile, particularly nausea, vomiting and other gastrointestinal effects. Topical administration of PDE4 inhibitors by inhalation may provide a wider therapeutic range (Barnes, 2003a, 2005).

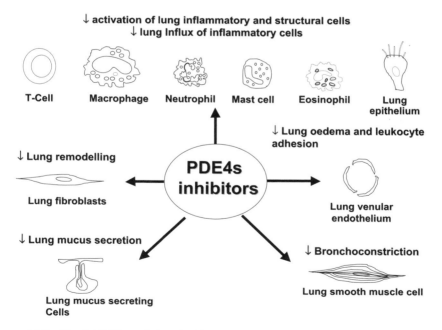

Figure 11.3 The inhibition of phosphodiesterase 4 (PDE4) in the inflammatory and structural cells of the lung has a variety of anti-inflammatory effects

The human PDE4 family is comprised of four isoenzymes (PDE4-A–D) and each has several splice variants. The four isoenzymes are differentially expressed among tissue and cells and it might be possible to develop isoenzyme-subtype-selective inhibitors in the future that could preserve the anti-inflammatory effect while having less propensity to side effects (Barnes, 2003a, 2005). PDE4-D appears to be of particular importance in nausea and vomiting and is expressed in the chemosensitive trigger zone in the brain stem. In mice, deletion of the gene for PDE4-D prevents a behavioural equivalent of emesis. This isoenzyme appears to be less important in anti-inflammatory effects and targeted gene disruption studies in mice indicate that PDE4-B is more important than PDE4-D in inflammatory cells (Barnes, 2003a, 2005). PDE4-B-selective inhibitors may, therefore, have a greater therapeutic to side-effect ratio and theoretically might be effective anti-inflammatory drugs (Barnes, 2003a, 2005). Cilomilast is selective for PDE4-D and this explains its propensity to cause emesis, whereas roflumilast, which is non-selective for PDE4 isoenzymes, has a more favourable therapeutic ratio. Several other potent PDE4 inhibitors with a more favourable therapeutic ratio are now in clinical development for COPD (Barnes, 2005; Chung, 2006a). Other problems with PDE4 inhibitors include an increased susceptibility to *Klebsiella pneumoniae* infections, possibly related to decreased TNFα production. This latter problem could potentially be detrimental in COPD patients who often have chronic bacterial colonisation of the lower airways (Barnes, 2005). Furthermore, the development of irreversible mesenteric arteritis in rodents was a major concern by the United States Food and Drug Administration's Pulmonary-Allergy Drug Advisory Committee in their review of cilomilast application for its use as a novel therapy for COPD (United States Food and Drug Administration, www.fda.gov/ohrms/dockets/ac/03/slides/3976s1.htm). Whether PDE4 inhibitors can cause mesenteric arteritis in humans, however, and whether this has any causal role in the gastrointestinal adverse effects of PDE4 inhibitors reported in humans have still not been established (Barnes, 2005).

Asthma

In asthma, roflumilast taken as a once-daily oral dose of 500 µg has been shown to improve clinical symptoms and lung function, prevent exercise- and allergen-induced asthma and decrease bronchial airway hyper-responsiveness. Once-daily oral roflumilast 500 µg is comparable with inhaled twice-daily beclomethasone (400 µg/day) in improving pulmonary function and asthma symptoms, and reducing rescue medication use in patients with persistent asthma (Chung, 2006a; Lipworth, 2005). However, there are no data on the steroid-sparing role of roflumilast in asthmatic patients. Interestingly, the development of cilomilast as an anti-asthma drug has been suspended.

COPD

Cilomilast and roflumilast are effective bronchodilators in COPD patients, giving greater reduction in dyspnoea than placebo. Cilomilast and roflumilast have been shown to reduce the exacerbation rate and to improve quality of life in patients with COPD (Chung, 2006a; Lipworth, 2005). Cilomilast has been shown to reduce the number of macrophages, $CD4^+$ and $CD8^+$ T lymphocytes and neutrophils in the bronchial biopsies of patients with COPD (Jeffery, 2005). As with asthma, there are no data available on the steroid-sparing role of roflumilast or cilomilast in COPD patients.

11.4 Modulators of the Synthesis or Action of Key Inflammatory Mediators

More than 100 pro- or anti-inflammatory mediators have now been implicated in asthmatic and/or COPD inflammation, including multiple cytokines, chemokines and growth factors (Barnes, 2004a; Barnes et al., 1998). Blocking a single mediator is therefore unlikely to be very effective in these complex diseases and single-mediator antagonists/agonists have so far not proved to be very effective compared with drugs that have a broad spectrum of anti-inflammatory effects, such as glucocorticoids or theophylline (Barnes, 2004a; Barnes et al., 1998).

11.5 Anticholinergics

Bronchodilators are the mainstay of current drug therapy for COPD (Global Initiative for COPD (GOLD), 2005). Bronchodilators cause only a small increase in forced expiratory volume in one second (FEV_1) in patients with COPD, but these drugs may improve symptoms by reducing hyperinflation and thus dyspnoea, and they may improve exercise tolerance (GOLD, 2006; Tennant et al., 2003). COPD appears to be more effectively treated by anticholinergic drugs than by $ß_2$-agonists, in sharp contrast to asthma, for which ß2-agonists are more effective (Tennant et al., 2003). Tiotropium is a novel anticholinergic drug with prolonged and selective antagonism at the muscarinic receptor subtype 3 (M_3) (Figure 11.4). Importantly, tiotropium decreases the number of hospital admissions for severe COPD exacerbations, suggesting the presence of non-bronchodilatating effects (Barr et al., 2006; Caramori and Adcock, 2003). Recent studies have demonstrated that acetylcholine is produced both in cholinergic nerves and non-neuronal cells in the lower airways. These cells include bronchial epithelial cells, endothelial cells, smooth muscle, lymphocytes

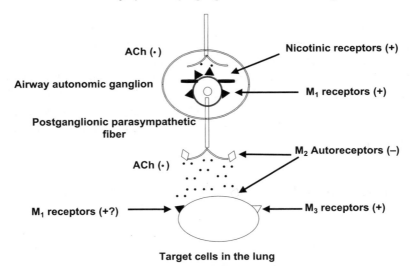

Figure 11.4   Acetylcholine (ACh) is produced and released in cholinergic nerves in the lower airways. ACh has strong bronchoconstrictor activity and stimulates mucus release in the lower airways through the stimulation of M_1, M_2 and M_3 muscarinic receptors located on its target cells. The activation of M_1 and M_3 receptors causes bronchoconstriction and mucus release. M_2 receptors act as autoreceptors, located mainly pre-junctionally on post-ganglionic parasympathetic nerve fibres, limiting the release of ACh and reducing airway smooth-muscle contraction and mucus release

and macrophages, configuring a true extra-neuronal airway cholinergic system (Racke and Matthiesen, 2004). This suggests the possibility that anticholinergic drugs might have inhibitory effects on inflammatory cells and that this may account for the 25% reduction in exacerbations of COPD seen in long-term studies with tiotropium (Barnes, 2004b).

There is clear evidence for additive effects of inhaled short-acting anticholinergics with inhaled short-acting $ß_2$-agonists, leading to the introduction of combination inhalers. There is emerging evidence that long-acting ß-agonists (LABA) and tiotropium may also have additive effects, suggesting that a combination of LABA and tiotropium or other long-acting anticholinergics may be useful (Tennant et al., 2003). A once-daily inhaler with a once-daily $ß_2$-agonist (many compounds in this class are in development; see Chapter 10 in this book) and a once-daily anticholinergic would, therefore, be ideal. The potential steroid-sparing activity of tiotropium alone or in combination (with LABA and/or low-dose theophylline) in asthma and COPD deserves to be investigated in controlled clinical trials, some of which are already underway.

11.6   Leukotriene Synthesis Inhibitors and Leukotriene Receptor Antagonists

Arachidonate 5-lipoxygenase (ALOX5; 5-LO) catalyses the two-step conversion of arachidonic acid to leukotriene A_4 (LTA$_4$), through the oxidation of arachidonic acid to the intermediate 5-hydroperoxyeicosatetraenoic acid (5-HPETE) followed by dehydration of 5-HPETE to form LTA$_4$ (Jampilek et al., 2006; Peters-Golden and Brock, 2003).

The gene ALOX5 is mapped on chromosome 10q11.21. ALOX5 action is regulated at many levels, including regulation of ALOX5 gene transcription and translation and of the activity of the mature protein (Jampilek et al., 2006). The ALOX5 promoter has a unique G+C-rich sequence, located between 176 and 147 bp upstream of the ATG translation start site, which contains five tandem Sp1 (a zinc-finger transcription factor) consensus binding sites overlapping five tandem Egr-1 (a zinc-finger transcription factor) consensus binding sites (Caramori and Adcock, 2003; Kalayci et al., 2006). There is a family of alleles in the promoter of the ALOX5 gene that is characterized by the deletion or addition of consensus Sp1 (5'GGGCGG3') and Egr-1 (-GCGGGGGCG-) binding motifs. Each of the variant alleles can bind Sp1 and Egr-1 protein. These alleles are less effective than the wild-type allele in initiating ALOX5 expression (Caramori and Adcock, 2003; Kalayci et al., 2006). ALOX5 is expressed in the lung in many cells involved in the asthmatic inflammation, such as eosinophils, mast cells and macrophages. Zileuton selectively and reversibly inhibits ALOX5 activity and is the only ALOX5 inhibitor currently marketed for the treatment of asthma (McGill and Busse, 1996).

ALOX5 activity depends on another protein named arachidonate 5-lipoxygenase-activating protein (ALOX5AP; FLAP), an arachidonic acid binding protein critical in the biosynthesis of leukotrienes. The ALOX5AP gene is mapped to the chromosome 13q12 region. After activation of the cell a stable complex between ALOX5, ALOX5AP and probably other enzymes is formed in the cellular membrane and this can translocate to the nucleus (Peters-Golden and Brock, 2003). 5-Lipoxygenase-activating protein inhibitors have not yet reached the market, because of their toxicity.

Leukotriene A_4 subsequently becomes a substrate for one of two enzymes, leukotriene A_4 epoxide hydrolase (LTA$_4$H) that catalyses the formation of LTB$_4$, or LTC$_4$ synthase that catalyses the formation of the cysteinyl leukotriene LTC$_4$.

The LTA$_4$H gene is located on chromosome 12q22. There are single nucleotide polymorphisms in the LTA$_4$H gene (such as rs2660845) that may downregulate the activity of LTA$_4$H, shunting LTA$_4$ away from the LTA$_4$H pathway and increasing the formation of Cysteinyl Leukotrienes (CysLTs) (Lima et al., 2006).

The gene coding for LTC$_4$S, the enzyme controlling CysLT biosynthesis, is located on chromosome 5q35 and exists as two common alleles distinguished by an adenine (A) to cytosine (C) transversion at a site 444 nucleotides upstream of the ATG translation start (C-444A) (Lam, 2003).

LTC_4 is transported to the extracellular space mainly by the multidrug resistance protein 1 (MRP1), a member of the ABC family of transmembrane transport proteins. MRP1 is highly expressed in human bronchial epithelial cells. The MRP1 gene is located on 16p13.12 and is highly polymorphic. A mutation in the last transmembrane segment influences LTC_4 transport and it is possible that MRP1 genetic variants (such as rs119774, which is located in intron 1) could have significant effects on LTC_4 transport and response to anti-leukotrienes (Lima et al., 2006). LTC_4 is converted to LTD_4 and LTE_4 by γ-glutamyltransferase and dipeptidase enzymes.

Neutrophils and alveolar macrophages prevalently produce LTB_4, whereas eosinophils prevalently produce LTC_4. Human lung mast cells produce LTC_4 and LTB_4 in response to stimulation from IgE, however the major eicosanoids released are prostaglandins (i.e. PGD_2) (Caramori and Adcock, 2003).

Leukotrienes induce their biological effects by stimulating specific receptors located on the plasma membrane of target cells. There are distinct receptors for LTB_4 and CysLTs, with no ligand cross-reactivity between these receptors. There are two subtypes of receptors (with high and low affinity) for LTB_4, respectively known as BLT1, expressed predominantly on the plasma membrane of the leukocytes (coupled via a G-protein to phospholipase C), and BLT2, which is more ubiquitous (Tager and Luster, 2003). Chemotactic LTB_4 activity is mediated by BLT1, while the inactivation of LTB_4 is promoted by peroxisome proliferator-activated receptor alpha (PPARα).

The actions of the CysLTs (LTC_4, LTD_4 and LTE_4) are mediated in humans through at least two distinct but related CysLT G-protein-coupled receptors, named respectively $CysLT_1$ and $CysLT_2$ (Capra et al., 2006). The human $CysLT_1$ receptor gene is a 337-amino-acid protein and its gene is mapped to the long arm of the X chromosome. $CysLT_2$ is a 346-amino-acid protein with 38% amino acid identity to the $CysLT_1$ receptor, and its gene is mapped to chromosome 13q14 (Capra et al., 2006).

In normal human lung, expression of the $CysLT_1$ receptor mRNA and protein is confined to smooth-muscle cells and tissue macrophages (Figueroa et al., 2001). $CysLT_1$ receptor is also expressed in most peripheral blood eosinophils and pre-granulocytic $CD34^+$ cells, and in subsets of monocytes and B lymphocytes (Figueroa et al., 2001).

Stimulation of the $CysLT_1$ and $CysLT_2$ receptors activates a guanosine triphosphate binding protein (GTBP) that regulates the receptor affinity for ligands and intracellularly transduces the signal. The major intracellular signalling pathway for the $CysLT_1$ receptor is via calcium release (Capra et al., 2006). Montelukast, zafirlukast and pranlukast are $CysLT_1$ receptor-selective antagonists with low potency as antagonists of $CysLT_2$ receptor signalling.

Recent studies suggest that genetic variation in the leukotriene synthesis pathway (such as ALOX5, LTA_4H, LTC_4S) and $CysLT_1$ receptor genes may contribute significantly to the variability in the clinical response to anti-leukotriene therapy in asthmatic patients (Lima et al., 2006).

Asthma

Whereas the role of LTB_4 in the pathogenesis of bronchial asthma, if any, remains controversial, the role of CysLTs in the pathogenesis of asthma is well established. Cysteinyl leukotrienes mediate a number of pathways relevant to the pathogenesis of asthma, including smooth-muscle contraction, increased vascular permeability and mucus secretion, decreased mucociliary clearance and recruitment of eosinophils in the airways (Caramori and Adcock, 2003). Cysteinyl leukotrienes can also play a role in maintaining the chronic airway inflammatory response, in airway neurogenic inflammation and in airway remodelling (Holgate et al., 2003). Patients with aspirin-intolerant asthma have significant basal overproduction of CysLTs and within their biosynthetic pathway the terminal enzyme leukotriene C_4 synthase (LTC_4S) is overexpressed (Holgate et al., 2003; Lam, 2003).

Leukotriene receptor antagonists and synthesis inhibitors reduce the severity of bronchial hyper-responsiveness and can reduce the inflammatory effect of allergen challenge (Caramori and Adcock, 2003).

Montelukast, pranlukast and zafirlukast also significantly reduce sputum as well as peripheral blood eosinophil counts in asthmatic patients. In addition, pranlukast causes a significant reduction in activated eosinophils in bronchial biopsy specimens and zileuton reduces circulating blood eosinophil numbers and bronchoalveolar eosinophils following allergen challenge (Caramori and Adcock, 2003).

Cysteinyl leukotriene receptor antagonists and leukotriene synthesis inhibitors are clinically effective in some groups of asthmatic patients and are a second-choice option in the treatment of mild persistent asthma, as an alternative to inhaled glucocorticoids (GINA, 2006; Ng et al., 2004). In fact in patients with mild persistent asthma low doses of inhaled glucocorticoids are more effective than anti-leukotrienes (GINA, 2006; Ng et al., 2004). There is now strong evidence to support the use of licensed doses of anti-leukotrienes as add-on therapy to inhaled glucocorticoids. Addition of anti-leukotrienes after glucocorticoid tapering has a glucocorticoid-sparing effect (Ducharme et al., 2004). In patients with moderate persistent asthma anti-leukotrienes have the same efficacy as LABA as an add-on treatment to inhaled glucocorticoids in the long-term control of asthma (GINA, 2006). Addition of a LABA seems to be superior to an anti-leukotriene in improving lung function. However, addition of LABA and anti-leukotriene may be equal with respect to asthma exacerbations (Kankaanranta et al., 2004). However, the clinical response to CysLT receptor antagonists varies widely among the asthmatic groups studied, with the best responders being not only the aspirin-intolerant asthmatics but also those treated with the highest doses of inhaled glucocorticoids. Single doses of the currently available leukotriene receptor antagonists provide a prompt, effective and persistent defence against exercise-induced asthma that equals that seen with a LABA (Drazen et al., 1999). The synthesis inhibitor zileuton affords a comparable magnitude of prophylaxis but has a considerably shorter duration of action.

COPD

Preliminary clinical observations suggest that 5-lipoxygenase inhibitors (such as zileuton, which is available in some countries for asthma therapy) significantly improve lung function in stable COPD patients, in contrast to CysLT receptor antagonists. This may be secondary to the reduction of LTB_4 production by 5-lipoxygenase inhibitors (Caramori and Adcock, 2003). However, in a placebo-controlled study in patients with stable COPD, 2 weeks of treatment with an oral FLAP inhibitor did not decrease chemotactic activity and myeloperoxidase levels in sputum despite a reduction in median LTB_4 levels (Gompertz and Stockley, 2002). Long-term controlled clinical trials in a large number of COPD patients are required to determine their potential clinical efficacy. A 5-lipoxygenase inhibitor ZD4407 (AstraZeneca, Loughborough, UK) entered phase I trials in patients with COPD a few years ago, but the results are still unpublished. LTB_4 receptor antagonists are particularly appealing because there are compounds available that are active with once-daily oral administration. However the preliminary results from the first controlled clinical trials using selective LTB_4 receptor antagonists in COPD are disappointing.

In a small uncontrolled study of COPD patients with severe COPD the long-term addition to their treatment of montelukast decreased the number of COPD exacerbations, and in a short-term study the same drug improved lung function and symptoms in stable COPD (Celik et al., 2005; Rubinstein et al., 2004). Again, long-term, placebo-controlled studies are necessary to clarify a potential role for CysLT receptor antagonists in the treatment of COPD.

11.7   Anti-IgE Therapy

Omalizumab is a non-immunogenic, non-anaphylactogenic, recombinant humanized monoclonal antibody that specifically binds to the binding site for high-affinity IgE receptors (FcɛRI) on the Fc fragment of the IgE molecule. Omalizumab does not bind to IgE bound to cells bearing the FcɛRI or the FcɛRII, thereby avoiding their activation. This is because the epitope on IgE against which they are directed is already attached to those receptors and as a consequence is masked (Chung, 2004; Strunk and Bloomberg, 2006). Parenteral administration of omalizumab induces a marked decrease in serum free IgE, whilst the serum total IgE concentration becomes elevated (Strunk and Bloomberg, 2006). This is due to the formation of IgE–anti-IgE complexes, which have a longer serum half-life. The decrease in free IgE correlates with a reversible downregulation of the FcɛRI density on mast cells, basophils and dendritic cells and a decrease of their responsiveness to allergens (Strunk and Bloomberg, 2006). Omalizumab therapy protects atopic asthmatic patients against allergen-induced bronchoconstriction (Chung, 2004). In addition, omalizumab is effective in reducing asthma exacerbations when used as an adjunctive therapy to inhaled glucocorticoids and during the glucocorticoid tapering phase of clinical trials (Walker et al., 2006) and is significantly more effective than placebo at increasing the numbers of asthmatic patients who are able to reduce or withdraw their inhaled glucocorticoids (Strunk and Bloomberg, 2006). But the clinical value of the reduction in glucocorticoid consumption has to be considered in the light of the high cost of omalizumab (Walker et al., 2006). Furthermore, studies are needed to determine the cause of the considerable variability of the clinical response to omalizumab therapy (Strunk and Bloomberg, 2006). Additionally, the efficacy and safety of omalizumab have not been established for durations of treatment that exceed 1 year, and it is not known how long clinical effects may persist after therapy is discontinued (Strunk and Bloomberg, 2006). There is a complete absence of published clinical trials of omalizumab in COPD.

11.8   Macrolides/Ketolides

Small uncontrolled serological studies suggest also that in a subgroup of adults with severe persistent asthma a chronic infection with *Chlamydia pneumoniae* may amplify the inflammation that occurs in asthma and will improve with antibiotic therapy effective against *Chlamydia pneumoniae* (Caramori and Adcock, 2003). However, other studies have shown that seropositivity to *Chlamydia pneumoniae* is common in older adults and does not correlate with asthma, and another study performed with methods (e.g. culture and polymerase chain reaction) that are more specific for persistent *Chlamydia pneumoniae* infection than serology could not find any evidence of *Chlamydia pneumoniae* infection in the airways of adults with persistent asthma in the stable phase (Caramori and Adcock, 2003).

A recent study shows that *Mycoplasma pneumoniae* is present by polymerase chain reaction (but not culture) in the lower airways (bronchoalveolar lavage and/or bronchial biopsies) of 9/18 adults with stable persistent asthma in the stable phase and only 1/11 control subjects (Kraft et al., 1998). Asthmatics with lower airway *Mycoplasma pneumoniae* infection have increased expression of substance P and/or neurokinin 1 in their lower airways, especially in the bronchial epithelium, compared with normal control subjects and asthmatics without *Mycoplasma pneumoniae* infection (Chu et al., 2000). Asthmatic patients treated with clarithromycin (a macrolide antibiotic active against *Mycoplasma pneumoniae*) show a reduction of substance P, neurokinin 1 and mucus in the epithelium. Reduction of epithelial neurokinin 1 expression is more prominent in asthmatics with *Mycoplasma pneumoniae* than in those without this infection (Chu et al., 2000). Clarithromycin treatment in asthmatics also reduces the aedematous area, as identified by α_2-macroglobulin staining, which may lead to airway tissue shrinkage and cause an artificial increase in the number of blood vessels (Chu et al., 2001).

In addition, a recent study has shown telithromycin, a macrolide-like antibiotic, to be effective in the treatment of asthmatic exacerbations, although the mechanisms of action were not determined (Johnston, 2006).

Macrolide/ketolide antibiotics also have some direct anti-inflammatory/immunomodulatory effects (Shinkai et al., 2005) and it is not possible to exclude the fact that these results in stable and acute asthma may be due to these effects and not to their antibacterial activity.

Telithromycin, like macrolides, is also a strong inhibitor of cytochrome P-450 (CYP) isoenzyme 3A4. Two inhaled glucocorticoids commonly used in clinical practice (budesonide and fluticasone) are metabolized to inactive catabolites predominantly by CYP3A enzymes in the liver. CYP3A4 is also responsible for aliphatic oxidation of the LABA bronchodilator salmeterol, which is extensively metabolized by hydroxylation. Drug interactions may reduce CYP3A4 activity through direct inhibition or increase metabolic activity through induction. Such interactions can expand the range of variability of its activity to about 400-fold (Caramori and Papi, 2006).

Further controlled clinical trial studies are required to assess the role of macrolides/ketolides in the treatment of severe stable asthma and in asthmatic exacerbations.

The majority (54–77%) of patients with COPD show serological evidence of past infection with *Chlamydia pneumoniae*, however in some studies this is not significantly greater than that found in control subjects of similar age and sex without lung disease (Caramori and Adcock, 2003).

Studies using immunohistochemistry and PCR have also provided inconclusive evidence that chronic *Chlamydia pneumoniae* infection is a major risk factor for progressive airflow obstruction. Clearly, further studies are necessary to determine whether chronic infection with *Chlamydia pneumoniae* is important in the pathogenesis of COPD or whether the organism is simply a "bystander" (Caramori and Adcock, 2003).

11.9 TNFα Inhibitors

Tumour necrosis factor alpha (TNFα) is codified by a gene located on chromosome 6p21.3. Certain polymorphisms in the 5'-regulatory region of the TNFα gene, particularly at 308 bp, are associated with increased production of TNFα and may predispose to the development of asthma or COPD in selected populations (Gao et al., 2006; Hersh et al. 2005). TNFα exists in a membrane-bound form and a soluble form (Idriss and Naismith, 2000). TNFα is released in the airways from epithelial and smooth-muscle cells, mast cells, alveolar macrophages and T lymphocytes. TNFα exerts its effects through binding to the type 1 TNF receptor (p55; TNFR1; CD120b) and the type 2 TNF receptor (p75; TNFR2; CD120a). Both receptors are found on immune, inflammatory and structural cells of the lung (Ermert et al., 2003; Idriss and Naismith, 2000).

TNFα is an important chemotactic protein for neutrophils and in fact the inhalation of TNFα induces sputum neutrophilia and airway hyper-responsiveness in normal subjects (Thomas et al., 1995). *In vitro*, TNFα also induces CCL13 [monocyte chemoattractant protein (MCP)-4] expression, a chemokine with potent chemotactic activities for eosinophils, monocytes, T lymphocytes and basophils. TNFα also activate structural (such as epithelial and smooth-muscle cells) and inflammatory cells of the airways to release inflammatory mediators (such as oxidants) (Barnes, 2003b; Chung, 2006b).

Additional data indicate that TNFα can stimulate the secretion of MUC5AC from bronchial epithelial cells, upregulate adhesion molecule expression on inflammatory, epithelial and endothelial cells, facilitate the migration of inflammatory cells into the lower airways and activate pro-fibrotic mechanisms involved in airway remodelling (Barnes, 2003b; Chung, 2006b).

TNFα inhibitors may, therefore, represent new potential pharmacological agents for the treatment of severe asthma and COPD. Interestingly, glucocorticoids, low-dose theophylline, PDE4 inhibitors and p38-MAPK inhibitors potently inhibit TNFα production *in vitro* and/or *in vivo* (Caramori and Adcock, 2003).

Selective TNFα inhibitors in clinical development include non-human or chimeric antibodies (infliximab, afelimomab and CytoTab), humanized antibodies [adalimumab and certolizumab pegol (CDP870)], human TNFR (onercept) and TNFR fusion protein (etanercept). TNFα converting enzyme (TACE/ADAM17) is a matrix metalloproteinase (MMP)-related enzyme required for the release of soluble TNFα that might be another attractive target. Small-molecule TACE inhibitors, some of which are also MMP inhibitors, are in development as oral TNFα inhibitors (Barnes, 2003b; Barnes and Stockley, 2005).

Infliximab, etanercept and adalimumab are already on the market for the treatment of inflammatory bowel disease, rheumatoid arthritis, ankylosing spondylitis and psoriasis. Their efficacy is now being tested in ongoing controlled clinical trials both in severe asthma and in COPD.

TNFα inhibitors are expensive drugs and may cause serious adverse effects such as injection-site reactions, increased susceptibility to tuberculosis and other severe infections (bacterial pneumonia, aspergillosis, candidiasis, histoplasmosis, listeriosis, *Pneumocystis jirovecii* pneumonia, reactivation of latent hepatitis B virus infection), demyelinating disorders, non-Hodgkin lymphoma and heart failure (Bongartz et al., 2006; Calabrese, 2006). For these reasons long-term controlled clinical studies monitoring safety and cost-effectiveness are warranted before the use of TNFα inhibitors should be recommended for severe asthma or COPD.

Asthma

Many *in vitro* and *in vivo* studies suggest that activation of the TNFα axis may be fundamental to the pathogenesis of airflow obstruction and airway hyper-responsiveness in glucocorticoid-dependent asthmatics (Erzurum, 2006). Elevated levels of TNFα have been demonstrated in the bronchial biopsies and sputum from asthmatic patients, and TNFα levels in bronchoalveolar lavage increase after allergen challenge in atopic asthmatics (Caramori and Adcock, 2003).

Furthermore, the level of TNFα expression in the lower airways is greater in glucocorticoid-dependent asthmatics compared with patients with mild asthma (Howarth et al., 2005). Glucocorticoid-dependent asthmatics also have an increased expression of membrane-bound TNFα, TNFα receptor 1 and TNFα-converting enzyme by peripheral blood monocytes as compared to patients with mild to moderate asthma (Berry et al., 2006). *In vitro*, in isolated tracheal-ring models administration of TNFα increases human airway smooth-muscle contractility to acetylcholine and allergen and impairs airway smooth-muscle relaxation to isoproterenol (Townley and Horiba, 2003). The inhalation of TNFα induces sputum neutrophilia and airway hyper-responsiveness in patients with mild asthma (Thomas et al., 1995).

TNFα inhibitors are promising new compounds for the treatment of moderate persistent asthma and oral glucocorticoid-dependent severe persistent asthma (Berry et al., 2006; Erin et al., 2006) and large controlled clinical trials are underway. Their results are awaited with interest in the scientific community.

COPD

The concentration of TNFα is increased in the blood and sputum of COPD patients (Gan et al., 2004; Keatings et al., 1996). They also have significantly higher levels of soluble TNFR1 in sputum and TNFR2 in blood. In addition, sputum sTNF receptors, but not blood sTNF receptors, are inversely related to the FEV_1 in patients with COPD (Vernnoy et al., 2002). COPD patients also show an increased TNFα gene expression in their skeletal muscles (Montes de Oca et al., 2005). The severe weight loss present in some patients with advanced COPD might also be due to skeletal-muscle cell apoptosis (muscle cachexia), as a result of increased levels of circulating TNFα (Barnes, 2003b; Lewis, 2002). TNFα and its receptors TNFR1 and TNFR2 have a pathogenetic role in animal models of pulmonary emphysema and lower airways inflammation (Chung, 2006b; Churg et al., 2004; Lucey et al., 2002; Lundblad et al., 2005).

However, TNFα inhibitors do not appear to be effective in the short-term treatment of stable COPD (van der Vaart et al., 2005).

11.10   Conclusions

Current asthma therapies are not cures and symptoms return soon after treatment is stopped, even after long-term therapy. Although glucocorticoids are highly effective in controlling the inflammatory process in asthma, they appear to have little effect on the remodelling processes that appear to play a role in the pathophysiology of asthma at currently prescribed doses. The development of novel drugs, particularly steroid-sparing agents, may allow resolution of these changes. In addition, severe glucocorticoid-dependent and-resistant asthma presents a great clinical burden and reducing the side effects of glucocorticoids using novel steroid-sparing agents will prove immensely beneficial.

With few exceptions, COPD is caused by tobacco smoking, and smoking cessation is the only truly effective treatment of COPD. Once smoking has caused COPD, the disease is still largely irreversible and progressive. Current pharmacological treatment of COPD is unsatisfactory, as it does not significantly influence the severity of the disease or its natural course. Bronchodilators, including inhaled LABA, improve symptoms and lung function in stable COPD patients but they do not significantly influence the natural course of the disease. Apart from the prevention of exacerbations, inhaled glucocorticoids have not been shown to be consistently effective in COPD, either in reducing symptoms or for improving lung function and the course of the disease. Steroid-sparing strategies are desperately needed. New anti-inflammatory drugs for COPD that are in the pipeline may prove more beneficial as add-on steroid-sparing agents rather than monotherapies and this should be considered during clinical development.

Acknowledgements

Work in our group is supported by Altana, Associazione per la Ricerca e la Cura dell'Asma (ARCA, Padova, Italy), Asthma UK, AstraZeneca, Boehringer Ingelheim, The British Lung Foundation, Chiesi Farmaceutici (Parma, Italy), The Clinical Research Committee (Brompton Hospital), Fondazione Carife (Ferrara, Italy), GlaxoSmithKline (UK), MerckSharp and Dohme (Italy), Ministero dell'Istruzione, dell'Università e della Ricerca (Italy), Mitsubishi (Japan), The National Institutes of Health (USA) and Università di Ferrara (Italy).

References

Barnes PJ. Theophylline:new perspectives for an old drug. *Am J Respir Crit Care Med* 2003a; **167**: 813–818.

Barnes PJ. Cytokine-directed therapies for the treatment of chronic airway diseases. *Cytokine Growth Factor Rev* 2003b; **14**: 511–522.

Barnes PJ. Mediators of chronic obstructive pulmonary disease. *Pharmacol Rev* 2004a; **56**; 515–548.

Barnes PJ. Distribution of receptor targets in the lungs. *Proc Am Thorac Soc* 2004b; **1**: 345–351.

Barnes PJ. Theophylline in chronic obstructive pulmonary disease:new horizons. *Proc Am Thorac Soc* 2005; **2**: 334–341.

Barnes PJ. Reduced histone deacetylase in COPD:clinical implications. *Chest* 2006; **129**: 151–155.

Barnes PJ, Stockley RA. COPD:current therapeutic interventions and future approaches. *Eur Respir J* 2005; **25**: 1084–1106.

Barnes PJ, Adcock IM, Ito K. Histone acetylation and deacetylation: importance in inlammatory lung diseases. *Eur Respir J* 2005; **253**: 552–563.

Barnes PJ, Chung KF, Page CP. Inflammatory mediators of asthma:an update. *Pharmacol Rev* 1998; **50**: 515–596.

Barr RG, Bourbeau J, Camargo Jr CA, Ram FS. Tiotropium for stable chronic obstructive pulmonary disease:a meta-analysis. *Thorax* 2006; **61**: 854–862.

Berry MA, Hargadon B, Shelley M, Parker D et al. Evidence of a role of tumor necrosis factor alpha in refractory asthma. *New Engl J Med* 2006; **354**: 697–708.

Bongartz T, Sutton AJ, Sweeting MJ, Buchan I, Matteson EL, Montori V. Anti-TNF antibody therapy in rheumatoid arthritis and the risk of serious infections and malignancies:systematic review and meta-analysis of rare harmful effects in randomized controlled trials. *J Am Med Assoc* 2006; **295**: 2275–2285 [Erratum on p. 2482].

Calabrese L. The yin and yang of tumor necrosis factor inhibitors. *Cleveland Clin J Med* 2006; **73**: 251–256.

Capra V, Thompson MD, Sala A, Cole DE, Folco G, Rovati GE. Cysteinyl-leukotrienes and their receptors in asthma and other inflammatory diseases:critical update and emerging trends. *Med Res Rev* 2007; **27**: 469–527.

Caramori G, Adcock I. Pharmacology of airway inflammation in asthma and COPD. *Pulmon Pharmacol Ther* 2003; **16**: 247–277.

Caramori G, Papi A. Telithromycin in acute exacerbations of asthma. *N Engl J Med* 2006; **355**: 96.

Celik P, Sakar A, Havlucu Y, Yuksel H, Turkdogan P, Yorgancioglu A. Short-term effects of montelukast in stable patients with moderate to severe COPD. *Respir Med* 2005; **99**: 444–450.

Chu HW, Kraft M, Krause JE, Rex MD, Martin RJ. Substance P and its receptor neurokinin 1 expression in asthmatic airways. *J Allergy Clin Immunol* 2000; **106**: 713–722.

Chu HW, Kraft M, , Rex MD, Martin RJ. Evaluation of blood vessels and edema in the airways of asthma patients:regulation with clarithromycin treatment. *Chest* 2001; **120**: 416–422.

Chung KF. Anti-IgE monoclonal antibody, omalizumab: a new treatment for allergic asthma. *Exp Opin Pharmacother* 2004; **5**: 439–446.

Chung KF. Phosphodiesterase inhibitors in airways disease. *Eur J Pharmacol* 2006a; **533**: 110–117.

Chung KF. Cytokines as targets in chronic obstructive pulmonary disease. *Curr Drug Targ* 2006b; **7**: 675–681.

Churg A, Wang RD, Tai H, Wang X, Xie C, Wright JL. Tumor necrosis factor-alpha drives 70% of cigarette smoke-induced emphysema in the mouse. *Am J Respir Crit Care Med* 2004; **170**: 492–498.

Drazen JM, Israel E, O'Byrne PM. Treatment of asthma with drugs modifying the leukotriene pathway. *New Engl J Med* 1999; **340**: 197–206 [Erratum in: **340**: 663; **341**: 1632].

Ducharme F, Schwartz Z, Hicks G, Kakuma R. Addition of anti-leukotriene agents to inhaled corticosteroids for chronic asthma. *Cochrane Database of Systematic Reviews* 2004; **2**: CD003133.

Erin EM, Leaker BR, Nicholson GC, Tan AJ et al. The effects of a monoclonal antibody directed against tumour necrosis factor-alpha (TNF-α) in asthma. *Am J Respir Crit Care Med* 2006; **174**: 753–762.

Ermert M, Pantazis C, Duncker HR, Grimminger F, Seeger W, Ermert L. In situ localization of TNFalpha/beta, TACE and TNF receptors TNF-R1 and TNF-R2 in control and LPS-treated lung tissue. *Cytokine* 2003; **22**: 89–100.

Erzurum SC. Inhibition of tumor necrosis factor alpha for refractory asthma. *New Engl J Med* 2006; **354**: 754–758.

Evans DJ, Taylor DA, Zetterstrom O, Chung KF, O'Connor BJ, Barnes PJ. A comparison of low-dose inhaled budesonide plus theophylline and high-dose inhaled budesonide for moderate asthma. *N Engl J Med* 1997; **337**: 1412–1418.

Figueroa DJ, Breyer RM, Defoe SK, Kargman S et al. Expression of the cysteinyl leukotriene 1 receptor in normal human lung and peripheral blood leukocytes. *Am J Respir Crit Care Med* 2001; **163**: 226–233.

Gan WQ, Man SF, Senthilselvan A, Sin DD. Association between chronic obstructive pulmonary disease and systemic inflammation:a systematic review and a meta-analysis. *Thorax* 2004; **59**: 574–580.

Gao J, Shan G, Sun B, Thompson PJ, Gao X. Association between polymorphism of tumour necrosis factor alpha-308 gene promoter and asthma:a meta-analysis. *Thorax* 2006; **61**: 466–471.

Global Initiative for Asthma (GINA). *Global Strategy for Asthma Management and Prevention*, Publication no. 02-3569. Bethesda, MD: National Institute of Health, last updated 2006.

Global Initiative for Chronic Obstructive Lung Disease (GOLD). *Global Strategy for the Diagnosis, Management and Prevention of Chronic Obstructive Pulmonary Disease*, Publication no. 2701. Bethesda, MD: National Institutes of Health, last updated 2006.

Gompertz S, Stockley RA. A randomized, placebo-controlled trial of a leukotriene synthesis inhibitor in patients with COPD. *Chest* 2002; **122**: 289–294.

Hersh CP, Demeo DL, Lange C, Litonjua AA et al. Attempted replication of reported chronic obstructive pulmonary disease candidate gene associations. *Am J Respir Cell Mol Biol* 2005; **33**: 71–78.

Holgate ST, Peters-Golden M, Panettieri RA, Henderson WR Jr. Roles of cysteinyl leukotrienes in airway inflammation, smooth muscle function, and remodeling. *J Allergy Clin Immunol* 2003; **111**: S18–S6.

Howarth PH, Babu KS, Arshad HS, Lau L et al. Tumour necrosis factor (TNFalpha) as a novel therapeutic target in symptomatic corticosteroid dependent asthma. *Thorax* 2005; **60**: 1012–1018.

Idriss HT, Naismith JH. TNF alpha and the TNF receptor superfamily: structure-function relationship(s). *Microsc Res Tech* 2000; **50**: 184–195.

Jampilek J, Dolezal M, Opletalova V, Hartl J. 5-Lipoxygenase, leukotrienes biosynthesis and potential antileukotrienic agents. *Curr Med Chem* 2006; **13**: 117–129.

Jeffery P. Phosphodiesterase 4-selective inhibition: novel therapy for the inflammation of COPD. *Pulmon Pharmacol Ther* 2005; **18**: 9–17.

Johnston SL. Macrolide antibiotics and asthma treatment. *J Allergy Clin Immunol* 2006; **117**: 1233–1236.

Kalayci O, Birben E, Sackesen C, Keskin O et al. ALOX5 promoter genotype, asthma severity and LTC4 production by eosinophils. *Allergy* 2006; **61**: 97–103.

Kankaanranta H, Lahdensuo A, Moilanen E, Barnes PJ. Add-on therapy options in asthma not adequately controlled by inhaled corticosteroids:a comprehensive review. *Respir Res* 2004; **5**: 17–43.

Keatings VM, Collins PD, Scott DM, Barnes PJ. Differences in interleukin-8 and tumor necrosis factor–alpha in induced sputum from patients with chronic obstructive pulmonary disease or asthma. *Am J Respir Crit Care Med* 1996; **153**: 530–534.

Kraft M, Cassell GH, Henson JE, Watson H et al. Detection of Mycoplasma pneumoniae in the airways of adults with chronic asthma. *Am J Respir Crit Care Med* 1998; **158**: 998–1001 [Erratum on p. 1692].

Lam BK. Leukotriene C(4) synthase. *Prostagland Leukotr Ess Fatty Acids* 2003; **69**: 111–116.

Lewis MI. Apoptosis as a potential mechanism of muscle cachexia in chronic obstructive pulmonary disease. *Am J Respir Crit Care Med* 2002; **166**: 434–436.

Lima JJ, Zhang S, Grant A, Shao L et al. Influence of leukotriene pathway polymorphisms on response to montelukast in asthma. *Am J Respir Crit Care Med* 2006; **173**: 379–385.

Lipworth BJ. Phosphodiesterase-4 inhibitors for asthma and chronic obstructive pulmonary disease. *Lancet* 2005; **365**: 167–175.

Lucey EC, Keane J, Kuang PP, Snider GL, Goldstein RH. Severity of elastase-induced emphysema is decreased in tumor necrosis factor-alpha and interleukin-1b,eta receptor-deficient mice. *Lab Invest* 2002; **82**: 79–85.

Lundblad LK, Thompson-Figueroa J, Leclair T, Sullivan MJ, Poynter ME, Irvin CG, Bates JH. Tumor necrosis factor-alpha overexpression in lung disease:a single cause behind a complex phenotype. *Am J Respir Crit Care Med* 2005; **171**: 1363–1370.

McGill KA, Busse WW. Zileuton. *Lancet* 1996; **348**: 519–524.

Montes de Oca M, Torres SH, De Sanctis J, Mata A, Hernandez N, Talamo C. Skeletal muscle inflammation and nitric oxide in patients with COPD. *Eur Respir J* 2005; **26**: 390–397.

Ng D, Salvio F, Hicks G. Anti-leukotriene agents compared to inhaled corticosteroids in the management of recurrent and/or chronic asthma in adults and children. *Cochrane Database of Systematic Reviews* 2004; **2**: CD002314.

Peters-Golden M, Brock TG. 5-Lipoxygenase and FLAP. *Prostagland Leukotr Ess Fatty Acids* 2005; **69**: 99–109.

Racke K, Matthiesen S. The airway cholinergic system:physiology and pharmacology. *Pulmon Pharmacol Ther* 2004; **17**: 181–198.

Rubinstein I, Kumar B, Schriever C. Long-term montelukast therapy in moderate to severe COPD–a preliminary observation. *Respir Med* 2004; **98**: 134–138.

Shah L, Wilson AJ, Gibson PJ, Coughlan J. Long acting beta-agonists versus theophylline for maintenance treatment of asthma. *Cochrane Database of Systematic Reviews* 2003; **3**: CD001281.

Shinkai M, Park CS, Rubin BK. Immunomodulatory effects of macrolide antibiotics. *Clin Pulmon Med* 2005; **12**: 341–348.

Strunk RC, Bloomberg GR. Omalizumab for asthma. *New Engl J Med* 2006; **354**: 2689–2695.

Tager AM, Luster AD. BLT1 and BLT2:the leukotriene B(4) receptors. *Prostagland Leukotr Ess Fatty Acids* 2003; **69**: 123–134.

Tennant RC, Erin EM, Barnes PJ, Hansel TT. Long-acting beta 2-adrenoceptor agonists or tiotropium bromide for patients with COPD: is combination therapy justified? *Curr Opin Pharmacol* 2003; **3**: 270–276.

Thomas PS, Yates DH, Barnes PJ. Tumor necrosis factor-alpha increases airway responsiveness and sputum neutrophilia in normal human subjects. *Am J Respir Crit Care Med* 1995; **152**: 76–80.

Townley RG, Horiba M. Airway hyperresponsiveness: a story of mice and men and cytokines. *Clin Rev Allergy Immunol* 2003; **24**: 85–110.

Ukena D, Harnest U, Sakalauskas R, Magyar P, Vetter N, Steffen H, Leichtl S, Rathgeb F, Keller A, Steinijans VW. Comparison of addition of theophylline to inhaled steroid with doubling of the dose of inhaled steroid in asthma. *Eur Respir J* 1997; **10**: 2754–2760.

Van der Vaart H, Koeter GH, Postma DS, Kauffman HF, ten Hacken NH. First study of infliximab treatment in patients with chronic obstructive pulmonary disease. *Am J Respir Crit Care Med* 2005; **172**: 465–469.

Vernnoy JH, Kucukaycan M, Jacobs JA, Chavannes NH, Buurman WA, Dentener MA, Wouters EF. Local and systemic inflammation in patients with chronic obstructive pulmonary disease: soluble tumor necrosis factor receptors are increased in sputum. *Am J Respir Crit Care Med* 2002; **166**: 1218–1224.

Walker S, Monteil M, Phelan K, Lasserson TJ, Walters EH. Anti-IgE for chronic asthma in adults and children. *Cochrane Database of Systematic Reviews* 2006; **2**: CD003559.

12

Kinases as Anti-inflammatory Targets for Respiratory Disease

Iain Kilty

12.1   Introduction

Kinases play a critical role in cellular signal transduction and in the inflammatory signalling characteristic of respiratory disease. Inflammation is a hallmark of respiratory diseases such as asthma and chronic obstructive pulmonary disease (COPD). In both of these diseases, a differing population of inflammatory cells is activated and recruited to the lung in addition to a range of inflammatory mediators being synthesized in structural cells such as the epithelium, fibroblasts and smooth muscle (Busse and Lemanske, 2001; MacNee, 2005; O'Donnell et al., 2006). This inflammatory cascade is characterized by increased expression of chemokines, cytokines, adhesion molecules, growth factors, enzymes and receptors, all of which can be regulated by kinases (Busse and Lemanske, 2001; MacNee, 2005; O'Donnell et al., 2006).

Recognition by a cell of external inflammatory stimuli, such as bacterial coat proteins, viral particles, allergens and cytokines, can activate a kinase cascade through the activity of a variety of receptors. These intracellular signalling networks amplify the inflammatory signal, activating a range of transcription factors such as nuclear factor kappa B (NF-κB) through inhibitor of kappa B kinases (IKKs), activator protein 1 (AP-1) through mitogen-activated protein kinases (MAPKs), STATs through Janus kinases (JAKs) and phosphoinositol signalling through phosphoinositide 3 kinases (PI3Ks), amongst others. Small molecule inhibitors of kinases may therefore represent an attractive means by which to modulate inflammatory signalling in these diseases (Adcock et al., 2006).

Overcoming Steroid Insensitivity in Respiratory Disease   Edited by Ian M. Adcock and Kian Fan Chung
© 2008 John Wiley & Sons, Ltd.

12.2   Pharmacological Targeting of Kinases

The protein kinase family consists of 518 members, all of which catalyse the transfer of the gamma phosphate of ATP onto a protein substrate. This substrate can be another kinase, amplifying the initial signal, or other proteins such as transcription factors, inducing gene transcription (Manning et al., 2002). These enzymes can be split into three families, serine threonine kinases such as the MAPKs and IKKs, non-receptor tyrosine kinases such as IL-2-inducible kinase (ITK) and receptor tyrosine kinases such as the epidermal growth factor receptor (EGFR) (Manning et al., 2002). Each of these kinase families represent potential therapeutic targets and will be discussed below. A further interesting family of kinases are the lipid kinases that similarly transfer the gamma phosphate of ATP onto lipid substrates. The best characterized of these are the PI3Ks that phosphorylate phosphatidyl-inositides and are involved in the regulation of a wide variety of processes from cellular proliferation to insulin signalling (Vanhaesebroeck, 2001; Vanhaesebroeck et al., 2005).

Considering the key role of kinases in inflammatory signalling, there is a paucity of kinase inhibitors that have been advanced to clinical trials for chronic inflammatory diseases (Adcock et al., 2006). Moreover, whilst kinase research has been ongoing in industry for over 20 years (Cohen, 2002), there are currently only six widely marketed compounds, each for oncology indications: Gleevec (Novartis), Rapamycin (Wyeth-Ayerst), Irresa (AstraZeneca), Tarceva (OSI Pharmaceuticals, Roche, Genentech), Sutent (Pfizer) and Sorafenib (Bayer).

The key challenge for kinase inhibitor development is the identification of small-molecule inhibitors that are selective for one kinase over the rest of the kinase family in addition to other enzymes that use ATP as their substrate (Cohen, 2002). With the exception of atypical kinases, protein kinases adopt a conserved conformation with an N-terminal domain connected via the hinge region to a larger C-terminal domain, with the substrate binding site between (Figure 12.1). The majority of kinase

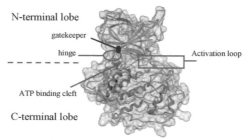

Figure 12.1   Molecular model of GSKb-3 as a template to indicate standard kinase nomenclature. A ribbon diagram (green) showing secondary structure elements (helices in red, strands in cyan). The molecular surface is represented in grey. A full-colour version of this figure appear in the colour plate section of this book. A full-colour version of this figure can be found in the colour plate section of this book.

inhibitors bind competitively with ATP in this pocket and selectivity is sought by exploiting small differences in the ATP pocket (Fabian et al., 2005; Luo, 2005). Indeed ATP competition itself can represent an issue with poor translation of potency to whole cells, where ATP concentrations can be up to 4 mM.

A number of selective kinase inhibitors have been identified by exploiting differences in a highly variable hydrophobic pocket at the back of the ATP binding site, access to which is determined by the so-called "gatekeeper" residue (Blencke et al., 2004). Approximately 20% of the kinome contains a threonine at this position, all other kinases containing amino acids with a larger side chain, which in turn can restrict access to this pocket. Interestingly, most kinase inhibitors in clinical studies gain at least some of their selectivity through binding in this pocket (e.g. Irresa: EGFR; Gleevec: Abl, PDGFR and *c*-kit; BAY 43-9006: Raf). Moreover, mutation of threonine 315 to isoleucine in Abl, effectively blocking access to this pocket, is one of the most common mechanisms of resistance to Gleevec (Gorre et al., 2001).

In certain kinases the N-terminal region of the activation loop containing an aspartic acid – phenylalanine – glycine motif (DFG) is able to move to a "DFG out" conformation, opening up a deep binding pocket adjacent to the ATP binding site. This DFG out conformation has only been reported for a small number of kinases, such as c-abl (Schindler, 2000), *c*-kit (Mol et al., 2004), p38α (Pargellis et al., 2002), B-RAF (Wan et al., 2004) and VEGF-R2 (Manley et al., 2004), and tends to have low sequence homology between these enzymes. Selective targeting of the DFG out conformation of these kinases, and investigating the potential for a similar conformation in other kinases, may therefore offer an exciting opportunity for the development of selective kinase inhibitors. Indeed Gleevec has been shown to bind Abl and *c*-kit in this conformation (Mol et al., 2004; Schindler, 2000), stabilizing the inactive form of these enzymes.

In the case of EGFR, the dual erbB1/erbB2 inhibitor Lapatinib stabilizes the enzyme in an inactive conformation not through movement of the DFG loop, but instead through rotation of an α helix that displaces a conserved glutamic acid side chain from the active site. Of 119 kinases tested, this compound only weakly inhibited two kinases in addition to the intended targets (Wood et al., 2004).

There are also examples of non-ATP competitive kinase inhibitors that either bind an allosteric site, such as the MEK inhibitor CI-1040 (Ohren et al., 2004), or the protein substrate binding site, such as the BCR-ABL inhibitor ONO12380 (Gumireddy et al., 2005). These compounds generally have an improved selectivity profile versus ATP site binders due to the high degree of heterogeneity of kinase amino acid sequences outside the ATP binding site. However, despite the obvious advantages of these types of inhibitors – high selectivity and avoiding issues with high intracellular ATP concentrations – there are relatively few examples of such inhibitor sites being identified within the kinome.

Therefore, whilst generating highly selective kinase inhibitors is challenging, there are precedents by which this can be achieved. The application of these strategies to the identification of kinase inhibitors targeted at inflammatory pathways important in respiratory disease is reviewed below.

12.3 Targeting NF-κB Activation

NF-κB is a redox-sensitive transcription factor that exists as a heterodimeric complex commonly consisting of p50 and p65/RelA subunits. There is a wide body of evidence to suggest that NF-κB plays a key role in the normal physiological induction of inflammatory gene expression, resulting in the expression of cytokines, chemokines, adhesion molecules, growth factors and enzymes. Importantly, this includes factors such as tumour necrosis factor α (TNFα), interleukins IL-1β, IL-6 and IL-8, macrophage inflammatory protein 1β (MIP-1β) and matrix metalloproteases (MMPs), thought to be important in the pathogenesis of respiratory disease (Barnes and Karin, 1997; Li and Verma, 2002).

Recently, Di Stefano and colleagues have demonstrated increased expression of the p65 protein of NF-κB in bronchial epithelium of smokers and patients with COPD (Di Stefano et al., 2002). The increased expression of p65 in epithelial cells was correlated with the degree of airflow limitation in patients with COPD. A lung resection study has also been carried out by Szulakowski et al., in which again p65 activation was observed in smokers and COPD patients but there were no significant differences between these groups (Szulakowski et al., 2006). Interestingly, an induction of nuclear p65 is also seen in smoke exposed rats, suggesting that smoke-exposure *per se* and the oxidative stress that this causes may result in NF-κB activation in the lung (Marwick et al., 2004).

Caramori and co-workers have shown that the p65 subunit of NF-κB was increased in sputum macrophages but not in sputum neutrophils during exacerbations of COPD, suggesting cell-specific activation of this factor (Caramori et al., 2003). The activation of NF-κB in monocytes/macrophages can then trigger the release of pro-inflammatory mediators in lung epithelial fluid, which would then amplify the inflammatory cascade by activation of epithelial cells as well as recruitment of neutrophils to the airways. Activation of NF-κB by oxidative stress is inhibited by co-incubation with the antioxidant N-acetyl cysteine *in vitro*, providing evidence for activation of this transcription factor in these patients being due to oxidative stress (Schreck and Baeuerle, 2002).

A large variety of inflammatory stimuli can activate NF-κB-dependent gene transcription, such as oxidative stress, bacterial coat proteins (e.g. lipopolysaccharide, LPS), double-stranded RNA and inflammatory cytokines such as IL-1β and TNFα (Li and Verma, 2002). Whilst such a broad range of stimuli can induce NF-κB activity, these can signal through only two activation pathways, the canonical or alternative pathways (Bonizzi and Karin, 2004) (Figure 12.2). The alternative signalling pathway affects only RelB/p52 dimers via phosphorylation-induced processing of the p100 precursor protein (Bonizzi and Karin, 2004). This pathway

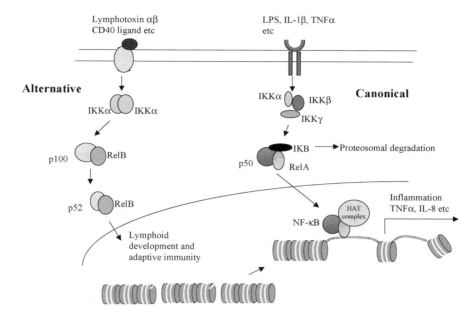

Figure 12.2 The NF-κB signalling pathway. The classical or canonical NF-κB pathway is activated by inflammatory stimuli such as lipopolysaccharide, IL-1 and TNFα binding to their cell-surface receptors, leading to phosphorylation and activation of the IKKβ subunit. This subunit resides in the cytoplasm in a complex with other IKK proteins (α and γ). IKKβ phosphorylates IκB, which is tagged for subsequent proteasomal degradation. This releases the classic NF-κB dimer of p50 and p65 monomers to enable nuclear translocation and binding to specific NF-κB response elements in the promoter regions of pro-inflammatory genes such as TNFα and IL-8. Gene induction requires recruitment of transcriptional coactivator proteins that contain intrinsic histone acetyltransferase (HAT) activity, which tags histones, leading to the recruitment of chromatin remodelling enzymes and changes in the chromatin structure. In contrast, stimulation of cells by lymphotoxin or CD40 binding to receptors leads to phosphorylation and activation of IKKα. This leads to phosphorylation of the p100 NF-κB subunit, which is cleaved to form a p52 submit. The p52 subunit translocates to the nucleus as a dimer with RelB and upregulates a distinct set of NF-κB-responsive genes involved in lymphoid development and adaptive immunity

is involved in secondary lymphoid organ development and adaptive immunity, but is not the primary signalling pathway for the pro-inflammatory effects of NF-κB activation and will not be considered further in this chapter.

In contrast there is a wealth of evidence for the canonical activation pathways playing a key role in both acute and chronic inflammatory signalling, suggesting that modulation of this pathway may have therapeutic benefits. In unstimulated cells NF-κB is found in the cytoplasm as an inactive non-DNA binding form, associated with an inhibitor protein called inhibitor of κB (IκB), which masks the nuclear translocation signal and so prevents NF-κB from entering the nucleus. Inflammatory stimuli such as LPS cause the phosphorylation and activation of the IκB kinase (IKK) signalling complex, consisting of at least three subunits: the catalytic units IKKα and IKKβ, plus the non-catalytic regulatory subunit IKKγ. Depending on the inflammatory stimuli and cell type, these can form part of a much larger protein complex with multiple regulatory units (Courtois et al., 2001; Karin, 1999). Activation of the IKK complex results in phosphorylation and ubiquitination of IκB proteins, ultimately leading to the destruction of IκB by the proteosome. The released NF-κB dimer can then translocate into the nucleus and activate target genes by binding with high affinity to κB elements in their promoters (Karin, 1999). Whilst both IKKα and IKKβ can directly phosphorylate IκB, IKKβ is the predominant catalytic subunit in inflammatory signalling (Mercurio et al., 1997). In addition, IKKβ can also directly phosphorylate the p65 subunit of NF-κB, resulting in its acetylation and modulation of pro-transcriptional properties (Sakurai et al., 2003). Pharmacological modulation of IKKβ activity is therefore an exciting potential therapeutic approach to treating NF-κB-dependent inflammatory signalling.

A variety of mechanisms have been investigated with a view to modulating NF-κB activation (Karin et al., 2004). Indeed a number of known anti-inflammatory compounds, such as aspirin, thalidomide, sulindac, resveratrol and glucocorticoids, gain part of their efficacy through their activity on NF-κB (Barnes and Karin, 1997; Yamamoto and Gaynor, 2001). Inhibitors of ubiquitin ligase (Wertz et al., 2004), peptide inhibitors of IKKγ (Choi et al., 2003) and direct inhibition of NF-κB transport through nuclear pores are being investigated in pre-clinical studies (Yamamoto and Gaynor, 2001). Interestingly, modification of the activation loop of IKKβ on a critical cysteine by arsenic trioxide has been shown to inhibit NF-κB activation and has shown efficacy in some haematological malignancies (Kapahi et al., 2000; Orlowski and Baldwin, 2002)

Targeting IKKβ with small-molecule inhibitors

A number of IKKβ inhibitors have been identified throughout the pharmaceutical industry, although no compounds specifically targeting IKKβ have as yet progressed to testing in humans (Coish et al., 2006). Unfortunately there is no crystal structure available for IKKβ at present to guide the chemical design of selective inhibitors. Indeed a key challenge with the identification of potential drug-like compounds has been gaining good selectivity over the highly homologous IKKα (Coish et al., 2006). However, inhibitors with a degree of selectivity have been claimed by a number of companies. For example, the GlaxoSmithKline inhibitor TPCA-1 is approximately 22-fold more selective for IKKβ over IKKα (Podolin et al., 2005) and encouragingly Bayer have claimed a series of pyridines, examples of which have up to 67-fold more selectivity for IKKβ over IKKα (Coish et al., 2006). These series, and indeed those exemplified in the majority of published patents, are thought to bind in the ATP binding site of IKKβ as they are competitive with ATP. Interestingly, Bristol

Myers Squib have also patented a series of imidazoquinoxalines, exemplified by BMS-354451, that are claimed to bind to an allosteric site on both IKKβ and IKKα (Burke et al., 2003). Whilst these compounds are fairly weak (0.3 μM IC_{50} versus IKKβ) and only show approximately 10-fold selectivity over IKKα, the presence of such an allosteric site on IKKβ may offer exciting opportunities for the development of highly selective IKKβ inhibitors in the future.

As predicted from gene knockout and kinase dead overexpression studies, IKKβ inhibitors show a broad anti-inflammatory profile *in vitro*. TPCA-1 shows a concentration-dependent inhibition of LPS-induced cytokine (IL-1β, IL-6, IL-8, TNFα, MIP-1α) production from the monocytic cell line THP-1 and primary human macrophages (Birrell et al., 2006). Similarly other data have been published showing that IKKβ inhibitors can modulate adhesion molecule upregulation, MMP expression and cytokine expression in human endothelial cells, lung epithelium, T lymphocytes and synovial fibroblasts, amongst other cell types (Birrell et al., 2005; Frelin et al., 2003; Kishore et al., 2003).

A number of these compounds have been screened in *in vivo* inflammation models, with encouraging data being released to the public domain. TPCA-1 has been shown to be active in a mouse arthritis model, reducing paw oedema and cytokine expression (Podolin et al., 2005). Similarly, BMS-345541 and the Celegene/ Serono compound AS602868 have been reported to have anti-inflammatory effects in a mouse and rat model of arthritis, respectively (Burke et al., 2003; Grimshaw, 2001). In addition, AS602868 has also been reported to have anti-inflammatory effects, reducing cytokine expression and tissue damage in a mouse dextran sulphate salt-induced colitis model (Karin, 2005). A tool IKKβ inhibitor from Pharmacia, SC-514, has also been reported to dose dependently reduce systemic LPS-induced TNFα production in the rat (Kishore et al., 2003).

At present there is limited information relating directly to *in vivo* lung inflammation models, however Bayer have recently reported that their selective IKKβ inhibitor reduces airway hyper-reactivity and inflammation in mouse carageenan and rat ova models of airway inflammation (Ziegelbauer et al., 2005). Moreover, TPCA-1 has been reported to reduce lung levels of TNFα, IL-1β, MMP-9, eosinophils and neutrophils in response to aerosolized LPS challenge (Birrell et al., 2006). Whilst these *in vivo* results are encouraging, it will be interesting to see how these compounds perform in models such as chronically smoke-exposed mice, which may undergo an inflammatory response more akin to COPD.

Efficacy in steroid-insensitive inflammation

As part of the mechanism by which steroids gain their efficacy is via modulation of NF-κB signalling, it is important to consider whether novel approaches to modulating this transcription factor via IKKβ inhibition are likely to be efficacious in steroid-insensitive respiratory inflammation. It has been suggested that oxidative stress may play a role in the poor efficacy of corticosteroids in COPD (Barnes, 2004). Tightly bound DNA around a nucleosome core (histone proteins) suppresses gene transcription by decreasing the accessibility of transcription factors such as NF-κB and AP-1 to the transcriptional complex. Acetylation of lysine residues in the N-terminal tails of the core histone proteins results in uncoiling of the DNA, allowing increased accessibility for transcription factor binding. Histone acetylation is reversible and is regulated by a group of histone acetyltransferases (HATs) that promote acetylation and histone deacetylases (HDACs) that promote deacetylation. Ito and co-workers have shown a role for histone acetylation and deacetylation in IL-1β-induced TNFα release in alveolar macrophages derived from cigarette smokers (Ito et al., 2001). They have also suggested that oxidants may play an important role in the modulation of the HDACs and inflammatory cytokine gene transcription. Furthermore, it has been reported that cigarette smoke/H_2O_2 and TNFα cause an increase in histone acetylation (HAT activity) leading to IL-8 expression in monocytes and alveolar epithelial cells both *in vitro* and *in vivo* in rat lungs (Marwick et al., 2004; Moodie et al., 2004).

Glucocorticoid suppression of inflammatory genes requires recruitment of HDAC2 to the NF-κB transcription activation complex by the glucocorticoid receptor (Barnes et al., 2004; Rahman et al., 2004). This results in deacetylation of histones and a decrease in inflammatory gene transcription. A reduced level of HDAC2 was associated with increased pro-inflammatory response and reduced responsiveness to glucocorticoids in alveolar macrophages obtained from smokers (Ito et al., 2001; Rahman et al., 2004). Culpitt and co-workers have shown that cigarette smoke solution stimulated the release of IL-8 and GM-CSF, which was not inhibited by dexamethasone, in alveolar macrophages obtained from patients with COPD compared to that of smokers (Culpitt et al., 2003). They suggested that the lack of efficacy of corticosteroids in COPD might be due to steroid insensitivity of macrophages in the respiratory tract via reduction in HDAC activity. Thus, the cigarette smoke/oxidant-mediated reduction in HDAC2 levels in alveolar epithelial cells and macrophages will not only increase inflammatory gene expression but will also cause a decrease in glucocorticoid function in patients with COPD (Barnes et al., 2004). As IKKβ inhibitors work via inhibition of NF-κB nuclear translocation, their efficacy should be independent of HDAC2 levels and specific activity. In support of this, Rahman and co-workers have developed a steroid-insensitive cigarette smoke condensate (CSC)-induced IL-8 production model in the human monocyte cell line MM6 (Yang et al., 2006). IL-8 production in this model is induced by oxidative stress-dependent activation of NF-κB-mediated transcription and deactivation of HDAC1, 2 and 3 via nitro-tyrosine and aldehyde adduct formation. Whilst dexamethasone shows poor efficacy in this model, the Pfizer IKKβ inhibitor UK436303 maintains both its efficacy and potency irrespective of the loss of HDAC activity (Yang et al., 2006).

Recent data from Birrell et al. does however sound a note of caution (Birrell et al., 2006). TPCA-1 efficacy was compared in rat LPS and neutrophil elastase-induced lung inflammation models. As previously discussed, this compound was active in the steroid-sensitive LPS model but inactive in the steroid-insensitive elastase model, although NF-κB activation was not seen with elastase (Birrell et al., 2006). Whilst the relevance of the elastase model to disease is unclear, this does demonstrate that inhibition of IKKβ does not represent a pan anti-inflammatory mechanism. Again, analysis of IKKβ inhibitors in the steroid-insensitive smoke-exposed mice model will help to build confidence as to whether we can expect efficacy of these agents in COPD.

Potential safety concerns for IKKβ inhibitors

In addition to regulating inflammatory gene expression, NF-κB plays a major role in the regulation of cellular apoptosis (Karin and Lin, 2002). This is exemplified in the p65, IKKβ and IKKγ knockout mice, which die *in utero* due to major liver apoptosis mediated by TNFα (Beg et al., 1995; Li et al., 1999; Li, 1999; Makris, 2000). Deletion of IKKβ in intestinal epithelial cells greatly increased their susceptibility to various apoptosis-inducing stimuli (Egan et al., 2004) and loss of mature B cells (Pasparakis et al., 2002b). Similarly, deletion of IKKβ in macrophages increases their susceptibility to LPS-induced apoptosis, potentially compromising host defence and increasing the risk of developing septic shock (Ruocco et al., 2005). Interestingly, however, conditional knockout of IKKβ in hepatocytes did not lead to a similar TNFα-dependent apoptosis, but instead protected these animals from ischaemia reperfusion injury (Luedde et al., 2005).

Activation of NF-κB also plays a key role in the regulation of skin homeostasis. Whilst epidermal proliferation seems primarily to be IKKα dependent and NF-κB independent (Hu et al., 2001), deletion of IKKβ in epidermal cells results in a severe TNFα-mediated skin inflammation, suggesting that this kinase plays an important role in immune homeostasis (Pasparakis et al., 2002a). Given the challenge in gaining a high degree of selectivity for IKKβ over IKKα, potential effects on skin biology are a concern for future therapeutic approaches

These data plus others are all generated in genetic models where IKKβ is either completely knocked out, potentially affecting the whole protein complex, or IKKβ is replaced with a kinase dead form of the enzyme in certain cell types. Neither of these models would be expected to fully represent the profile one would see with a small-molecule inhibitor of this enzyme. Unfortunately, at present there are few disclosed toxicity data for small-molecule inhibitors on chronic dosing *in vivo* and consequently the degree of concern we should have about these potential adverse events is unknown.

Table 12.1   The IKK and MAPK inhibitors exemplified in the text

Compound	Structure	Target	Development stage	Company
TPCA-1		IKKβ	Discovery	GSK
BMS-354451		IKKβ	Discovery	BMS
SC-514		IKKβ	Research tool	Pfizer
AS602868		IKKβ	Discovery	Celgene/ Serono
Bayer IKKβ selective series	Patent example:	IKKβ	Discovery	Bayer AG
SB203580		p38	Research tool	GSK
FR-167653		p38	Research tool	Fujisawa Pharmaceutical Co Ltd
VX745		p38	Discontinued Phase 2	Vertex
VX702	No published structure	p38	Phase 2 for RA	Vertex
SCIO-469	No published structure	p38	Phase 2 for RA	Scios Inc
SCIO-323	No published structure	p38	Phase 1	Scios Inc

Table 12.1 (*Continued*)

Compound	Structure	Target	Development stage	Company
RWJ67657		p38	Discontinued Phase 1	RW Johnson Pharmacutical Research Institute
BIRB796		p38	No development reported Phase 2b/3 psoriasis, 2a RA	Boehringer Ingelheim
SP600125		JNK	Research tool	Celgene
CC-401	No published structure	JNK	Phase 1	Celgene

12.4 Targeting the MAPKs

The MAPKs are stress-activated protein kinases comprising three families of enzymes: the p38 kinases (α, β, δ, γ), the *c*-jun-NH$_2$ terminal kinases (JNK-1, -2 and -3) and the extracellular signal-regulated kinases (ERK-1 and -2) (Chang and Karin, 2001; Johnson and Lapadat, 2002). These enzymes are activated via a phosphorylation cascade by a wide range of stimuli and they activate a range of downstream kinases and transcription factors. Whilst both the p38 and JNK enzymes are involved in inflammatory signalling, ERK signalling is primarily involved in the regulation of cellular proliferation (Chang and Karin, 2001; Johnson and Lapadat, 2002). Indeed the upstream activator of ERK, MEK, is a target for oncology, with the a number of compounds now being progressed towards clinical trials, such as the Pfizer allosteric MEK inhibitor PD-0325901 (Thompson and Lyons, 2005). Recently a role for ERK in LPS-induced TNFα release from alveolar macrophages has been reported, with inhibition of ERK activation resulting in impaired transport of TNFα mRNA from the nucleus to the cytoplasm (Dumitru et al., 2000). These results may suggest that ERKs play a greater role in inflammatory signalling than originally thought, however at present no specific inhibitors of this enzyme have been reported and further studies will be required to confirm the importance of ERK in respiratory inflammation. In contrast, a number of specific inhibitors have been reported for both p38 and JNK, with these kinases representing promising targets for the treatment of inflammation (Kumar et al., 2003; Manning and Davis, 2003).

Targeting p38 MAPK

There is a large body of evidence that p38-MAPK-mediated signalling may be involved in the inflammation associated with respiratory diseases such as asthma and COPD (Newton and Holden, 2006). p38 MAPK was first identified as the molecular target for the SmithKline and French anti-inflammatory pyridinyl imidazole compounds, including derivatives of SK&F 86002, which had been shown to effectively inhibit LPS-induced IL-1β and TNFα secretion from human peripheral blood monocytes (Han et al., 1994; Lee et al., 1994). From this initial compound a number of more potent and selective ATP-competitive pyridinyl imidazole compounds were identified, such as SB203580. The activity of this tool compound has been widely studied and used to build our understanding of p38 as a key point of conversion for multiple inflammatory signalling pathways (Figure 12.3).

There are four p38 isozymes: α, β, δ and γ. Each of these enzymes are serine/threonine kinases activated by MAPKs (MKK3 or MKK6) but they differ in their

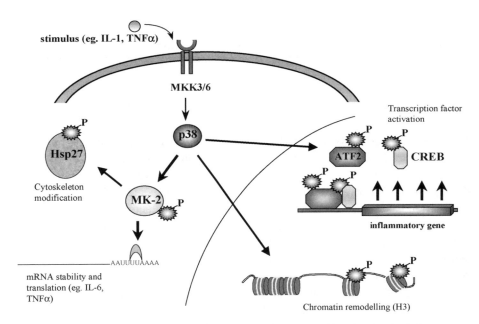

Figure 12.3 Central role of p38a in inflammatory signalling. Cell activation by inflammatory stimuli such as interleukin IL-1 and TNFα binding to their cell-surface receptors can stimulate p38 mitogen-activated protein kinase (MAPK) through a cascade of MAPKs. Activation of p38 MAPK can stimulate phosphorylation of downstream effector molecules, including transcription factors such as ATF2 and cAMP response element binding protein (CREB), thereby enhancing inflammatory gene expression. Activation of p38 MAPK can also lead to phosphorylation of MAPk-activated MK2, which controls mRNA stability and translation by binding to AU-rich regions in the 3′ region of some inflammatory genes. In addition, MK2 is able to regulate cytoskeletal structure by altering the phosphorylation status of hsp27

tissue distribution, regulation of activation and downstream substrates (Kumar et al., 2003; Saklatvala, 2004). p38α and p38β are widely expressed, with p38α being the dominant isoform in monocytes, macrophages and neutophils, and p38β being highly expressed in endothelial cells. In contrast the other isozymes have more restricted expression, with p38γ being expressed in skeletal muscle along with heart, lung, thymus and testis and p38δ being expressed in lung, pancreas, small intestine, kidney, testis and epidermis (Saklatvala, 2004). p38α and p38β are targets for the pyridinyl imidazole compounds such as SB203580, whilst these compounds show greater than 100× reduction in potency versus the δ and γ isozymes due to specific amino acid differences in the ATP binding site at the position equivalent to Thr-106 in p38α (Young et al., 1997). Consequently the majority of data supporting a key role for p38 enzymes in inflammatory signalling relate to p38α/β, and it is these enzymes that have been targeted therapeutically for the treatment of inflammatory diseases. p38α/β regulate inflammatory gene expression at multiple stages in gene induction, transcription and translation (Figure 12.3). There is evidence that p38 indirectly activates a range of transcription factors involved in AP-1-dependent transcription, such as CREB, ATF1, ATF2 and myocyte enhancer factor 2C (MEF2C) (Saklatvala, 2004). AP-1 expression has been reported to be upregulated in asthma and is required for the expression of a range of inflammatory mediators thought to be important in COPD, such as TNFα, IL-6, IL-8, monocyte chemoattractant protein (MCP)-1, MIP-1β and the T-cell cytokines IL-12, interferon (IFN)β and IFNγ. In support of this, SB203580 effectively inhibits expression of these cytokines from a range of cell types, including LPS-induced cytokine production from peripheral blood monocytes, IL-12-induced IFNγ-expression from T cells and IFNγ-induced arachidonic acid release from bronchial epithelial cells (Hedges et al., 2000; Marie et al., 1999; Wu et al., 2004; Zhang and Kaplan, 2000).

p38α/β can also regulate translation and stability of mRNA through activation of MK2 and MK3 (Newton and Holden, 2006). Whilst pyridinyl imidazole inhibitors effectively inhibit LPS-induced TNFα production from macrophages, this is not reflected in a reduction of mRNA (Lee, 1994). In addition, targeted mutation of MK2 effectively inhibited TNFα biosynthesis but not mRNA expression (Kotlyarov et al., 1999). A number of inflammatory genes have now been shown to contain AU-rich elements (AREs) in their 3' untranslated regions (3'UTR), which bind proteins regulating both mRNA stability and translation (Caput et al., 1986). Indeed deletion of these elements in TNFα mRNA results in TNFα protein expression that is independent of MK2 activity (Neininger et al., 2002). Regulation of a range of mediators via p38-dependent phosphorylation of ARE binding proteins has been reported for a number of inflammatory mediators and enzymes, such as TNFα, IL-3, IL-6, IL-8, GM-CSF and COX-2 (Newton and Holden, 2003).

MK2 and MK3 also both phosphorylate the small heat shock protein hsp27, which is involved in actin reorganization and stress fibre formation (McLaughlin et al., 1996; Stokoe et al., 1992). Hsp27 has been reported to play a role in both cellular movement and apoptosis, suggesting that activation of the p38 cascade may rapidly modulate these end points, and has recently been reported to modulate neutrophil chemotaxis via this mechanism (Jog et al., 2007).

It has also been reported that p38 signalling may facilitate inflammatory gene transcription via NF-κB through phosphorylation of the nucleosomal protein histone H3 and the non-histone structural protein HMG14 (Hazzalin et al., 1996; Thomson et al., 1999). It has been suggested that phosphorylation of these proteins causes a change in the chromatin structure, facilitating NF-κB binding and hence inflammatory gene expression (Saccani et al., 2002). Given the suggested key role of NF-κB-mediated gene expression in asthma and COPD, this provides further confidence that p38 inhibitors may have therapeutic benefit for these diseases.

Various p38 inhibitors have been shown to be active in *in vivo* models of lung inflammation. p38α is activated upon lung LPS exposure both in animal models and also in humans (Haddad et al., 2001; Roos-Engstrand et al., 2005). SB203580 has been reported to attenuate both IL-1β and neutrophilia in the bronchoalveolar lavage (BAL) from aerosolized LPS lung challenge model in Wistar rats (Haddad et al., 2001). Interestingly, in these studies SB203580 also significantly inhibited the acute systemic increase in TNFα in response to aerosolized LPS, but did not affect BAL TNFα levels. Similarly, LPS challenge studies in guinea pig with the related compound SB239063 have shown that inhibition of p38 results in attenuation of BAL neutrophilia, IL-6 and MMP-9 activity (Underwood et al., 2000a). Whilst BAL TNFα levels were not reported in this study, SB239063 significantly inhibited serum TNFα production in response to intraperitoneal administration of LPS in Lewis rats. In addition, it has also been reported that SB239063 effectively inhibits ozone-induced BAL neutrophilia, KC and IL-6 production in BALB/c mice and importantly has activity in a mouse cigarette smoke-induced airway neutrophilia model (Underwood et al., 2001). Therefore p38 inhibitors have been shown to have a range of anti-inflammatory properties in *in vivo* models that represent elements of the inflammation characteristic of COPD.

A number of compounds have also been reported to be active in respiratory models of asthma-like inflammation. Birrell et al. have reported that SB203580 significantly inhibited lung oedema, but not BAL TNFα or eosinophilia, in an intratracheal Sephadex-induced inflammation Sprague-Dawley rat model (Birrell et al., 2000). However further studies with the more potent and selective inhibitor SB239063 showed a dose-dependent inhibition of lung eosinophil and lymphocyte recruitment in the Brown Norway ovalbumin challenge model (Underwood et al., 2000b). In addition, Matsuoka and co-workers have reported that a systemically available p38 inhibitor FR-167653, attenuates bleomycin-induced increases in TNFα and lung fibrosis (Matsuoka et al., 2002). Underwood et al. also profiled SB239063 in the bleomycin lung fibrosis model and showed that this compound effectively inhibited increases in hydroxyproline levels and right ventricular hypertrophy (Underwood et al., 2000a). These results suggest that p38 inhibitors may have utility in treating inflammatory cell recruitment and, importantly, lung remodelling in asthma.

Efficacy in steroid-insensitive inflammation

As p38 inhibitors work at multiple levels that are not dependent on recruitment and activation of HDAC enzymes, a similar argument can be made as for IKKβ inhibitors, that they should maintain efficacy in steroid-insensitive inflammation. Indeed, supporting evidence comes from the recent report from Smith et al. showing that in contrast to glucocorticoids there is no difference in efficacy of TNFα inhibition by SB239063 in macrophages from COPD patients and controls (Smith et al., 2006). Recently we have also reported that p38 inhibitors maintain their efficacy in the MM6 oxidative stress model, as previously discussed for inhibitors of IKKβ (Campwala and Kilty, 2006; Yang et al., 2006). In addition to these data, there are a number of properties specific to p38 biology that would support differentiation from steroids in diseases such as COPD.

Activation of the glucocorticoid receptor (GR) results in upregulation of the phosphatase MKP-1 that de-phosphorylates p38α, and in so doing converts it to its inactive form (Lasa et al., 2002). Inhibition of GR activity will therefore result in net induction of p38α activity and therefore increase inflammatory signalling.

Interestingly, it has also been reported that p38α can directly phosphorylate GR, modulating its anti-inflammatory activity (Irusen et al., 2002). Therefore one can hypothesize that inhibition of p38α will both reduce direct inflammatory signalling through this enzyme and also potentially turn off one of the mechanisms that can serve to reduce steroid efficacy.

It has also been suggested that a potential reason for the poor efficacy of steroids in COPD is that they are poor inhibitors of neutrophil function and that lung neutrophilia is a hallmark of this disease (Barnes, 2004). Indeed it has been reported that steroids actively inhibit neutrophil apoptosis, therefore potentially exacerbating neutrophil dependent inflammation. p38α activity also inhibits neutrophil apoptosis and it has been reported that inhibitors of p38α serve to increase the rate of neutrophil apoptosis *in vitro* (Alvarado Kristensson et al., 2004). Therefore both via the primary anti-inflammatory mechanism by which we anticipate efficacy for p38 inhibitors, in addition to the role of p38 in the regulation of GR activity and neutrophil apoptosis, it is reasonable to suggest that these compounds should be efficacious in steroid-insensitive inflammatory conditions such as COPD.

Small-molecule inhibitors of p38

From the initial identification of the pyridinyl imidazoles as potent inhibitors of p38α and p38β, there has been a large amount of interest in the pharmaceutical industry in identifying potent, selective and orally available inhibitors of this enzyme. A number of diverse chemotypes have been identified and optimization of these compounds has been greatly facilitated in the recent past through the availability of a p38α crystal structure (Dominguez et al., 2005a, b; Tong, 1997). The profile of the pyridinyl imidazole compounds has provided much of the confidence in rationale for p38α as an anti-inflammatory target and understanding of how to gain selectivity for this enzyme. SB203580 is highly selective for p38α/β over a wide range of kinases. Analysis of this compound bound into the p38α crystal has revealed that this selectivity is gained by binding the hydrophobic pocket adjacent to the ATP binding site (Tong, 1997). These compounds can access this site in p38α due to the small side chain of the gatekeeper residue Thr-106, and its mutation to a bulky amino acid as found in the majority of kinases prevents sensitivity to this inhibitor.

A number of structurally diverse inhibitors have now been taken to the clinic, providing compelling data for *in vivo* anti-inflammatory activity of p38α inhibitors (Kumar et al., 2003). The primary indications for the majority of p38 inhibitors profiled in the clinic have been rheumatoid arthritis (RA), with pain, psoriasis, cardiovascular disease and cancer also being targeted. However, at present there are no clinical data relating to efficacy in respiratory disease. The Vertex compound VX745 was reported to show efficacy in a Phase 2 study for RA, giving the first compelling evidence that p38 inhibitors are anti-inflammatory in humans (Haddad, 2001). However, this compound was also reported to have some neuronal toxicities, the details of which have not been released, and its development was consequently discontinued (Dominguez et al., 2005a). A second generation compound VX702 entered Phase 2 trials for cardiovascular disease in 2003 and RA in 2005 (Dominguez et al., 2005a). Preliminary results from the RA trial were released in March 2006, reporting an improvement in swollen joints, disease activity and morning stiffness versus placebo, further providing encouraging data for anti-inflammatory efficacy in humans. Similarly, the Scios compound SCIO-469 has been reported to show efficacy in RA trials in combination with methotrexate as measured by ACR20 score and is currently in Phase 2b studies (Dominguez et al., 2005a). In addition, this compound has been reported to show efficacy in a clinical study of post-surgery dental pain, suggesting a role for p38 in the treatment of inflammatory pain (Tong et al., 2004). Scios are now also progressing a second generation p38 inhibitor SCIO-323, with greater potency and selectivity than SCIO-469, through Phase 1 trials.

Anti-inflammatory effects of p38 inhibition in a human endotoxic shock model have been reported for a number of compounds, such as the R. W. Johnson compound RWJ67657 (Fijen et al., 2002) and Boehringer Ingelheim compound BIRB796 (Branger et al., 2001), in addition to conference reports of similar studies being successful for compounds under investigation at Pfizer, Amgen and other companies (Dominguez et al., 2005a). In the BIRB796 studies, 24 healthy male volunteers received a single dose of compound prior to LPS challenge. Systemic LPS challenge was shown to induce activation of p38α, which was in turn inhibited by BIRB796. Moreover, there was a dose-dependent reduction of fever, systemic inflammatory mediator production (TNFα, IL-6, IL-10 and IL1R antagonist), adhesion molecule expression (CD11b) and leukocyte responses, including neutrophilia (Branger et al., 2001). Given the important role of these mediators and cell types in COPD, this provides encouraging confidence in the rationale for p38α inhibition as a therapeutic target in this disease. BIRB796 has a distinct binding mechanism to the other p38 compounds that have been taken forward to date (Pargellis et al., 2002). Whilst this compound is partially competitive with ATP, it gains most of its binding affinity through movement of the DFG loop in p38α, opening a large pocket adjacent to the ATP binding site (Pargellis et al., 2002). There is precedent for movement of the DFG loop in a number of tyrosine kinases, however this was the first example of a serine/threonine kinase with this activity and offers new opportunities for obtaining greater kinase selectivity. Indeed, BIRB796 has good selectivity over a broad range of kinases, although there is still some crossover to JNK-2 (Regan et al., 2002). A consequence of this mode of binding is that the compounds have very slow onset and offset kinetics, which in turn essentially negate the effect of high intracellular ATP concentrations (Regan et al., 2003). Interestingly Boehringer Ingelheim have also published a series of substrate-selective p38α inhibitors (Davidson et al., 2004). These compounds potently inhibit p38α-dependent phosphorylation of MK2, but not ATF2. Interestingly, the compounds do not compete with ATP and, whilst the detail of the compound binding site has not been disclosed, it suggests that there may be an allosteric binding site on p38α that may offer the potential to gain greater selectivity and provide a different biological profile than ATP binding-site inhibitors (Davidson et al., 2004).

Potential safety concerns for p38 inhibitors

A number of p38 inhibitor chemotypes have now been reported to cause elevations in liver transaminases and sporadic skin rash upon chronic dosing (Dominguez et al., 2005a). Whether this effect is mechanism related is still debateable and the fact that there are compounds progressing through Phase 2 trials at present suggests that there may be a therapeutic window between anti-inflammatory efficacy and dose-limiting adverse events. Topical delivery of these compounds limiting systemic exposure, targeting of specific downstream pathways through the use of substrate-selective inhibitors or targeting kinases such as the MKs may provide alternative means to increase the therapeutic index of these approaches.

Targeting JNK

There are three JNK enzymes, with a number of splice variants resulting in a total of 10 JNK isoforms (Gupta, 1996). JNK-1 and -2 are broadly expressed, whereas JNK-3 expression is mainly restricted to neuronal tissue. Activation of JNK enzymes by a wide range of inflammatory stimuli results in phosphorylation of a number of transcription factors, most notably *c*-jun that forms part of the AP-1 transcription factor complex (Hibi et al., 1993), therefore inhibitors of these enzymes will be targeting part of the mechanism modulated by p38 inhibitors. In addition, JNKs have also been associated with stress-induced apoptosis through phosphorylation of proteins such as p53 and Bd2 (Eferl, 2003; Schreiber, 1999).

The JNKs are activated by MKK4- and MKK7- mediated phosphorylation, with maximal enzymatic activity being achieved under conditions of dual phosphorylation (Lawler et al., 1998). These kinases are in turn phosphorylated by a wide variety of MAPKKKs, resulting in a range of stimuli from cytokines such as TNFα to mitogens such as EGF and cellular stresses such as osmotic shock activating this pathway (Manning and Davis, 2003).

LPS-mediated induction of TNFα from macrophages and IgE-stimulated induction of TNFα from mast cells are both dependent upon JNK signalling (Ishizuka, 1997; Swantek et al., 1997). JNK isozymes also play a key role in T-cell maturation and signalling. JNK-1 null CD4$^+$ T-cells selectively differentiate into Th-2 effector cells, moreover JNK-2 null CD4$^+$ cells produce only low levels of IFNγ and fail to differentiate into the Th-1 subtype (Dong, 2000; Yang, 1998). Interestingly, JNK-1 and JNK-2 seem to have opposing roles with respect to CD8$^+$ T-cell expansion, with JNK-1 null mice having an impaired and JNK-2 null mice a greatly increased CD8 cell response (Arbour, 2002; Conze, 2002). The non-JNK isozyme selective inhibitor SP600125 (Celgene) has been used as a tool to build our understanding of JNK signalling both *in vitro* and *in vivo*. This compound is reported to show good selectivity over other MAPKs and IKKs, however recent broader profiling data suggested that there may be crossover to other kinases and therefore data with this tool should be interpreted with caution (Bain et al., 2003). However, SP600125 mimics JNK-1 ablation in mice, suggesting that this may be the predominant activity and also that inhibitors of JNK may have potential for the treatment of autoimmune disease (Conze, 2002). In cellular assays SP600125 inhibited TNFα production from monocytes and IL-2 production from Jurkat T cells, again supporting the role of JNK in these cell types suggested from genetic experiments (Manning and Davis, 2003). Cytokines such as TNFα and also a bias to a CD8$^+$ inflammation have both been implicated in the pathogenesis of COPD. Recently it has also been reported that nicotine also induces JNK-mediated induction of IL-8 from lung epithelial cells, providing another link to this disease, as the vast majority of sufferers are current or ex-smokers (Tsai et al., 2006). Interestingly, in severe glucocorticoid-resistant asthma it has been reported that there is an increase in JNK activity and also in AP-1 transcription factor complex components (Sousa et al., 1999).

SP600125 reduces BAL eosinophilia and serum IgE in the sensitized rat ova-induced airway inflammation model (Eynott et al., 2001) and smooth-muscle proliferation in a chronic allergen exposure model (Nath et al., 2005). This compound has also been reported to show activity in the bleomycin-induced lung fibrosis model in mice (Blease et al., 2003). These studies provide exciting preliminary evidence that JNK inhibitors may show efficacy versus a number of key endpoints characteristic of severe steroid-insensitive asthma. SP600125 administration reduced paw swelling plus bone and cartilage damage in a rat adjuvant-induced arthritis model and these results were reproduced with a JNK-2 null mouse (Han, 2001; Han et al., 2002). In rats, a related JNK inhibitor attenuated systemic LPS-induced TNFα expression when administered 15 min prior to challenge (Manning and Davis, 2003). These studies, coupled with the *in vitro* profile of JNK inhibition, provide some confidence that JNK inhibitors will also be active in non-allergic inflammation. However, at present there is little information available about the efficacy of these compounds in models representing elements of COPD.

Small-molecule inhibitors of JNK

Celgene have identified a second generation inhibitor CC-401 that successfully completed a Phase 1 trial with ascending intravenous dosing in 2003. This compound is now being progressed through a Phase 1 study for acute myelogenous leukaemia (Manning and Davis, 2003). Further studies are also planned to see if CC-401 is steroid-sparing in humans (Adcock et al., 2006). Previous reports from Celgene had suggested that this compound would also be progressed for psoriasis, but no development in this area has been reported. A number of other companies are also developing JNK inhibitors in the Discovery phase, with a range of chemotypes being described in the patent literature (Manning and Davis, 2003). Due to the central role of JNKs in a number of pathways, specifically their link to cellular apoptosis, there are a number of concerns around the likely safety of a chronic treatment targeting these enzymes. This may be reflected in the refocusing of the Celgene clinical studies to oncology endpoints. A number of companies, including Celgene, are consequently investigating whether other points in this signal transduction pathway, such as inhibition of MKK4 or MKK7, may represent safer future therapies (Manning and Davis, 2003). Ongoing clinical studies with CC-401 may help us to better understand the therapeutic potential of JNK inhibitors.

12.5 Targeting PI3K

The phosphoinositide 3-kinases (PI3Ks) are a large family of primarily lipid kinases involved in a range of cellular functions from mitogenesis to insulin signalling (Vanhaesebroeck, 2001; Vanhaesebroeck et al., 2005). These kinases are classified according to their primary sequence, domain structure, regulation and substrate specificity. Of this family of enzymes, the class 1 PI3Ks are the best characterized largely due to the availability of the pharmacological inhibitors wortmanin and LYS294002. The class 1 PI3Ks are composed of two subgroups, class 1A containing PI3Kα, -β and -δ, and class 1B in which the sole representative is PI3Kγ. All of these enzymes catalyse the conversion of phosphatidylinositol (4, 5)-diphosphate (PI(4,5)P2) to PI(3,4,5)P3 (Vanhaesebroeck, 2001). PI(3,4,5)P3 acts as a second

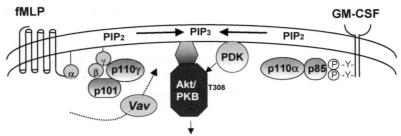

PI3Kγ → shape change, chemotaxis, respiratory burst, protease-release

Figure 12.4   Class 1 PI3Ks: linking cell-surface receptors to signaling networks and cell functions. After cell stimulation, all class I phosphoinositide 3-kinases (PI3Ks) are recruited to the inner face of the plasma membrane, where they generate phosphatidylinositol (PI) trisphosphate (PIP$_3$) by direct phosphorylation of PI bisphosphate (PIP$_2$). Class 1A PI3K iso-forms (p110α, p110β and p110δ) bind directly or indirectly to receptors through the interaction of their regulatory subunits (p85) with phosphotyrosine residues in the receptors or soluble adaptor proteins (SAPs). The only class 1B PI3K isoform, PI3Kγ, is recruited to G-protein-cou-pled receptors such as that for fMet-Leu-Phe (fMLP) by direct interaction with G-protein βγ subunits, through both the catalytic p110 and the regulatory subunits. Activation of all class 1 PI3Ks leads to the generation of the lipid second messenger PIP$_3$ at the cell membrane; this serves as a docking platform for protein kinase B (PKB/Akt), which is phosphorylated at two residues (T308 and S473) by phosphoinositide-dependent kinase (PDK). This leads to a cas-cade of downstream phosphorylating events, protein–protein interactions and the regulation of multiple biological processes

messenger, recruiting proteins that contain a pleckstrin homology domain, and it-self is the substrate for the 3′ phosphate PTEN and 5′ phosphatases such as SHIP-1 (Vanhaesebroeck, 2001). Through PI(3,4,5)P3, PI3Ks activate PDK1 and AKT. This PI3K signalling pathway is involved in a wide variety of cellular activities, including inflammatory signalling, proliferation, survival, adhesion, motility and NADPH-oxidase activation (Vanhaesebroeck, 2001).

The class 1A PI3Ks are heterodimers composed of a p85 regulatory subunit and a p110 catalytic subunit. The class 1B enzyme PI3Kγ is also a heterodimer of a p101 regulator subunit and a p110 catalytic subunit, and is biologically distinct from the class 1A enzymes as it is involved in G-protein-coupled receptor (GPCR) signal transduction (Vanhaesebroeck, 2001) (Figure 12.4).

Whereas PI3Kα and -β are ubiquitously expressed, PI3Kδ and -γ expression is primarily restricted to leukocytes and both of these enzymes may represent interest-ing therapeutic targets for steroid-insensitive respiratory inflammation.

PI3Kδ and PI3Kγ as anti-inflammatory targets

Whilst wortmanin and LYS294002 have been invaluable tools in developing our understanding of the role of PI3Ks in inflammation, these compounds are not subtype selective and also have activity on a number of other lipid kinases, complicating the interpretation of results (Knight et al., 2006). However, knockout mice for both PI3Kδ and -γ are viable, and have been important in defining the role of these kinases in inflammatory signalling (Vanhaesebroeck et al., 2005).

The PI3Kγ heterodimer is activated via interaction with the Gβγ subunit that is released from the Gαβγ trimer post-stimulation of GPCRs such as the IL-8 chemokine receptor CXCR-2. Consequently it has been shown to be involved in cellular chemotaxis of a range of inflammatory cells, such as neutrophils (Thomas et al., 2005), T lymphocytes (Reif et al., 2004), dendritic cells (Del Prete, 2004) and eosinophils (Walker et al., 2006). In addition, PI3Kγ has been reported to be involved in neutrophil degranulation (Hannigan et al., 2004) and mast cell signalling in response to adenosine and a range of chemokines (Laffargue, 2002). Interestingly there is also a growing body of evidence that PI3Kγ is involved in the regulation of MMPs, such as MMP-9, which have been associated with the pathogenesis of COPD. Therefore PI3Kγ signalling is involved in multiple processes important in COPD, from recruitment of cells to production of inflammatory mediators.

PI3K p110γ KO mice are healthy and show no overt adverse phenotype. Intranasal instillation of MIP-2 or KC results in a reduced lung neutrophilia in KO mice (Thomas et al., 2005). Moreover, in an intratracheal LPS model, these mice showed reduced BAL neutrophilia relative to littermate controls (Puri et al., 2005). Interestingly, Puri et al. also showed that PI3Kγ has a critical role in endothelial cell upregulation of adhesion molecules (Puri et al., 2005). Currently there are no published data for these mice in smoking models representing elements of COPD-like inflammation, but these data will be important in building our confidence in the rationale for PI3Kγ inhibitors as therapies for this disease. Interestingly, intratracheal administration of LYS294002 results in inhibition of ova-induced increases in BAL eosinophilia, IL-5, IL-13 and eotaxin levels. PI3Kγ KO mice also show a reduced BAL eosinophilia in an allergen challenge model 48 h after stimulation, but not at earlier time points (Pinho et al., 2005), suggesting a role for the other PI3Ks in this response.

Currently there is relatively little information about isozyme-selective small-molecule inhibitors in *in vivo* models. However, Camps et al. have recently published studies with a selective PI3Kγ inhibitor AS605240 in rat collagen-induced arthritis and αCII-induced arthritis models (Camps et al., 2005). In these studies oral administration of a PI3Kγ inhibitor reduced paw swelling, synovial inflammation and cartilage erosion with similar efficacy to the PI3Kγ KO mice. In addition, this compound also showed efficacy in a model of systemic lupus, further providing evidence of an *in vivo* anti-inflammatory profile for PI3Kγ inhibitors (Barber et al., 2005). Assessment of this tool compound in models of respiratory inflammation would be very interesting.

The recent publication of a selective inhibitor of PI3Kδ, IC87114 (ICOS Corporation), has greatly increased our understanding of this enzyme, complementing knockout mouse studies. PI3Kδ plays a key role in both T- and B-lymphocyte antigen receptor signalling and allergen-IgE-induced mast cell degranulation (Ali, 2004; Puri et al., 2004). *In vivo* administration of IC87114 protected mice from FcεRI-mediated allergic responses in a passive cutaneous anaphylaxis model in mouse (Ali, 2004). In an ova challenge model in BALB/c mice, intratracheal administration of IC87114 significantly attenuated BAL eosinophils, neutrophils and lymphocytes as well as a range of cytokines including IL-4, IL-5, IL-13 and RANTES (Lee et al., 2006). Moreover, IC87114 also significantly inhibited serum IgE, tissue eosinophilia, tissue mucus production and airway hyper-responsiveness to methacholine. As for PI3Kγ, there are no published data describing the activity of this PI3Kδ inhibitor or knockout mice in *in vivo* models of COPD-like inflammation.

PI3Kδ and PI3Kγ in steroid-insensitive inflammation

Lung neutrophilia and oxidative stress are characteristic of the steroid-insensitive inflammation in COPD and severe asthma. Indeed, a potential reason for poor efficacy of corticosteroids in COPD is that they are ineffective at inhibiting neutrophil function (Barnes, 2004). As a major role of PI3Kγ signalling is the chemotaxis and hence recruitment of inflammatory cells, including neutrophils, it is reasonable to hypothesize that inhibition of this enzyme would be anti-inflammatory in these diseases.

There is a growing body of evidence that PI3Ks are activated by and involved in the production of reactive oxygen species (ROS), which contribute to the oxidative stress in these diseases. PI3K signalling is activated in various cell types in response to H_2O_2 via deactivation of PTEN phosphatase, causing a net increase in PI(3,4,5)P3 levels (Leslie et al., 2003). Interestingly, LY294002 abolishes chemokine-induced ROS generation in phagocytes and similar inhibition has also been reported in neutrophils from PI3Kγ KO mice (Qin and Chock, 2003). In contrast, recent data also suggest that PI3Ks may have a role in the production of the antioxidant enzyme haeme oxygenase-1, suggesting a role for PI3Ks in both the production of ROS and the inhibition of the downstream effects of this pro-inflammatory stimulus (Rojo et al., 2006).

As previously described, a potential reason for poor efficacy of corticosteroids under conditions of oxidative stress is the downregulation of HDAC proteins, specifically HDAC2. Interestingly, it has been reported that LY294002 and an AKT inhibitor (SH-5) can restore defective HDAC2 expression in these models (Ito et al., 2006). Further studies to determine the isozyme responsible for this activity will be interesting and may offer an opportunity to re-sensitize patients to corticosteroids to some degree.

Small-molecule inhibitors of PI3Kδ and PI3Kγ

There are currently no PI3K inhibitors in the clinic, although there is significant interest in these potential targets throughout the pharmaceutical industry, with a number of molecules in pre-clinical development (Ito et al., 2006). Selectivity of these compounds over the closely related PI3Kα and -β enzymes will be critical for the likely safety profile of PI3K inhibitors. These enzymes are thought to be important for a number of processes such as cellular proliferation and insulin signalling (Vanhaesebroeck et al., 2005), inhibition of which would be incompatible with chronic treatment of respiratory disease.

Recent identification of selective PI3Kγ inhibitors such as AS-605240 (Serono) has been greatly facilitated by the crystal structure of p110γ (Walker et al., 1999; Walker, 2000). Indeed, analysis of a variety of PI3K inhibitors in recombinant assays and modelled into crystal structures has led to the identification of various pockets within the ATP binding site that have the potential to provide selectivity within this kinase family and, importantly, against the much larger protein kinase family (Knight et al., 2006). These studies and the publication of PI3Kγ (AS-605240)- and PI3Kδ (IC87114)-selective compounds suggest that it will be possible to identify isozyme-selective inhibitors for future clinical assessment.

12.6   Further Potential Kinase Targets

In addition to the NF-κB, MAPK and PI3K pathways, there are a number of other potential kinase targets for the treatment of steroid-insensitive respiratory inflammation for which preliminary data have been reported.

EGFR antagonists such as Irresa have been developed for the treatment of epidermal cancers, but may also suppress airway mucus secretion (Wakeling, 2002). Moreover, EGFR expression in the airway is associated with airway remodelling and is enhanced with increased asthma severity, providing circumstantial evidence for a role of this receptor in these processes (Puddicombe et al., 2000). Interestingly this expression is insensitive to glucocorticoid therapy. The treatment of COPD or severe asthma may therefore represent alternative indications for inhibitors such as Irresa and it would be interesting if these were to be studied further in the clinic, whilst accepting that the safety profile of this compound may limit its suitability for the chronic treatment of respiratory disease.

The Janus kinases (JAK1, -2 and -3) are primary mediators of cytokine signalling, activating STAT transcription factors such as STAT6 that are associated with T-cell differentiation to a Th-2 phenotype. A number of JAK3 inhibitors are in development for transplant rejection, effectively blocking IL-2-mediated T-cell function and resulting in immunosupression (Papageorgiou and Wilkman, 2004). The JAK3-selective compound WHI-P131 also inhibits IgE-mediated FcεR cross-linking-induced mast cell degranulation and cytokine release (Malaviya et al., 1999). In addition this compound shows efficacy in a mouse anaphylaxis model (Malaviya et al., 1999). Interestingly, immunosuppressive agents such as cyclosporin and rapamycin have been studied clinically in patients with oral steroid-dependent asthma (Kon and Kay, 1999; Niven and Argyros, 2003). Whilst these compounds showed

Table 12.2 Further kinase inhibitors exemplified in the text

Compound	Structure	Target	Development Stage	Company
Wortmanin		PI3K	Research tool	–
LYS294002		PI3K	Research tool	–
AS-605240		PI3Kγ	Discovery	Serono
IC87114		PI3Kδ	Discovery	ICOS Corp.
Irresa		EGFR	Launched cancer treatment	AstraZeneca

Compound	Target	Phase	Company
WHI-P131	JAK3	Discovery	Hughes Institute
BAY 61-3606	SYK	Discovery (possibly discontinued)	Bayer AG
R-112 (No published structure)	SYK	Phase 2 allergic rhinitis	Rigel
R406	SYK	Phase 2 RA	Rigel
BMS-509744	ITK	Discovery	BMS

significant beneficial effects, they were outweighed by the adverse events reported upon chronic dosing and it is likely that there may be similar issues with oral JAK inhibitors, limiting the utility of this approach.

Spleen tyrosine kinase (SYK) is a tyrosine kinase that is critical for IgE-mediated mast cell degranulation, B- and T-cell lymphocyte signal transduction and eosinophil survival (Wong et al., 2004). The potent selective SYK inhibitor BAY 61-3606 suppresses antigen-induced passive cutaneous anaphylactic reaction, bronchoconstriction and bronchial oedema in rat, in addition to inhibiting ova-induced airway inflammation in a sensitized rat model (Yamamoto et al., 2003). Rigel currently have two SYK inhibitors in clinical development. R-112 delivered intranasally was reported to show efficacy in the Phase 2 park study of allergic rhinitis, although recent press releases suggest that this efficacy was not reproduced in a blinded crossover allergen challenge study (Meltzer et al., 2005). R406 is an oral SYK inhibitor that is currently undergoing Phase 2 clinical trials for rheumatoid arthritis. A third compound, R343, is currently being developed by Pfizer under licence with Rigel as an inhaled therapy for asthma and is in late pre-clinical testing. The IL-2-inducible T-cell kinase ITK may also offer potential as a target for asthma via modulation of mast cell and T-cell signalling. ITK KO mice show reduced tissue eosinophilia, cytokine expression and mast cell degranulation in comparison to littermate controls (Forssell et al., 2005; Mueller and August, 2003). Moreover, a selective ITK inhibitor published by Bristol Myers Squib (BMS-509744) has been reported to have a similar phenotype to the knockout mice in these models (Lin et al., 2004). Relatively little information is currently available about inhibitors of this kinase, although a variety of companies such as Bristol Myers Squib, Aventis and AstraZeneca have published patents describing ITK inhibitors.

Various other kinases such as the SRC kinase LCK or the protein kinase C family of enzymes have been suggested to play roles in both asthma and COPD (Adcock et al., 2006). As selective inhibitors for each of these enzymes become available it will be interesting to test their efficacy pre-clinically in models of inflammation, or preferentially clinically in the true disease states.

12.7   Conclusions

The central role of kinases in mediating inflammatory signalling and amplification of the inflammatory response makes them attractive therapeutic targets for the treatment of respiratory diseases such as asthma and COPD. There is compelling evidence that NF-κB, MAPK and PI3K signalling pathways are activated in these diseases and emerging data to provide evidence that modulation of these pathways via small-molecule kinase inhibitors is anti-inflammatory in a range of *in vitro* and *in vivo* models. Moreover, whilst these pathways share some similar mechanisms of action to glucocorticoids, there is evidence to suggest that they may still be effective in glucocorticoid-insensitive inflammation and, in the case of PI3Ks, re-sensitize cells to glucocorticoids.

A key hurdle to the progression of these potential anti-inflammatory therapies is the development of highly selective compounds that have a suitable safety profile for chronic administration. Our knowledge of how to obtain selective kinase inhibitors has expanded greatly over recent years, facilitated by the availability of a growing number of kinase crystal structures. However, this is still a significant hurdle. The central role of these kinases in signalling pathways involved in a variety of processes such as cell proliferation, apoptosis and homeostasis also provides a challenge with regard to gaining maximal anti-inflammatory efficacy whilst avoiding side effects. Investigating alternative kinase targets with a more restricted signalling role or the potential to deliver kinase inhibitors specifically to their intended site of action may represent the means by which to overcome these challenges.

A large number of kinase inhibitors are now in pre-clinical development for the treatment of inflammatory diseases, or in the case of p38 MAPK in clinical development. As more information is released about these compounds with regard to their safety on chronic dosing and efficacy in disease models, or indeed the clinic, we will get a clearer view of the potential for this exciting class of therapeutic targets, which offer the potential to be highly efficacious treatments for a disease area that is poorly treated with current therapies.

Acknowledgements

I would like to thank Dr Chris Phillips and Dr Russell Lewthwaite of PGRD Sandwich, for their help with crystallography and chemistry, respectively, and Dr Nandini Kishore of PGRD St. Louis for critical reading of this manuscript.

References

Adcock IM, Chung KF, Caramori G, Ito K. Kinase inhibitors and airway inflammation. *Eur J Pharmacol* 2006; **533**: 118–132.

Ali K. Essential role for the p110delta phosphoinositide 3-kinase in the allergic response. *Nature* 2004; **431**: 1007–1011.

Alvarado Kristensson M, Leandersson F, Ronnstrand K, Wernstedt L, Tommy CA. p38-MAPK signals survival by phosphorylation of caspase-8 and caspase-3 in human neutrophils. *J Exp Med* 2004; **199**: 449–458.

Arbour N. c-Jun NH2-terminal kinase (JNK)1 and JNK2 signaling pathways have divergent roles in CD8+ T cell-mediated antiviral immunity. *J Exp Med* 2002; **195**: 801–810.

Bain J, McLauchlan H, Elliott M, Cohen P. The specificities of protein kinase inhibitors: an update. *Biochem J* 2003; **371**: 199–204.

Barber DF, Bartolome A, Hernandez C, Flores JM et al. PI3Kγ inhibition blocks glomerulonephritis and extends lifespan in a mouse model of systemic lupus. *Nat Med* 2005; **11**: 933–935.

Barnes PJ. Corticosteroid resistance in airway disease. *Proc Am Thoracic Soc* 2004; **1**: 264–268.

Barnes PJ, Karin M. Nuclear factor-κB – a pivotal transcription factor in chronic inflammatory diseases. *N Engl J Med* 1997; **336**: 1066–1071.

Barnes PJ, Ito K, Adcock IM. Corticosteroid resistance in chronic obstructive pulmonary disease: inactivation of histone deacetylase. *Lancet* 2004; **363**: 731–733.

Beg AA, Sha WC, Bronson RT, Ghosh S, Baltimore D. Embryonic lethality and liver degeneration in mice lacking the RelA component of NF-κB. *Nature* 1995; **376**: 167–169.

Birrell MA, Hardaker E, Wong S, Mccluskie K et al. IκB kinase-2 inhibitor blocks inflammation in human airway smooth muscle and a rat model of asthma. *Am J Respir Crit Care Med* 2005; **172**: 962–971.

Birrell M, Hele D, Mccluskie K, Webber S, Foster M, Belvisi MG. Effect of the p38 kinase inhibitor, SB 203580, on sephadex induced airway inflammation in the rat. *Eur Respir J* 2000; **16**: 947–950.

Birrell MA, Wong S, Hardaker EL, Catley MC et al. I kappa B kinase-2-independent and -dependent inflammation in airway disease models: Relevance of IKK-2 inhibition to the clinic. *Mol Pharm* 2006; **69**: 1791–1800.

Blease K, Leisten JC, Pai S, Groessl T, Shirley M, Raymon HK. The small molecule JNK inhibitor, SP600125, attenuates bleomycin-induced pulmonary fibrosis. *Inflamm Res* 2003; **52**: S153.

Blencke S, Zech B, Engkvist O, Greff Z et al. Characterization of a conserved structural determinant controlling protein kinase sensitivity to selective inhibitors. *Chem Bio* 2004; **11**: 691–701.

Bonizzi G, Karin M. The two NF-κB activation pathways and their role in innate and adaptive immunity. *Trends Immunol* 2004; **25**: 280–288.

Branger J, Blink BVD, Weijer S, Madwed J et al. Anti-inflammatory effects of a p38 mitogen activated protein kinase inhibitor (BIRB 796 BS) during human endotoxemia. *Arthritis Rheum* 2001; **44**: S164.

Burke JR, Pattoli MA, Gregor KR, Brassil PJ et al. BMS-345541 is a highly selective inhibitor of I kappa B kinase that binds at an allosteric site of the enzyme and blocks NF-κB-dependent transcription in mice. *J Biol Chem* 2003; **278**: 1450–1456.

Busse WW, Lemanske RF Jr. Asthma. *N Engl J Med* 2001; **344**: 350–362.

Camps M, Ruckle T, Ji H, Ardissone V et al. Blockade of PI3Kγ suppresses joint inflammation and damage in mouse models of rheumatoid arthritis. *Nat Med* 2005; **11**: 936–943.

Campwala H, Kilty I. Development of a steroid-insensitive cytokine release assay in the human monocytic MM6 cell line. *Am. J. Resp. Crit. Care Med* 2006; **173**: A357.

Caput D, Beutler B, Hartog K, Thayer R, Brown-Shimer S, Cerami A. Identification of a common nucleotide sequence in the 3′-untranslated region of mRNA molecules specifying inflammatory mediators. *Proc Nat Acad Sci USA* 1986; **83**: 1670–1674.

Caramori G, Romagnoli M, Casolari P, Bellettato C et al. Nuclear localisation of p65 in sputum macrophages but not in sputum neutrophils during COPD exacerbations. *Thorax* 2003; **58**: 348–351.

Chang L, Karin M. Mammalian MAP kinase signalling cascades. *Nature* 2001; **410**: 37–40.

Choi M, Rolle S, Wellner M, Cardoso MC, Scheidereit C, Luft FC, Kettritz R. Inhibition of NF-{kappa}B by a TAT-NEMO-binding domain peptide accelerates constitutive apoptosis and abrogates LPS-delayed neutrophil apoptosis. *Blood* 2003; **102**: 2259–2267.

Cohen P. Protein kinases–the major drug targets of the twenty-first century? *Nature Rev Drug Discov* 2002; **1**: 309–315.

Coish PDG, Wickens PL, Lowinger TB. Small molecule inhibitors of IKK kinase activity. *Expert Opin Ther Pat* 2006; **16**: 1–12.

Conze D. c-Jun NH$_2$-terminal kinase (JNK)1 and JNK2 have distinct roles in CD8$^+$ T cell activation. *J Exp Med* 2002; **195**; 811–823.

Courtois G, Smahi A, Israel A. NEMO/IKKγ: linking NF-κB to human disease. *Trends Mol Med* 2001; **7**: 427–430.

Culpitt SV, Rogers DF, Shah P, De Matos C, Russell REK, Donnelly LE, Barnes PJ. Impaired inhibition by dexamethasone of cytokine release by alveolar macrophages from patients with chronic obstructive pulmonary disease. *Am J Respir Crit Care Med* 2003; **167**: 24–31.

Davidson W, Frego L, Peet GW, Kroe RR et al. Discovery and Characterization of a substrate selective p38 inhibitor. *Biochemistry* 2004; **43**: 11658–11671.

Del Prete A. Defective dendritic cell migration and activation of adaptive immunity in PI3K-gamma-deficient mice. *EMBO J* 2004; **23**: 3505–3515.

Di Stefano A, Caramori G, Oates T, Capelli A et al. Increased expression of nuclear factor-κB in bronchial biopsies from smokers and patients with COPD. *Eur Respir J* 2002; **20**: 556–563.

Dominguez C, Powers DA, Tamayo N. p38 MAP kinase inhibitors: Many are made, but few are chosen. *Curr Opin Drug Discov Dev* 2005a; **8**: 421–430.

Dominguez C, Tamayo N, Zhang D. p38 Inhibitors: beyond pyridinylimidazoles. *Expert Opin Ther Pat* 2005b; **15**: 801–816.

Dong C. JNK is required for effector T-cell function but not for T-cell activation. *Nature* 2000; **405**: 91–94.

Dumitru CD, Ceci JD, Tsatsanis C, Kontoyiannis D et al. TNF-α induction by LPS is regulated posttranscriptionally via a Tpl2/ERK-dependent pathway. *Cell* 2000; **103**: 1071–1083.

Eferl R. Liver tumor development. c-Jun antagonizes the proapoptotic activity of p53. *Cell* 2003; **112**: 181–192.

Egan LJ, Eckmann L, Greten FR, Chae S et al. IκB-kinaseβ-dependent NF-κB activation provides radioprotection to the intestinal epithelium. *Proc Natl Acad Sci USA* 2004; **101**: 2452–2457.

Eynott PR, Adcock IM, Chung P. The effects of selective c-Jun N-terminal kinase inhibition in a sensitized Brown Norway rat model of allergic asthma. *Am J Respir Crit Care Med* 2001; **49**: S102–S102.

Fabian MA, Biggs WH 3rd, Treiber DK, Atteridge, CE et al. A small molecule-kinase interaction map for clinical kinase inhibitors. *Nature biotechnol* 2005; **23**: 329–336.

Fijen JW, Tulleken JE, Kobold ACM, De Boer P et al. Inhibition of p38 mitogen-activated protein kinase: dose-dependent suppression of leukocyte and endothelial response after endotoxin challenge in humans. *Crit Care Med* 2002; **30**: 841–845.

Forssell J, Sideras P, Eriksson C, Malm-Erjefalt M, Rydell-Tormanen K, Ericsson P-O, Erjefalt JS. Interleukin-2-inducible T cell kinase regulates mast cell degranulation and acute allergic responses. *Am J Respir Cell Mol Biol* 2005; **32**: 511–520.

Frelin C, Imbert V, Griessinger E, Loubat A, Dreano M, Peyron J-F. AS602868, a pharmacological inhibitor of IKK2, reveals the apoptotic potential of TNF-alpha in Jurkat leukemic cells. *Oncogene* 2003; **22**: 8187–8194.

Gorre ME, Mohammed M, Ellwood K, Hsu N, Paquette R, Rao PN, Sawyers CL. Clinical resistance to STI-571 cancer therapy caused by BCR-ABL gene mutation or amplification. *Science* 2001; **293**: 876–880.

Grimshaw CE. Identification of a potent, orally active small molecule IKK2 inhibitor. *Inflamm Res* 2001; **50**: S149.

Gumireddy K, Baker SJ, Cosenza SC, John P et al. A non-ATP-competitive inhibitor of BCR-ABL overrides imatinib resistance. *Proc Natl Acad Sci USA* 2005; **102**: 1992–1997.

Gupta S. Selective interaction of JNK protein kinase isoforms with transcription factors. *EMBO J* 1996; **15**: 2760–2770.

Haddad EB, Birrell M, McCluskie K, Ling A, Webber SE, Foster ML. Role of p38 MAP kinase in LPS-induced airway inflammation in the rat. *Br J Pharmacol* 2001; **132**: 1715–1724.

Haddad JJ. VX-745. Vertex Pharmaceuticals. *Curr Opin Invest Drugs* 2001; **2**: 1070–1076.

Han J, Lee JD, Bibbs L, Ulevitch R J. A MAP kinase targeted by endotoxin and hyperosmolarity in mammalian cells. *Science* 1994; **265**: 808–811.

Han Z. c-Jun N-terminal kinase is required for metalloproteinase (MMP) expression in synoviocytes and regulates bone destruction in adjuvant arthritis. *J Clin Invest* 2001; **108**: 73–81.

Han Z, Chang L, Yamanishi Y, Karin M, Firestein GS. Joint damage and inflammation in c-Jun N-terminal kinase 2 knockout mice with passive murine collagen-induced arthritis. *Arthritis Rheum* 2002; **46**: 818–823.

Hannigan MO, Huang CK, Wu DQ. Roles of PI3K in neutrophil function. *Book title: Phosphoinositides in Subcellular Targeting and Enzyme Activation.* New York: Springer-Verlag.

Hazzalin CA, Cano E, Cuenda A, Barratt MJ, Cohen P, Mahadevan LC. p38/RK is essential for stress-induced nuclear responses: JNK/SAPKs and c-Jun/ATF-2 phosphorylation are insufficient. *Curr Biol* 1996; **6**: 1028–1031.

Hedges JC, Singer CA, Gerthoffer WT. Mitogen-activated protein kinases regulate cytokine gene expression in human airway myocytes. *Am J Respir Cell Mol Biol* 2000; **23**: 86–94.

Hibi M, Lin A, Smeal T, Minden A, Karin M. Identification of an oncoprotein- and UV-responsive protein kinase that binds and potentiates the c-Jun activation domain. *Genes Dev* 1993; **7**: 2135–2148.

Hu Y, Baud V, Oga T, Kim KI, Yoshida K, Karin M. IKKα controls formation of the epidermis independently of NF-κB. *Nature* 2001; **410**: 710–714.

Irusen E, Matthews JG, Takahashi A, Barnes PJ, Chung KF, Adcock IM. p38 Mitogen-activated protein kinase-induced glucocorticoid receptor phosphorylation reduces its activity: role in steroid-insensitive asthma. *J Allergy Clin Immunol* 2002; **109**: 649–657.

Ishizuka T. Mast cell tumor necrosis factor [alpha] production is regulated by MEK kinases. *Proc Natl Acad Sci USA* 1997; **94**: 6358–6363.

Ito K, Caramori G, Adcock IM. Therapeutic potential of PI3K inhibitors in inflammatory respiratory disease. *J Pharmacol Exp Ther* 2006; **106**: 1166–1174.

Ito K, Lim S, Caramori G, Chung KF, Barnes PJ, Adcock IM. Cigarette smoking reduces histone deacetylase 2 expression, enhances cytokine expression, and inhibits glucocorticoid actions in alveolar macrophages. *FASEB J* 2001; **15**: 1110–1112.

Jog NR, Jala VR, Ward RA, Rane MJ, Haribabu B, Mcleish KR. Heat shock protein 27 regulates neutrophil chemotaxis and exocytosis through two independent mechanisms. *J Immunol* 2007; **178**: 2421–2428.

Johnson GL, Lapadat R. Mitogen-activated protein kinase pathways mediated by ERK, JNK, and p38 protein kinases. *Science* 2002; **298**: 1911–1912.

Kapahi P, Takahashi T, Natoli G, Adams SR, Chen Y, Tsien RY, Karin M. Inhibition of NF-kappa B activation by arsenite through reaction with a critical cysteine in the activation loop of Ikappa B kinase. *J Biol Chem* 2000; **275**: 36062–36066.

Karin M. The beginning of the end: Ikappa B kinase (IKK) and NF-kappa B activation. *J. Biol Chem* 1999; **274**: 27339–27342.

Karin M. Inflammation-activated protein kinases as targets for drug development. *Proc Am Thorac Soc* 2005; **2**: 386–390.

Karin M, Lin A. NF-κB at the crossroads of life and death. *Nat Immunol* 2002; **3**: 221–227.

Karin M, Yamamoto Y, Wang QM. The IKK NF-kappaB system: a treasure trove for drug development. *Nature Rev Drug Discov* 2004; **3**: 17–26.

Kishore N, Sommers C, Mathialagan S, Guzova J et al. A selective IKK-2 inhibitor blocks NF-kappa B-dependent gene expression in interleukin-1 beta-stimulated synovial fibroblasts. *J Biol Chem* 2003; **278**: 32861–32871.

Knight ZA, Gonzalez B, Feldman ME, Zunder ER et al. A pharmacological map of the PI3-K family defines a role for p110α in insulin signaling. *Cell* 2006; **125**: 733–747.

Kon OM, Kay AB. Anti-T cell strategies in asthma. *Inflamm Res* 1999; **48**: 516–523.

Kotlyarov A, Neininger A, Schubert C, Eckert R, Birchmeier C, Volk HD, Gaestel M. MAP-KAP kinase 2 is essential for LPS-induced TNF-alpha biosynthesis. *Nature Cell Biol* 1999; **1**: 94–97.

Kumar S, Boehm J, Lee JC. p38 MAP kinases: key signalling molecules as therapeutic targets for inflammatory diseases. *Nat Rev Drug Discov* 2003; **2**: 717–726.

Laffargue M. Phosphoinositide 3-kinase gamma is an essential amplifier of mast cell function. *Immunity* 2002; **16**: 441–451.

Lasa M, Abraham SM, Boucheron C, Saklatvala J, Clark AR. Dexamethasone causes sustained expression of mitogen-activated protein kinase (MAPK) phosphatase 1 and phosphatase-mediated inhibition of MAPK p38. *Mol Cell Biol* 2002; **22**: 7802–7811.

Lawler S, Fleming Y, Goedert M, Cohen P. Synergistic activation of SAPK1/JNK1 by two MAP kinase kinases in vitro. *Curr Biol* 1998; **8**: 1387–1390.

Lee JC. A protein kinase involved in the regulation of inflammatory cytokine biosynthesis. *Nature* 1994; **372**: 739–746.

Lee JC, Laydon JT, McDonnell PC, Gallagher TF et al. A protein kinase involved in the regulation of inflammatory cytokine biosynthesis. *Nature* 1994; **372**: 739–746.

Lee KS, Lee HK, Hayflick JS, Lee YC, Puri KD. Inhibition of phosphoinositide 3-kinase {delta} attenuates allergic airway inflammation and hyperresponsiveness in murine asthma model. *FASEB J* 2006; **20**: 455–465.

Leslie NR, Bennett D, Lindsay YE, Stewart H, Gray A, Downes CP. Redox regulation of PI 3-kinase signalling via inactivation of PTEN. *EMBO J* 2003; **22**: 5501–5510.

Li Q, Verma IM. NF-κB regulation in the immune system. *Nature Rev Immunol* 2002; **2**: 725–734.

Li Q, Van Antwerp D, Mercurio F, Lee KF, Verma IM. Severe liver degeneration in mice lacking the IκB kinase 2 gene. *Science* 1999; **284**: 321–325.

Li ZW. The IKKβ subunit of IκB kinase (IKK) is essential for NF-κB activation and prevention of apoptosis. *J Exp Med* 1999; **189**: 1839–1845.

Lin TA, McIntyre KW, Das J, Liu C et al. Selective Itk inhibitors block T-cell activation and murine lung inflammation. *Biochemistry* 2004; **43**: 11056–11062.

Luedde T, Assmus U, Wustefeld T, Meyer Zu Vilsendorf A et al. Deletion of IKK2 in hepatocytes does not sensitize these cells to TNF-induced apoptosis but protects from ischemia/reperfusion injury. *J Clin Invest* 2005; **115**: 849–859.

Luo Y. Selectivity assessment of kinase inhibitors: strategies and challenges. *Curr Opin Mol Ther* 2005; **7**: 251–255.

MacNee W. Pathogenesis of chronic obstructive pulmonary disease. *Proc Am Thorac Soc* 2005; **2**: 258–266.

Makris C. Female mice heterozygote for IKK[gamma]/NEMO deficiencies develop a genodermatosis similar to the human X-linked disorder Incontinentia Pigmenti. *Mol Cell* 2000; **15**: 969–979.

Malaviya R, Zhu D, Dibirdik I, Uckun FM. Targeting Janus kinase 3 in mast cells prevents immediate hypersensitivity reactions and anaphylaxis. *J Biol Chem* 1999; **274**: 27028–27038.

Manley PW, Bold G, Bruggen J, Fendrich G et al. Advances in the structural biology, design and clinical development of VEGF-R kinase inhibitors for the treatment of angiogenesis. *Biochim Biophys Acta* 2004; **1697**: 17–27.

Manning AM, Davis RJ. Targeting JNK for therapeutic benefit: from junk to gold? *Nature Rev Drug Discov* 2003; **2**: 554–565.

Manning G, Whyte DB, Martinez R, Hunter T, Sudarsanam S. The protein kinase complement of the human genome. *Science* 2002; **298**: 1912–1934.

Marie C, Roman-Roman S, Rawadi G. Involvement of mitogen-activated protein kinase pathways in interleukin-8 production by human monocytes and polymorphonuclear cells stimulated with lipopolysaccharide or Mycoplasma fermentans membrane lipoproteins. *Infect Immun* 1999; **67**: 688–693.

Marwick JA, Kirkham PA, Stevenson CS, Danahay H et al. Cigarette smoke alters chromatin remodeling and induces proinflammatory genes in rat lungs. *Am J Respir Cell Mol Biol* 2004; **31**: 633–642.

Matsuoka H, Arai T, Mori M, Goya S et al. A p38 MAPK inhibitor, FR-167653, ameliorates murine bleomycin-induced pulmonary fibrosis. *Am J Physiol Lung Cell Mol Physiol* 2002; **283**: L103–112.

McLaughlin MM, Kumar S, Mcdonnell PC, Van Horn S, Lee JC, Livi GP, Young PR. Identification of mitogen-activated protein (MAP) kinase-activated protein kinase-3, a novel substrate of CSBP p38 MAP kinase. *J Biol Chem* 1996; **271**: 8488–8492.

Meltzer EO, Berkowitz RB, Grossbard EB. An intranasal Syk-kinase inhibitor (R112) improves the symptoms of seasonal allergic rhinitis in a park environment. *J Allergy Clin Immunol* 2005; **115**: 791–796.

Mercurio F, Zhu H, Murray BW, Shevchenko A et al. IKK-1 and IKK-2: cytokine-activated IκB kinases essential for NF-κB activation. *Science* 1997; **278**: 860–866.

Mol CD, Dougan DR, Schneider TR, Skene RJ et al. Structural basis for the autoinhibition and STI-571 Inhibition of c-kit tyrosine kinase. *J Biol Chem* 2004; **279**: 31655–31663.

Moodie FM, Marwick JA, Anderson CS, Szulakowski P et al. Oxidative stress and cigarette smoke alter chromatin remodeling but differentially regulate NF-κB activation and proinflammatory cytokine release in alveolar epithelial cells. *FASEB J* 2004; **18**: 1897–1899.

Mueller C, August A. Attenuation of immunological symptoms of allergic asthma in mice lacking the tyrosine kinase ITK. *J Immunol* 2003; **170**: 5056–5063.

Nath P, Eynott P, Leung S-Y, Adcock IM, Bennett BL, Chung KF. Potential role of c-Jun NH2-terminal kinase in allergic airway inflammation and remodelling: effects of SP600125. *Eur J Pharmacol* 2005; **506**: 273–283.

Neininger A, Kontoyiannis D, Kotlyarov A, Winzen R et al. MK2 targets AU-rich elements and regulates biosynthesis of tumor necrosis factor and interleukin-6 independently at different post-transcriptional levels. *J Biol Chem* 2002; **277**: 3065–3068.

Newton R, Holden N. Inhibitors of p38 mitogen activated protein kinase. *Biodrugs* 2003; **17**: 113–129.

Newton R, Holden NS. New aspects of p38 mitogen activated protein kinase (MAPK) biology in lung inflammation. *Drug Discov Today: Disease Mech* 2006; **3**: 53–61.

Niven AS, Argyros G. Alternate treatments in asthma. *Chest* 2003; **123**: 1254–1265.

O'Donnell R, Breen D, Wilson S, Djukanovic R. Inflammatory cells in the airways in COPD. *Thorax* 2006; **61**: 448–454.

Ohren JF, Chen H, Pavlovsky A, Whitehead C et al. Structures of human MAP kinase kinase 1 (MEK1) and MEK2 describe novel noncompetitive kinase inhibition. *Nat Struct Mol Biol* 2004; **11**: 1192–1197.

Orlowski RZ, Baldwin JAS. NF-κB as a therapeutic target in cancer. *Trends Mol Med* 2002; **8**: 385–389.

Papageorgiou AC, Wikman LEK. Is JAK3 a new drug target for immunomodulation-based therapies? *Trends Pharmacol Sci* 2004; **25**: 558–562.

Pargellis C, Tong L, Churchill L, Cirillo PF et al. Inhibition of p38 MAP kinase by utilizing a novel allosteric binding site. *Nature Struct Biol* 2002; **9**: 268–272.

Pasparakis M, Courtois G, Hafner M, Schmidt-Supprian M et al. TNF-mediated inflammatory skin disease in mice with epidermis-specific deletion of IKK2. *Nature* 2002a; **417**: 861–866.

Pasparakis M, Schmidt-Supprian M, Rajewsky K. I{kappa}B kinase signaling is essential for maintenance of mature B cells. *J Exp Med* 2002b; **196**: 743–752.

Pinho V, Souza DG, Barsante MM, Hamer FP, De Freitas MS, Rossi AG, Teixeira MM. Phosphoinositide-3 kinases critically regulate the recruitment and survival of eosinophils in vivo: importance for the resolution of allergic inflammation. *J Leuk Biol* 2005; **77**: 800–810.

Podolin PL, Callahan JF, Bolognese BJ, Li YH et al. Attenuation of murine collagen-induced arthritis by a novel, potent, selective small molecule inhibitor of I{kappa}B kinase 2, TPCA-1 (2-[(aminocarbonyl)amino]-5-(4-fluorophenyl)-3-thiophenecarboxamide), occurs via reduction of proinflammatory cytokines and antigen-induced T cell proliferation. *J Pharmacol Exp Ther* 2005; **312**: 373–381.

Puddicombe SM, Polosa R, Richter A, Krishna MT, Howarth PH, Holgate ST, Davies DE. Involvement of the epidermal growth factor receptor in epithelial repair in asthma. *FASEB J* 2000; **14**: 1362–1374.

Puri KD, Doggett TA, Douangpanya J, Hou Y et al. Mechanisms and implications of phosphoinositide 3-kinase δ in promoting neutrophil trafficking into inflamed tissue. *Blood* 2004; **103**: 3448–3456.

Puri KD, Doggett TA, Huang C-Y, Douangpanya J et al. The role of endothelial PI3Kγ activity in neutrophil trafficking. *Blood* 2005; **106**: 150–157.

Qin S, Chock PB. Implication of phosphatidylinositol 3-kinase membrane recruitment in hydrogen peroxide-induced activation of PI3K and Akt. *Biochemistry* 2003; **42**: 2995–3003.

Rahman I, Marwick J, Kirkham P. Redox modulation of chromatin remodeling: impact on histone acetylation and deacetylation, NF-κB and pro-inflammatory gene expression. *Biochem Pharmacol* 2004; **68**: 1255–1267.

Regan J, Breitfelder S, Cirillo P, Gilmore T et al. Pyrazole urea-based inhibitors of p38 MAP kinase: from lead compound to clinical candidate. *J Med Chem* 2002; **45**: 2994–3008.

Regan J, Pargellis CA, Cirillo PF, Gilmore T et al. The kinetics of binding to p38 MAP kinase by analogues of BIRB 796. *Bioorg Med Chem Lett* 2003; **13**: 3101–3104.

Reif K, Okkenhaug K, Sasaki T, Penninger JM, Vanhaesebroeck B, Cyster JG. Cutting edge: differential roles for phosphoinositide 3-kinases, p110γ and p110δ, in lymphocyte chemotaxis and homing. *J Immunol* 2004; **173**: 2236–2240.

Rojo AI, Salina M, Salazar M, Takahashi S et al. Regulation of heme oxygenase-1 gene expression through the phosphatidylinositol 3-kinase/PKC-[zeta] pathway and Sp1. *Free Radic Biol Med* 2006; **41**: 247–261.

Roos-Engstrand E, Wallin A, Bucht A, Pourazar J, Sandstrom T, Blomberg A. Increased expression of p38 MAPK in human bronchial epithelium after lipopolysaccharide exposure. *Eur Respir J* 2005; **25**: 797–803.

Ruocco MG, Maeda S, Park JM, Lawrence T et al. IκB kinase (IKK)β, but not IKKα, is a critical mediator of osteoclast survival and is required for inflammation-induced bone loss. *J Exp Med* 2005; **201**: 1677–1687.

Saccani S, Pantano S, Natoli G. p38-dependent marking of inflammatory genes for increased NF-κB recruitment. *Nat Immunol* 2002; **3**: 69–75.

Saklatvala J. The p38 MAP kinase pathway as a therapeutic target in inflammatory disease. *Curr Opin Pharmacol* 2004; **4**: 372–377.

Sakurai H, Suzuki S, Kawasaki N, Nakano H et al. Tumor necrosis factor-α-induced IKK phosphorylation of NF-κB p65 on serine 536 is mediated through the TRAF2, TRAF5, and TAK1 signaling pathway. *J Biol Chem* 2003; **278**: 36916–36923.

Schindler T. Structural mechanism of STI-571 inhibition of Abelson tyrosine kinase. *Science* 2000; **289**: 1938–1942.

Schreck RAK, Baeuerle PA. Nuclear factor kappa B: an oxidative stress-responsive transcription factor of eukaryotic cells (a review). *Free Radic Res Commun* 2002; **17**: 221–237.

Schreiber M. Control of cell cycle progression by c-Jun is p53 dependent. *Genes Dev* 1999; **13**: 607–619.

Smith SJ, Fenwick PS, Nicholson AG, Kirschenbaum F et al. Inhibitory effect of p38 mitogen-activated protein kinase inhibitors on cytokine release from human macrophages. *Br J Pharmacol* 2006; **149**: 393–404.

Sousa AR, Lane SJ, Soh C, Lee TH. In vivo resistance to corticosteroids in bronchial asthma is associated with enhanced phosyphorylation of JUN N-terminal kinase and failure of prednisolone to inhibit JUN N-terminal kinase phosphorylation. *J Allergy Clin Immunol* 1999; **104**: 565–574.

Stokoe D, Engel K, Campbell DG, Cohen P, Gaestel M. Identification of MAPKAP kinase 2 as a major enzyme responsible for the phosphorylation of the small mammalian heat shock proteins. *FEBS Lett* 1992; **313**: 307–313.

Swantek JL, Cobb MH, Geppert TD. Jun N-terminal kinase/stress-activated protein kinase (JNK/SAPK) is required for lipopolysaccharide stimulation of tumor necrosis factor-α (TNF-α) translation: glucocorticoids inhibit TNF-[alpha] translation by blocking JNK/SAPK. *Mol Cell Biol* 1997; **17**: 6274–6282.

Szulakowski P, Crowther AJL, Jimenez LA, Donaldson K et al. The effect of smoking on the transcriptional regulation of lung inflammation in patients with chronic obstructive pulmonary disease. *Am J Respir Crit Care Med* 2006; **174**: 41–50.

Thomas MJ, Smith A, Head DH, Milne L et al. Airway inflammation: chemokine-induced neutrophilia and the class I phosphoinositide 3-kinases. *Eur J Immunol* 2005; **35**: 1283–1291.

Thompson N, Lyons J. Recent progress in targeting the Raf/MEK/ERK pathway with inhibitors in cancer drug discovery. *Curr Opin Pharmacol* 2005; **5**: 350–356.

Thomson S, Clayton AL, Hazzalin CA, Rose S, Barratt MJ, Mahadevan LC. The nucleosomal response associated with immediate-early gene induction is mediated via alternative MAP kinase cascades: MSK1 as a potential histone H3/HMG-14 kinase. *EMBO J* 1999; **18**: 4779–4793.

Tong L. A highly specific inhibitor of human p38 MAP kinase binds in the ATP pocket. *Nature Struct Biol* 1997; **4**: 311–316.

Tong SE, Daniels SE, Montano T, Chang S, Desjardins P. SCIO-469, a novel P38A MAPK inhibitor, provides efficacy in acute post-surgical dental pain. *Clin Pharm Ther* 2004; **75**: P3.

Tsai JR, Chong IW, Chen CC, Lin SR, Sheu CC, Hwang JJ. Mitogen-activated protein kinase pathway was significantly activated in human bronchial epithelial cells by nicotine. *DNA Cell Biol* 2006; **25**: 312–322.

Underwood D, Kotzer C, De-Bruin S, Wells G et al. Inhibition of inhaled cigarette smoke-induced airway neutrophilia, lung chemokine and cytokine production in mice by the p38 MAP kinase inhibitor, SB 239063. *Am J Respir Crit Care Med* 2001; **163**: A112 (Abstr).

Underwood DC, Osborn RR, Bochnowicz S, Webb EF et al. SB 239063, a p38 MAPK inhibitor, reduces neutrophilia, inflammatory cytokines, MMP-9, and fibrosis in lung. *Am J Physiol Lung Cell Mol Physiol* 2000a; **279**: L895–L902.

Underwood DC, Osborn RR, Kotzer CJ, Adams JL et al. SB 239063, a potent p38 MAP kinase inhibitor, reduces inflammatory cytokine production, airways eosinophil infiltration, and persistence. *J Pharm Exp Ther* 2000b; **293**: 281–288.

Vanhaesebroeck B. Synthesis and function of 3-phosphorylated inositol lipids. *Annu Rev Biochem* 2001; **70**: 535–602.

Vanhaesebroeck B, Ali K, Bilancio A, Geering B, Foukas LC. Signalling by PI3K isoforms: Insights from gene-targeted mice. *Trends Biochem Sci* 2005; **30**: 194–204.

Wakeling AE. Epidermal growth factor receptor tyrosine kinase inhibitors. *Curr Opin Pharmacol* 2002; **2**: 382–387.

Walker C, Thomas M, Edwards MJ. Phosphoinositide 3-kinase (PI3K) family of signalling enzymes and their role in asthma. *Drug Discov Today: Dis Mech* 2006; **3**: 63–69.

Walker EH, Pacold ME, Perisic O, Stephens L, Hawkins PT, Wymann MP, Williams RL. Structural determinants of phosphoinositide 3-kinase inhibition by wortmannin, LY294002, quercetin, myricetin, and staurosporine. *Mol Cell* 2000; **6**: 909–919.

Walker EH, Perisic O, Ried C, Stephens L, Williams RL. Structural insights into phosphoinositide 3-kinase catalysis and signalling. *Nature* 1999; **402**: 313–320.

Wan PTC, Garnett MJ, Roe SM, Lee S et al. Mechanism of activation of the RAF-ERK signaling pathway by oncogenic mutations of B-RAF. *Cell* 2004; **116**: 855–867.

Wertz IE, O'Rourke KM, Zhou H, Eby M et al. De-ubiquitination and ubiquitin ligase domains of A20 downregulate NF-κB signalling. *Nature* 2004; **430**: 694–699.

Wong BR, Grossbard EB, Payan DG, Masuda ES. Targeting Syk as a treatment for allergic and autoimmune disorders. *Expert Opin Invest Drugs* 2004; **13**: 743–762.

Wood ER, Truesdale AT, McDonald OB, Yuan D et al. A unique structure for epidermal growth factor receptor bound to GW572016 (lapatinib): relationships among protein conformation, inhibitor off-rate, and receptor activity in tumor cells. *Cancer Res* 2004; **64**: 6652–6659.

Wu T, Han C, Shelhamer JH. Involvement of p38 and p42/44 MAP kinases and protein kinase C in the interferon-gamma and interleukin-1alpha-induced phosphorylation of 85-kDa cytosolic phospholipase A(2) in primary human bronchial epithelial cells. *Cytokine* 2004; **25**: 11–20.

Yamamoto N, Takeshita K, Shichijo M, Kokubo T et al. The orally available spleen tyrosine kinase inhibitor 2-[7-(3,4-dimethoxyphenyl)-imidazo[1,2-c]pyrimidin-5-ylamino]nicotinamide dihydrochloride (BAY 61-3606) blocks antigen-induced airway inflammation in rodents. *J Pharm Exp Ther* 2003; **306**: 1174–1181.

Yamamoto Y, Gaynor RB. Therapeutic potential of inhibition of the NF-κB pathway in the treatment of inflammation and cancer. *J Clin Invest* 2001; **107**: 135–142.

Yang DD. Differentiation of CD4+ T cells to Th1 cells requires MAP kinase JNK2. *Immunity* 1998; **9**: 575–585.

Yang S-R, Chida AS, Bauter MR, Shafiq N et al. Cigarette smoke induces proinflammatory cytokine release by activation of NF-κB and posttranslational modifications of histone deacetylase in macrophages. *Am J Physiol Lung Cell Mol Physiol* 2006; **291**: L46–57.

Young PR, Mclaughlin MM, Kumar S, Kassis S et al. Pyridinyl imidazole inhibitors of p38 mitogen-activated protein kinase bind in the ATP site. *J Biol Chem* 1997; **272**: 12116–12121.

Zhang S, Kaplan MH. The p38 mitogen-activated protein kinase is required for IL-12-induced IFN-gamma expression. *J Immunol* 2000; **165**: 1374–1380.

Ziegelbauer K, Gantner F, Lukacs NW, Berlin A et al. A selective novel low-molecular-weight inhibitor of IkappaB kinase-beta (IKK-beta) prevents pulmonary inflammation and shows broad anti-inflammatory activity. *Br J Pharmacol* 2005; **145**: 178–192.

13

Pharmacokinetic/ Pharmacodynamic Factors and Steroid Sensitivity

Günther Hochhaus

13.1 Introduction

Corticosteroids administered locally to the lung remain the most efficient therapeutic approach for the treatment of asthma, as pulmonary inflammation can be controlled by providing high local pulmonary activity with minimized systemic side effects (pulmonary targeting). Several articles have evaluated the importance of specific pharmacokinetic and pharmacodynamic factors for establishing pulmonary targeting after pulmonary delivery (Edsbacker and Johansson, 2006; Hochhaus, 2007; Hochhaus et al., 1997). Glucocorticoid therapy is generally an efficient treatment of asthma but the benefits may vary among patients. While other sections of the book discuss in detail the biochemical and molecular pharmacological basis of glucocorticoid insensitivity, this chapter will limit its discussion on factors that relate to the clinical variability observed in patients after the administration of glucocorticoids through inhalation therapy.

13.2 What Factors are Important for Pulmonary Efficacy and Safety?

Based on the underlying pharmacokinetic/pharmacodynamic (PK/PD) relationships, a number of primary research and review articles have discussed factors

Overcoming Steroid Insensitivity in Respiratory Disease   Edited by Ian M. Adcock and Kian Fan Chung
© 2008 John Wiley & Sons, Ltd.

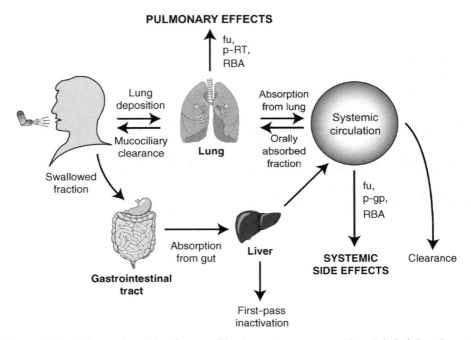

Figure 13.1   Scheme describing factors affecting pulmonary targeting. Inhaled drug is not just deposited in the lung but may be swallowed and absorbed through the gastrointestinal tract and inactivated by the liver or pass into the systemic circulation. In addition, lung-deposited drug can also be absorbed into the systemic circulation. Once in the systemic circulation the degree of side effects will depend upon the systemic availability (a composite of RBA, f_u and the volume of distribution) and the clearance rate. (f_u is the fraction unbound to plasma proteins; RBA is the receptor binding affinity)

modulating pulmonary selectivity (Edsbacker and Johansson, 2006; Hochhaus, 2007; Hochhaus et al., 1997). The model in Figure 13.1 depicts the relevant factors involved in pulmonary targeting and the nasal situation. After inhalation, a fraction of the delivered dose is deposited in the upper or lower part of the lung while the rest is deposited in the oropharyngeal region and swallowed. Unless the drug is given as a solution, it has to dissolve in the pulmonary lining fluid at a rate determined by the physicochemical properties of the deposited particles. When the inhaled corticosteroid is given as a suspension, the undissolved particles are subjected to mucociliary clearance and, as a result, can be removed from the lung and therefore would not be available to induce the desired local effects (Edsbacker and Johansson, 2006; Hochhaus, 2007; Hochhaus et al., 1997).

Once dissolved, the drug molecules can enter pulmonary cells and either interact with the relevant receptors (glucocorticoid receptors, GR) as determined by free drug levels and the receptor binding affinity to induce the desired effects or be captured in pulmonary cells as lipophilic ester derivatives. It needs to be stressed that once the drug is dissolved, the only way for the dissolved drug molecules to leave the lung and be distributed throughout the body is through systemic absorption into the blood stream. Drug molecules that were potentially able to induce local pulmonary effects are therefore also able to induce systemic side effects (Edsbacker and Johansson, 2006; Hochhaus, 2007; Hochhaus et al., 1997).

Drug that is deposited in the oropharyngeal region or is removed through the mucociliary transporter from the lung will be swallowed and subjected to systemic absorption. The amount of absorbed drug will be determined by the oral bioavailability. Orally absorbed drug together with the drug absorbed from the lung is responsible for the systemic side effects of inhaled glucocorticoids (Edsbacker and Johansson, 2006; Hochhaus, 2007; Hochhaus et al., 1997).

Table 13.1 lists the relevant pharmacokinetic and pharmacodynamic factors affecting the performance of inhaled glucocorticoids and potentially being involved in the interpatient variability observed in inhaled glucocorticoid therapy. Among these, the following factors are crucial in achieving distinct pulmonary selectivity. A high drug concentration should be present in the lung over an extended period of time to achieve pronounced pulmonary efficacy. A good inhaled glucocorticoid should exhibit low oral bioavailability and high systemic clearance, permitting efficient removal of drug from the systemic circulation through a systemic clearance mechanism (generally hepatic metabolism) (Edsbacker and Johansson, 2006; Hochhaus, 2007; Hochhaus et al., 1997).

Table 13.1 Pharmacodynamic and pharmacokinetic factors relevant for pulmonary selectivity

Pharmacodynamics[a]	• Receptor binding affinity and number • Transactivation to transrepression ratios • Interindividual differences in pharmacodynamics • Time of administration
Pulmonary pharmacokinetics	• Pulmonary deposition efficiency • Mucociliary transport • Pulmonary deposition (central versus peripheral) • Deactivation of drugs/activation of prodrugs • Lung residence time • Lung tissue binding/transporters • Local metabolism • Time of administration
Systemic pharmacokinetics	• Oral bioavailability • Systemic clearance (drug metabolism) • Protein/tissue binding/transporters • Plasma protein binding; volume of distribution • Stability in tissues

[a] See section 13.3.

13.3   Pharmacodynamic Aspects

Pharmacodynamic aspects of glucocorticoid actions are relatively well understood and have been reviewed in recent review articles (Barnes, 2006a; Ito et al., 2006). Due to the fact that significant portions of this book will focus in great detail on the pharmacodynamic aspects of glucocorticoid action as they relate to glucocorticoid insensitivity, this chapter will only briefly discuss certain aspects. After entering the cell, glucocorticoids will interact with the GR (α receptor isoform) in the cytosol, resulting in activation of the receptor and transportation into the nucleus. Activated receptor dimer complexes can induce protein synthesis, e.g. induction of proteins such as Annexin 1 (Barnes, 2006b) or scavenger receptors such as CD163 (Hogger et al., 1998), via transactivation pathways. Activated GRs are also able to prevent or reverse the induction of transcription (transrepression) by transcription factors such as nuclear factor-κB (NF-κB) or activator protein-1(AP-1) (Barnes, 2006a). NF-κB and AP-1, activated by tumour necrosis factor alpha (TNFα) for example, induce gene expression by interacting with nuclear cofactors that can acetylate histones. Acetylation of histones results in an opening up of the chromatin structure and allows RNA–polymerase to start the transcriptional processes. GR might prevent acetylation of histones (a step necessary for induction of transcription) by interacting with the histone acetyltransferase complex or can even reverse it through recruiting histone deacetylase 2 (HDAC2) (Barnes, 2006a). GR has also been shown to reduce the stability of certain mRNAs and prevent the activation of certain transcription factors (Barnes, 2006a).

It has been suggested that most of the inhaled corticosteroid-induced adverse effects are associated with transactivation processes, while the desired anti-inflammatory processes are related to transrepression. Newer dissociated GR ligands are able to preferentially activate the transrepression pathway in human cell lines (Schäcke et al., 2005). Clinical studies are needed to confirm whether or not such drugs show favourable therapeutic activity with reduced adverse effects. Current commercially available glucocorticoids do not seem to differentiate between these pathways in certain cells (Dirks et al., 2005) and therefore do not exhibit an advantage for selectivity. The affinity of commercial glucocorticoids for GR is therefore a major determinant for the activity at the site of action. This is also indicated by the observation that for a given effect or side effect a good correlation exists between the IC_{50} values determined by PK/PD analysis in humans and the receptor binding affinity (Derendorf et al., 1993; Wu et al., 2005).

While the rank order for a given effect is reflected in differences in receptor affinities, the actual sensitivity differs among effects. For example, the IC_{50} for cortisol suppression has been found to be lower than that observed for the decrease in blood lymphocytes (Stark et al., 2006). While the relative activity rank order for glucocorticoids is generally highly reproducible across individuals (e.g. relative binding activity), a distinct variability has been observed in the activity estimates (IC_{50} for a given glucocorticoid) across individuals. For example, across patients with lung cancer, the GR content as well as the affinity for dexamethasone of the receptor varied by ± 50% (Hochhaus et al., 1983). The IC_{50} determined in PK/PD studies showed a standard deviation of more than ± 50% (47–150%)(Wu et al., 2005). In addition to differences in GR number and affinity, other factors such as decreased DNA binding or reduced translocation to the nucleus might be the reason for glucocorticoid resistance. It has also been shown that increased numbers of GRβ (Lewis–Tuffin and Cidlowski, 2006), an isoform of the receptor, might be involved in steroid insensitivity. This isoform of the receptor seems to be able to reduce the activity of the classical functional GRα and an increased expression might be responsible for steroid resistance. In addition, differences in factors involved in the regulation of transactivation or transrepression pathways of glucocorticoid-sensitive genes have been observed between patients with sensitivity disorders (Russcher et al., 2006). Cytokines such as IL-2, IL-4 and IL-13, which show increased expression in asthma patients, decrease the affinity of glucocorticoids for GR, presumably due to phosphorylation of the receptor (Barnes, 2006a). A reduction in the HDAC activity due to smoking might be responsible for reduced glucocorticoid actions in smoking asthmatics (Barnes et al. 2005). Assuming that these and other inflammatory events are limited to the lung and not present in tissues relevant for the induction of side effects, a reduction in pulmonary activity and selectivity will be observed. In addition to these relationships, new tools in evaluating genetic regulation of asthma pathogenesis, such as gene expression profiling, will allow the identification of new asthma-related genes (ALOX15) and the possibility of identifying optimized personalized therapeutic approaches for individual asthmatics (Hansel and Diette, 2007; Tantisira and Weiss, 2006).

13.4   Pharmacokinetic Drug Properties

General covariates for pharmacokinetic variability

As reviewed elsewhere (Edsbacker and Johansson, 2006; Hochhaus et al., 1997), the pulmonary selectivity of an inhaled glucocorticoid is driven significantly by pharmacokinetic properties. These factors include pulmonary deposition efficiency, pulmonary residence time, oral systemic clearance and factors related to the distribution of the drug, such as the volume of distribution (V_d) and affinity to transporters. While some of these factors are relatively constant among patients and volunteers, other factors show significant interindividual variability.

Theoretically, differences in the pharmacokinetic behaviour of inhaled glucocorticoids could be the basis for the lack of clinical efficacy in non-responding patients (Horne, 2006). In order for pharmacokinetic properties to be a main reason for glucocorticoid insensitivity, glucocorticoid non-responders would have to: show an inability to absorb glucocorticoids; have the ability to metabolize drug much faster than "normal" patients (super-metabolizers); express transporter systems that would prevent the uptake of glucocorticoids into the pharmacologically relevant cells even at higher doses; or be unstable in the target cells. However, because most inhaled glucocorticoids exhibit maximum systemic clearance by the liver (clearance equals liver blood flow), and have the ability to enter relevant cells after absorption, the pharmacokinetic reasons for being a true non-responder are essentially non-existent.

Compliance

Compliance describes the ability or willingness of the patient to use the prescribed medication. Insensitivity of glucocorticoid treatment has been shown to be related to non-compliance of asthma patients (Horne, 2006). According to Bender and colleagues, because of concerns of drug safety and cost, only 30–70% of asthma patients adhere to the therapy (Bender and Bender, 2005; Bender et al., 1997). Holt and colleagues list a similar estimate (40–50%), while values as low as 15% have been reported (Holt et al., 2004). This is why a large number of practitioners believe that compliance is the major reason for steroid insensitivity. One major improvement in glucocorticoid therapy would be to develop drug delivery systems that would induce improved patient compliance. On the other hand, patient education has to become more effective.

Half-life

Half-life $(t_{1/2})$ is a secondary pharmacokinetic parameter that is determined by clearance and the V_d (Hubner et al., 2005):

$$t_{1/2} = 0.693 \times V_d/\text{clearance}$$

A short half-life, because of a high clearance, is beneficial for achieving pronounced pulmonary selectivity. However, a short half-life due to a small V_d does not affect the pulmonary selectivity (Hochhaus et al., 1997).

Clearance

Inhaled glucocorticoids are usually cleared by hepatic metabolism. Generally, systemic clearance depends on the activity of the enzymatic machinery to metabolize the drug, the liver blood flow and the degree of protein binding. Pronounced systemic clearance favours pulmonary targeting because the systemically absorbed drug is removed more efficiently (Hochhaus et al., 1997). All of the second and third generation inhaled glucocorticoids are efficiently cleared by hepatic metabolism (high extraction drugs), with clearance values very close to hepatic blood flow.

Population pharmacokinetic analysis revealed that, in general, race, gender, age and asthma severity do not influence the pharmacokinetics of inhaled glucocorticoids such as ciclesonide, budesonide and fluticasone propionate (Edsbacker and Andersson, 2004; Glaxo. Flovent HFA prescribing information. http://us.gsk. com/products/assets/us_flovent_hfa.pdf 2006; Rohatagi et al., 2003, 2005a). This indicates that while variability of pharmacokinetic properties of inhaled glucocorticoids does exist, the identification of specific covariates and the necessary change in treatment are challenges to predict.

Assuming that the intrinsic clearance (activity and number of enzymes available for metabolism is pronounced) remains high in a given patient, clearance values of high extraction drugs are mainly determined by liver blood flow. Based on this, factors modulating liver blood flow should also affect the clearance of inhaled glucocorticoids. A number of factors, including exercise, reduced liver blood flow (Schoemaker et al., 1998) and thus should lead to a reduction in pulmonary targeting. On the other hand, food intake increases liver blood flow (Okazaki et al., 1986) and consequently the clearance of steroids (Sangsritavong et al., 2002). Whilst direct clinical studies evaluating the effects of liver blood flow on the systemic clearance and pulmonary selectivity are lacking, the above examples make it very likely that differences in liver blood flow will influence the systemic load of inhaled glucocorticoids and consequently the pulmonary selectivity. A reduced systemic clearance might be based not only on reduced liver blood flow, but also on a reduced number of hepatic enzymes. In this case, systemic exposure to inhaled glucocorticoids is also increased and the degree of targeting is diminished (Hochhaus et al., 1997). Similarly, the clearance of budesonide is reduced in patients with certain liver diseases (Geier et al., 2003; Wiegand et al., 2005), presumably because of a reduced intrinsic clearance. In addition, liver cirrhosis influences the pharmacokinetics of the active metabolite of ciclesonide (Hartmann, 1998), resulting in a larger systemic exposure and potentially a reduced pulmonary selectivity.

A potential explanation for pharmacokinetically based steroid insensitivity might be a significant increase in systemic clearance. Such a relationship has been shown for prednisolone, which shows an increased clearance in the presence of the enzyme inducer rifampin (Lofdahl et al., 1984). While increased clearance might be an explanation for the lack of efficacy of systemically given drugs, this explanation is unlikely for inhaled glucocorticoids. First, the mode of action of inhaled glucocorticoids is based on local effects of the glucocorticoids in the lung. After inhalation, drug levels in the lung are predominantly modulated by the pulmonary fate of glucocorticoids. Thus, the interplay of pulmonary available drug (determined by pulmonary deposited dose and mucociliary clearance), dissolution rate, absorption rate into the relevant cells, potential "capture mechanism" such as esterification (Edsbacker and Brattsand, 2002) or the removal from lung cells into the systemic circulation due to absorption should determine the pulmonary drug levels after inhalation of the drug during the absorption phase. Even when the free pulmonary drug concentrations approach systemic drug levels (this is the case after all the pulmonary drug has been absorbed), an increased hepatic enzyme level (increased intrinsic clearance) in certain patients would not affect the total hepatic clearance because hepatic clearance of high extraction drugs is identical to the liver blood flow and not the number of enzymes present in the liver. Indeed, Lane and colleagues were unable to find any patients whose abnormally fast metabolism was the reason for non-responsiveness to glucocorticoids (Lane et al., 1990).

On the other hand, CYP3A4 inhibitors such as ketoconazole, ritonavir or grapefruit juice might increase the systemic availability of budesonide, fluticasone and similar glucocorticoids (Arrington-Sanders et al., 2006; Bolland et al., 2004; Chen et al., 1999; Clevenbergh et al., 2002; Edsbacker and Andersson, 2004; Glaxo. Flovent HFA prescribing information. http://us.gsk.com/products/assets/us_flovent_hfa.pdf 2006; Gupta and Dube, 2002; Naef et al., 2007; Raaska et al., 2002). An interaction between itraconazole and budesonide, a combination used in allergic bronchopulmonary aspergillosis, resulted in a patient developing symptoms of Cushing's disease, probably because of a cytochrome P-450-mediated interaction. Again, such drug interactions would decrease the pulmonary selectivity of inhaled glucocorticoids. Similarly, certain liver disease patients have significantly reduced cytochrome P-450 (CYP) 3A enzymes (Hubner et al., 2005) and patients with autoimmune hepatitis showed a significant increase in systemic exposure after oral administration of budesonide (Wiegand et al., 2005), presumably in part due to an increase in oral bioavailability and a decreased clearance (see below) (Stoilov et al., 2006).

Drug distribution/protein binding

The degree of drug distribution is quantified by V_d. The higher the V_d, the greater the amount of drug present in the tissues and the lower the plasma concentration. For drugs that can easily cross membranes, the V_d is determined by how much drug is bound to plasma proteins (fraction unbound in plasma: f_u; V_p, volume of the plasma, generally 3 l) and how much drug is bound to tissue components (fraction unbound but present in the tissue: (f_{ut}; V_t, volume of tissue compartment). This is indicated by the following equation:

$$V_d = V_p + V_t(f_u/f_{ut})$$

As tissue binding generally increases somewhat faster than plasma protein binding with lipophilicity, newer more lipophilic glucocorticoids show a larger volume of distribution. An increase in the terminal half-life due to increased non-pulmonary tissue binding does not affect the pulmonary selectivity (Hochhaus et al., 1997). Variability in the volume of distribution due to weight differences should not affect the degree of pulmonary selectivity.

It is also of interest to examine a somewhat different scenario, namely the case of two patients who differ both in tissue and plasma protein binding to the same degree.

Increased plasma protein binding has been stressed to be an important feature for the safety of an inhaled corticosteroid (Rohatagi et al., 2003, 2005b; Hochhaus, 2004). This is based on the fact that for high extraction inhalation drugs with low oral bioavailability, the clearance and consequently the area under the total concentration–time profile in the blood are relatively independent of plasma protein binding (Rowland and Tozer, 1995). Thus, differences in the plasma protein binding will not affect the total plasma levels but will affect the free drug plasma concentrations. Indeed, increased plasma protein binding (and, because of an increased volume of distribution, also increased tissue binding) is observed with newer glucocorticoids. Glucocorticoids with increased plasma protein binding have been shown to be safe at employed doses. For example, the high plasma protein binding of des-ciclesonide is responsible for the very low cortisol concentration. PK/PD-based simulations predict that the receptor occupancy in the lung will be reduced, assuming that an increased pulmonary tissue binding will also be reduced for such glucocorticoids. Thus, based on these calculations no selectivity advantage is observed (Rowland and Tozer, 1995). This contradicts statements from others (Lipworth and Jackson, 2000) who state that an increase in lipophilicity favours pulmonary activity or that plasma and non-specific tissue binding are not relevant for high affinity glucocorticoids because the bound steroid would be stripped from these sites by high affinity receptors (Daley-Yates et al., 2005).

These experiments and simulations are in agreement with the general pharmacological "rule" that because only free drug is able to interact with the receptors, lower free drug concentrations will reduce the systemic as well as pulmonary effects. In general, less lipophilic drugs show a relatively low plasma protein binding (80%). Newer lipophilic glucocorticoids, such as ciclesonide and mometasone furoate, show pronounced plasma protein binding (Rohatagi et al., 2003, 2005b; Hochhaus, 2004). It is this high plasma (tissue) binding that seems to be responsible for the relatively minor systemic side effects of ciclesonide, which is considered to be a major safety advantage (Rohatagi et al., 2005a). Pulmonary efficacy is also dependent on the free drug concentration in the lung. Drugs with high plasma protein binding have a V_d slightly higher than those with a lower plasma protein binding (Hochhaus, 2004). This indicates that the tissue binding of such steroids is also more pronounced. Thus, such drugs also will show a lower unbound fraction in tissues, resulting in a lower free drug concentration and reduced receptor occupancy in both pulmonary and systemic tissues. Modeling of these relationships using a further improved PK/PD model clarifies that differences in tissue and plasma protein binding can be adjusted by dose (Figure 13.2). Indeed, a recent study in rats that compared GR number after administration of ciclesonide and budesonide showed that while the total lung concentrations were equivalent, ciclesonide showed a lower degree of pulmonary receptor occupancy (Hochhaus et al., 2007). To date, differences in protein binding across different patient populations have not been studied. However it is likely that certain patient populations, such as liver disease patients, might show lower plasma protein binding. It is also more likely that very high protein binding drugs will

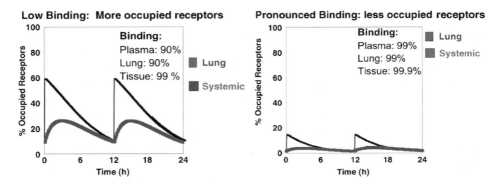

Figure 13.2 Relationship between lung tissue and plasma protein binding and the degree of pulmonary and systemic effects. The drug with the higher binding in plasma and lung tissue will show reduced occupancy of the lung receptors and the systemic receptors. However, increasing the dose of the higher bound drug (right figure) by a factor of 10 will result in the receptor occupancy profiles shown in figure on the left

produce more pronounced variability in free levels because even very small differences in the tissue and plasma protein binding will have a significant effect on free drug concentrations. The therapy for patients with differences in tissue and plasma protein binding can be adjusted by adjusting their dose.

Transporters

The importance of drug transporters in drug distribution has been increasingly recognized. The efflux transporter MDR1 (p-glycoprotein) is expressed in organs such as the kidney and liver, which are involved in the elimination of drugs. MDR1 has also been shown to modulate the absorption of drugs in the gastrointestinal tract and is responsible for the efficient function of the blood/brain barrier (Kerb, 2006). Because of their lipophilic character, inhaled glucocorticoids have been thought to be distributed throughout the body by passive diffusion. It was DeKloet and his group who first showed that dexamethasone is transported by p-glycoprotein (p-gp) and that this transporter is responsible for the lack of uptake of dexamethasone into the brain. More recent studies indicate that synthetic glucocorticoids are generally poorly taken up by the brain and that MDR1 (p-glycoprotein) is involved in the functioning of the blood/brain barrier for corticosteroids (Arya et al., 2005; Cooray et al., 2006). Concomitant administration of p-gp blockers might increase tissue levels of glucocorticoids and increase effectiveness and side effects. The relevance of p-gp transporters for the protection of the hypothalamic-pituitary-adrenal (HPA) axis has been shown by Muller and colleagues. They showed that blood levels of corticosterone and ACTH were significantly lower in knockout mice not expressing p-gp, presumably due to higher corticosterone levels in the brain that activate the HPA axis on a more central level (Muller et al., 2003).

The importance of an intact blood/brain barrier might also be indicated by the finding that neonatal rats (an animal model for preterm babies) allow uptake of glucocorticoids into the brain because of poor development of the transporters at the blood/brain barrier (Arya et al., 2006). If this finding is applicable to humans, it might explain the neurotoxicity seen in preterm babies upon treatment with high-dose glucocorticoids (Arya et al., 2006), especially as synthetic glucocorticoids are not subject to 11β-hydroxysteroid dehydrogenase (11β-HSD), which protects the brain from endogenous glucocorticoids (Seckl et al., 2002).

The expression of p-gp in the placenta has also been described as a way to protect the developing foetus (Ceckova-Novotna et al., 2006; Mark and Waddell, 2006). Excess glucocorticoids have been shown to reduce foetal and placental growth. The foetus is protected from endogenous glucocorticoids such as cortisol and corticosterone by a dual mechanism: 11β-HSD (Burton and Waddell, 1999) and p-gp (Mark and Waddell, 2006). Protection from synthetic glucocorticoids that are not substrates of 11β-HSD depends on the expression of the transporter. The use of synthetic glucocorticoids during pregnancy therefore seems to be justified as long as the activity of the transporter is warranted.

In addition, tissues with barrier function, including cells of the lung and the gastrointestinal tract, express a wide variety of transporters (van der Deen et al., 2005). It is interesting to note that drug treatment might induce changes in the number of transporters expressed and thereby modulate the distribution of other drugs. Glucocorticoids have been shown to affect the expression of transporters. The effects of dexamethasone on p-gp transporters are not uniform and are gene-, gender-, tissue- and cell-type specific (Demeule et al., 1999; van der Deen et al., 2005). An increase in p-gp transporters by dexamethasone was shown in the lungs and liver of rats. These findings might be of relevance for clinical studies, as glucocorticoids might modulate the distribution and absorption of drugs, including themselves. For example, the induction of p-glycoprotein by dexamethasone reduces the absorption of cyclosporin A (Jin et al., 2006; Yokogawa et al., 2002).

Kuzaya and co-workers described the induction of p-glycoproteins and other transporters (MDR and MRPs) by beclomethasone dipropionate in bronchial epithelial cells and hypothesize that the individual differences of expression of transporters and their transactivation by glucocorticoids (e.g. BDP) might contribute to the differences of reactivity of steroid treatment (Kuzuya et al., 2004). Further investigations are required in order to determine whether levels of glucocorticoids in pulmonary cells are affected by glucocorticoids and can be modulated by the overexpression of transporters. Overexpression of transporters in the gastrointestinal tract has been suggested to be a factor in determining the pharmacodynamic response to glucocorticoids in the treatment of bowel disease (Farrell and Kelleher, 2003; Farrell et al., 2000) because the pharmacodynamic levels in the target cells may be reduced (Dilger et al., 2004).

A change in the expression or activity of transporters might also be responsible for producing pharmacodynamic variability in the brain, lung, placenta and gastrointestinal tract. It is feasible that drug co-medication of verapamil, a p-gp inhibitor, results in a blockage of the transporter sites (Ejsing et al., 2006). This might be relevant by modulating the effects of glucocorticoids similar to events for drug–drug interaction on the transporter level (Aszalos, 2004; Balayssac et al., 2005; Hoffmann and Kroemer, 2004; Shitara et al., 2006).

Similarly, p-gp polymorphisms, associated with a reduced p-gp activity (Kerb, 2006; Marzolini et al., 2004), might affect the distribution of glucocorticoids and explain the variability in the pharmacodynamic response.

Tissue metabolism

The majority of inhaled glucocorticoids are inactivated through metabolism in the liver. Exceptions represent glucocorticoid prodrugs such as beclomethasone propionate and ciclesonide, two glucocorticoids with 21-ester functions. Esterases have to cleave these esters before the activated prodrugs can bind to GR. It has been shown for ciclesonide and beclomethasone dipropionate that a portion of the administered prodrug escapes activation in the lung and will enter the system in unactivated form (Daley-Yates et al., 2005). This portion of the drug is unable to induce direct pulmonary effects and reduces pulmonary selectivity. While direct data are missing, it is likely that differences in the location of drug deposition and differences in the esterase activity among patients affect the activation seen among patients (Daley-Yates et al., 2005).

Oral bioavailability

A low oral bioavailability is vital for a pronounced pulmonary selectivity, as the systemic spillover of swallowed glucocorticoids is controlled by this property. Newer inhaled glucocorticoids have been optimized for high hepatic clearance (high extraction drugs). Inhaled glucocorticoids such as budesonide and fluticasone propionate are biotransformed by CYP3A to metabolites with negligible glucocorticoid activity (Edsbacker and Andersson, 2004; Pearce et al., 2006).

Oral bioavailability is predominantly determined by the ability of the liver to inactivate swallowed drug during the first-pass effect in the liver. Therefore glucocorticoids such as moemetasone furoate, fluticasone propionate and ciclesonide, which are efficiently cleared by the liver, have a low oral bioavailability. For these drugs, the systemic load is mainly determined by drug that has been absorbed from the lung. The oral bioavailability of high extraction drugs is affected by plasma protein binding, intrinsic clearance and liver blood flow (Rowland and Tozer, 1995) and this phenomenon, in general, will also be of relevance for inhaled glucocorticoids.

Thus, increased liver blood flow, increased plasma protein binding and decreased intrinsic clearance should affect oral bioavailability. However, the systemic load of inhaled glucocorticoids depends on oral as well as pulmonary absorbed drug. In this special case, an increased oral bioavailability (e.g. from 0.2 to 0.6 %) will not significantly affect the systemic exposure over those induced by pulmonary absorbed drug, because the majority of systemically available drug is coming from pulmonary absorption. Differences in plasma protein binding and hepatic blood flow are unlikely to significantly affect the systemic exposure. The oral bioavailability of inhaled glucocorticoids that show a somewhat higher oral bioavailability (budesonide, triamcinolone acetonide and flunisolide) might be more sensitive to interpatient variability of these parameters.

As discussed earlier, strong CYP3A4 inhibitors such as ketoconazole, ritonavir and grapefruit juice might increase the systemic availability of inhaled glucocorticoids. This, in conjunction with a decreased clearance (see below) (Stoilov et al., 2006), may account for the significant increase in systemic exposure after oral administration of budesonide in patients with autoimmune hepatitis (Wiegand et al., 2005).

Pulmonary deposition

For glucocorticoids with low oral bioavailability, variability in the patient's deposition efficiency will affect the dose reaching the lung and consequently the pulmonary effects (assuming the existence of a dose–response relationship). Increased pulmonary deposition will increase pulmonary selectivity for inhaled glucocorticoids with distinct oral availability, as less drug will be swallowed and the ratio of inhaled to orally absorbed drug will be favoured.

Pulmonary deposition has been shown to be highly variable among patients and dependent on numerous factors, including coordination between the patient and the device (education, use of spacers) (Crompton, 1982; Newman, 2004; Newman et al., 1991), the breathing pattern (Smaldone, 2006), as well as lung function, for dry powder inhalers (Borgstrom, 1994; Borgstrom et al., 1994). Variability is also observed in the regional deposition, with a more pronounced central deposition seen in patients with poor lung function. Recent work has indicated that asthma is not only a disease of the upper but also of the lower alveolar region of the lung (Sutherland and Martin, 2005) and that inhaled glucocorticoids should also reach these portions of the lung. It is feasible that not only differences in the delivery device, but also differences in the disease severity will affect deposition in the alveolar region (Sutherland and Martin, 2005). More clinical studies are necessary in order to investigate the clinical benefit of peripheral deposition of glucocorticoids.

A low variability in inhalation efficiency is desired as it ensures a more constant dose for the patient over time and a constant pharmacodynamic profile. A recent study by Borgstrom and colleagues showed that variability in lung deposition is mainly determined by the efficiency of the device to deliver to the lung, with highly efficient devices also showing the lowest variability (Borgstrom et al., 2006). The degree of deposition depends on both the device and the throat geometry (with larger throat favouring lower degree of pulmonary deposition. Interestingly, differences between the devices (dry powder vs. metered dose inhalers) were rather small, although dry powder inhalers seem to show a somewhat smaller variability (Borgstrom et al., 2006). The same was true for subgroups of study participants. There was no significant difference in the variability of deposition between children and adults, healthy volunteers and asthmatics (Borgstrom et al., 2006), while the actual degree of lung deposition depends on the subgroups, e.g. the pulmonary deposition is often smaller in children than in adults, quite in agreement with their smaller throat geometry. Interestingly, variability of the device determined in *in vitro* tests is unrelated to the variability seen *in vivo*.

The fate of inhaled particles, whether dust or glucocorticoids, will be affected by the mucociliary transporter that removes solids from the upper part of the lung. Variability in this transporter is likely to affect the pulmonary fate of glucocorticoid drug particles. Indeed, the pulmonary pharmacokinetics of drugs with a relatively slow dissolution time are affected by pulmonary clearance. Lipophilic drugs, such as mometasone furoate and fluticasone propionate, are subject to significant mucociliary clearance. Fluticasone propionate has been shown to dissolve relatively slowly, with a half-life of pulmonary absorption of about 4 h (Krishnaswami et al., 2005). During the dissolution process remaining solid particles are subject to mucociliary removal from the lung. Variation of drug deposition into areas of the lung with low (peripheral lung) or high mucociliary clearance (more central lung areas) will affect pulmonary and systemically available dose.

Indeed, differences have been reported on the degree with which healthy volunteers and asthmatics were able to absorb fluticasone propionate (Harrison and Tattersfield, 2003), presumably due to a more central deposition (Brown et al., 2002; Saari et al., 1998) and more efficient mucociliary transport. Indeed, lower systemic availability in asthmatics seems to be directly linked to lung function (FEV$_1$ % predicted) (Mortimer et al., 2006).

The mucociliary transport rate is also affected by a number of factors, including the age of the patient (Incalzi et al., 1989) and beta-2-adrenergic or other drugs (Hasani et al., 1992, 2003, 2005). In addition, Del Donno and colleagues described a much higher variability in the mucociliary transport rate in smokers, asthmatics and bronchitics than in healthy volunteers (Del Donno et al., 2000). Thus, variability in the mucociliary transport rate should be involved in the variability in the pulmonary and systemic exposure to glucocorticoids with a slow dissolution rate.

Differences in esterification

The esterification of glucocorticoid 21-alcohols, such as budesonide, has been shown to extend the pulmonary residence times. Increasing the pulmonary residence time has been shown to be beneficial for improved pulmonary selectivity (Edsbacker and Johansson, 2006; Hochhaus, 2007; Hochhaus et al., 1997). In pulmonary cells, budesonide can be converted into a lipophilic ester that is trapped within the cells. Slow cleavage of the ester (re-activation) provides an extended presence of steroid in the lung. However, there is very little known about patient variability with respect to the esterification and ester hydrolysis. Variability in these processes could, however, affect the length and the degree of pulmonary selectivity.

Circadian factors

Plasma cortisol concentrations have been known to undergo a circadian rhythm. Ocular light seems to be the key factor in inducing the cortisol peak in the morning (Scheer and Buijs, 1999). Because of fluctuating cortisol levels, inflammatory cytokines and pain sensations also show a diurnal rhythm (Cutolo et al., 2006) in arthritis patients. Cutolo et al. (2006) recently reviewed that in healthy volunteers a diurnal rhythm between cellular (Th-1) and humoral (Th-2) immune response has been described that has been related to cortisol (Th-2) and melanocortin (Th-1) (Petrovsky and Harrison, 1997; Petrovsky et al., 1998). It is therefore of no surprise that diurnal variation in the effect of exogenous glucocorticoids have been suggested. PK/PD analysis has shown that administration of exogenous glucocorticoids in the evening results in optimum effects, as the combined effects of cortisol and exogenous glucocorticoids are maximized (Wu et al., 2005).

Clinical studies with once-daily administration of inhaled glucocorticoids have been performed with both a.m. and p.m. dosing of inhaled glucocorticoids (Bensch et al., 2006; D'Urzo et al., 2005; Nayak et al., 2000; Pearlman et al., 2005). In agreement with this finding, clinical studies for inhaled glucocorticoids have shown that once-daily administration of inhaled glucocorticoids in the evening is more efficacious than administration in the morning (McCormack and Plosker, 2006). While this seems to hold true for both desired effects and side effects, and therefore should not affect the degree of pulmonary selectivity, the time of administration might be another factor for variability in the overall activity of glucocorticoids.

13.5 Conclusion

While pharmacodynamic factors seem to be the major determinant of glucocorticoid insensitivity, pharmacokinetic factors have an impact and must be considered in explaining the variability in the response to glucocorticoids.

References

Arrington-Sanders R, Hutton N, Siberry GK. Ritonavir–fluticasone interaction causing Cushing syndrome in HIV-infected children and adolescents. *Pediatr Infect Dis J* 2006; **25**: 1044–1048.

Arya V, Demarco VG, Issar M, Hochhaus G. Contrary to adult, neonatal rats show pronounced brain uptake of corticosteroids. *Drug Metab Dispos* 2006; **34**: 939–942.

Arya V, Issar M, Wang Y, Talton JD, Hochhaus G. Brain permeability of inhaled corticosteroids. *J Pharm Pharmacol* 2005; **57**: 1159–1167.

Aszalos A. P-glycoprotein-based drug–drug interactions: preclinical methods and relevance to clinical observations. *Arch Pharm Res* 2004; **27**: 127–135.

Balayssac D, Authier N, Cayre A, Coudore F. Does inhibition of P-glycoprotein lead to drug–drug interactions? *Toxicol Lett* 2005; **156**: 319–329.

Barnes PJ. How corticosteroids control inflammation: Quintiles Prize Lecture 2005. *Br J Pharmacol* 2006b; **148**: 245–254.

Barnes PJ. Corticosteroids: the drugs to beat. *Eur J Pharmacol* 2006a; **533**: 2–14.

Barnes PJ, Adcock IM, Ito K. Histone acetylation and deacetylation: importance in inflammatory lung diseases. *Eur Respir J* 2005; **25**: 552–563.

Bender BG, Bender SE. Patient-identified barriers to asthma treatment adherence: responses to interviews, focus groups, and questionnaires. *Immunol Allergy Clin North Am* 2005; **25**: 107–130.

Bender B, Milgrom H, Rand C. Nonadherence in asthmatic patients: is there a solution to the problem? *Ann Allergy Asthma Immunol* 1997; **79**: 177–186.

Bensch GW, Prenner B, Berkowitz R, Galant S, Ramsdell J, Lutsky B. Once-daily evening administration of mometasone furoate in asthma treatment initiation. *Ann Allergy Asthma Immunol* 2006; **96**: 533–540.

Bolland MJ, Bagg W, Thomas MG, Lucas JA, Ticehurst R, Black PN. Cushing's syndrome due to interaction between inhaled corticosteroids and itraconazole. *Ann Pharmacother* 2004; **38**: 46–49.

Borgstrom L. Deposition patterns with Turbuhaler. *J Aerosol Med* 1994; **7**: S49–53.

Borgstrom L, Bondesson E, Moren F, Trofast E, Newman SP. Lung deposition of budesonide inhaled via Turbuhaler: a comparison with terbutaline sulphate in normal subjects. *Eur Respir J* 1994; **7**: 69–73.

Borgstrom L, Olsson B, Thorsson L. Degree of throat deposition can explain the variability in lung deposition of inhaled drugs. *J Aerosol Med* 2006; **19**: 473–483.

Brown JS, Zeman KL, Bennett WD. Ultrafine particle deposition and clearance in the healthy and obstructed lung. *Am J Respir Crit Care Med* 2002; **166**: 1240–1247.

Burton PJ, Waddell BJ. Dual function of 11beta-hydroxysteroid dehydrogenase in placenta: modulating placental glucocorticoid passage and local steroid action. *Biol Reprod* 1999; **60**: 234–240.

Ceckova-Novotna M, Pavek P, Staud F. P-glycoprotein in the placenta: expression, localization, regulation and function. *Reprod Toxicol* 2006; **22**: 400–410.

Chen F, Kearney T, Robinson S, Daley-Yates PT, Waldron S, Churchill DR. Cushing's syndrome and severe adrenal suppression in patients treated with ritonavir and inhaled nasal fluticasone. *Sex Transm Infect* 1999; **75**: 274.

Clevenbergh P, Corcostegui M, Gerard D, Hieronimus S et al. Iatrogenic Cushing's syndrome in an HIV-infected patient treated with inhaled corticosteroids (fluticasone propionate) and low dose ritonavir enhanced PI containing regimen. *J Infect* 2002; **44**: 194–195.

Cooray HC, Shahi S, Cahn AP, van Veen HW, Hladky SB, Barrand MA. Modulation of p-glycoprotein and breast cancer resistance protein by some prescribed corticosteroids. *Eur J Pharmacol* 2006; **531**: 25–33.

Crompton GK. Problems patients have using pressurized aerosol inhalers. *Eur J Respir Dis Suppl* 1982; **119**: 101–104.

Cutolo M, Sulli A, Pizzorni C, Secchi ME et al. Circadian rhythms: glucocorticoids and arthritis. *Ann NY Acad Sci* 2006; **1069**: 289–299.

Daley-Yates PT, Harker AJ, Taylor S, Daniel MJ. Plasma protein binding of corticosteroids: reappraisal of its significance in systemic pharmacological activity. *J Allergy Clin Immunol* 2005; **115**: S4 [Abstract 13].

Del Donno M, Bittesnich D, Chetta A, Olivieri D, Lopez-Vidriero MT. The effect of inflammation on mucociliary clearance in asthma: an overview. *Chest* 2000; **118**: 1142–1149.

Demeule M, Jodoin J, Beaulieu E, Brossard M, Beliveau R. Dexamethasone modulation of multidrug transporters in normal tissues. *FEBS Lett* 1999; **442**: 208–214.

Derendorf H, Hochhaus G, Mollmann H, Barth J, Krieg M, Tunn S, Mollmann C. Receptor-based pharmacokinetic-pharmacodynamic analysis of corticosteroids. *J Clin Pharmacol* 1993; **33**: 115–123.

Dilger K, Schwab M, Fromm MF. Identification of budesonide and prednisone as substrates of the intestinal drug efflux pump P-glycoprotein. Inflamm *Bowel Dis* 2004; **10**: 578–583.

Dirks NL, Li S, Hochhaus G, Yates CR, Meibohm B. *Glucocorticoid Transrepression and Transactivation Potencies as Measured by Inhibition of AP-1, NF-kB and Activation of GRE.* Nashville, TN: American Association of Pharmaceutical Scientists, 2005.

D'Urzo A, Karpel JP, Busse WW, Boulet LP, Monahan ME, Lutsky B, Staudinger H. Efficacy and safety of mometasone furoate administered once-daily in the evening in patients with persistent asthma dependent on inhaled corticosteroids. *Curr Med Res Opin* 2005; **21**: 1281–1289.

Edsbacker S, Andersson T. Pharmacokinetics of budesonide (Entocort EC) capsules for Crohn's disease. *Clin Pharmacokinet* 2004; **43**: 803–821.

Edsbacker S, Brattsand R. Budesonide fatty-acid esterification: a novel mechanism prolonging binding to airway tissue. Review of available data. *Ann Allergy Asthma Immunol* 2002; **88**: 609–616.

Edsbacker S, Johansson CJ. Airway selectivity: an update of pharmacokinetic factors affecting local and systemic disposition of inhaled steroids. *Basic Clin Pharmacol Toxicol* 2006; **98**: 523–536.

Ejsing TB, Hasselstrom J, Linnet K. The influence of P-glycoprotein on cerebral and hepatic concentrations of nortriptyline and its metabolites. *Drug Metabol Drug Interact* 2006; **21**: 139–162.

Farrell RJ, Kelleher D. Glucocorticoid resistance in inflammatory bowel disease. *J Endocrinol* 2003; **178**: 339–346.

Farrell RJ, Murphy A, Long A, Donnelly S et al. High multidrug resistance (P-glycoprotein 170) expression in inflammatory bowel disease patients who fail medical therapy. *Gastroenterology* 2000; **118**: 279–288.

Geier A, Gartung C, Dietrich CG, Wasmuth HE, Reinartz P, Matern S. Side effects of budesonide in liver cirrhosis due to chronic autoimmune hepatitis: influence of hepatic metabolism versus portosystemic shunts on a patient complicated with HCC. *World J Gastroenterol* 2003; **9**: 2681–2685.

Gupta SK, Dube MP. Exogenous cushing syndrome mimicking human immunodeficiency virus lipodystrophy. *Clin Infect Dis* 2002; **35**: E69–E71.

Hansel NN, Diette GB. Gene expression profiling in human asthma. *Proc Am Thorac Soc* 2007; **4**: 32–36.

Harrison TW, Tattersfield AE. Plasma concentrations of fluticasone propionate and budesonide following inhalation from dry powder inhalers by healthy and asthmatic subjects. *Thorax* 2003; **58**: 258–260.

Hartmann M. BY 9010/FHP018: Influence of liver cirrhosis on the pharmacokinetics of the active metaboite B9207-201 of ciclesonide in comparison to a control group of healthy volunteers. *Aventis Study Report* 1998; 210/2000.

Hasani A, Spiteri MA, Pavia D, Lopez-Vidriero MT, Agnew JE, Clarke SW. Effect of temazepam on tracheobronchial mucus clearance. *Thorax* 1992; **47**: 298–300.

Hasani A, Toms N, Agnew JE, Lloyd J, Dilworth JP. Mucociliary clearance in COPD can be increased by both a D2/beta2 and a standard beta2 agonists. *Respir Med* 2005; **99**: 145–151.

Hasani A, Toms N, O'Connor J, Dilworth JP, Agnew JE. Effect of salmeterol xinafoate on lung mucociliary clearance in patients with asthma. *Respir Med* 2003; **97**: 667–671.

Hochhaus G. New developments in corticosteroids. *Proc Am Thorac Soc* 2004; **1**: 269–274.

Hochhaus G. What pharmacokinetic and pharmacodynamic properties are important for inhaled glucocorticoids? *Ann Allergy, Asthma Immunol* 2007; **98**: S7–S15.

Hochhaus G, Mollmann H, Derendorf H, Gonzalez-Rothi RJ. Pharmacokinetic/pharmacodynamic aspects of aerosol therapy using glucocorticoids as a model. *J Clin Pharmacol* 1997; **37**: 881–892.

Hochhaus G, Rohdewald P, Mollmann H, Greschuchna D. Identification of glucocorticoid receptors in normal and neoplastic adult human lung. *Res Exp Med (Berl)* 1983; **182**: 71–78.

Hochhaus G, Wu K, Blomgren AL, Ekholm K, Edsbacker S. How do differences in tissue and protein binding affect pulmonary pharmacodynamics: ciclesonide vs budesonide. *Am J Respir Crit Care Med* 2007; **175**: A189.

Hoffmann U, Kroemer HK. The ABC transporters MDR1 and MRP2: multiple functions in disposition of xenobiotics and drug resistance. *Drug Metab Rev* 2004; **36**: 669–701.

Hogger P, Erpenstein U, Rohdewald P, Sorg C. Biochemical characterization of a glucocorticoid-induced membrane protein (RM3/1) in human monocytes and its application as model system for ranking glucocorticoid potency. *Pharm Res* 1998; **15**: 296–302.

Holt S, Masoli M, Beasley R. Increasing compliance with inhaled corticosteroids through the use of combination therapy. *J Allergy Clin Immunol* 2004; **113**: 219–220.

Horne R. Compliance, adherence, and concordance: implications for asthma treatment. *Chest* 2006; **130**: 65S–72S.

Hubner M, Hochhaus G, Derendorf H. Comparative pharmacology, bioavailability, pharmacokinetics, and pharmacodynamics of inhaled glucocorticosteroids. *Immunol Allergy Clin North Am* 2005; **25**: 469–488.

Incalzi RA, Maini CL, Fuso L, Giordano A, Carbonin PU, Galli G. Effects of aging on mucociliary clearance. *Compr Gerontol [A]* 1989; **3**: 65–68.

Ito K, Chung KF, Adcock IM. Update on glucocorticoid action and resistance. *J Allergy Clin Immunol* 2006; **117**: 522–543.

Jin M, Shimada T, Yokogawa K, Nomura M et al. Site-dependent contributions of P-glycoprotein and CYP3A to cyclosporin A absorption, and effect of dexamethasone in small intestine of mice. *Biochem Pharmacol* 2006; **72**: 1042–1050.

Kerb R. Implications of genetic polymorphisms in drug transporters for pharmacotherapy. *Cancer Lett* 2006; **234**: 4–33.

Krishnaswami S, Hochhaus G, Mollmann H, Barth J, Derendorf H. Interpretation of absorption rate data for inhaled fluticasone propionate obtained in compartmental pharmacokinetic modeling. *Int J Clin Pharmacol Ther* 2005; **43**: 117–122.

Kuzuya Y, Adachi T, Hara H, Anan A, Izuhara K, Nagai H. Induction of drug-metabolizing enzymes and transporters in human bronchial epithelial cells by beclomethasone dipropionate. *IUBMB Life* 2004; **56**: 355–359.

Lane SJ, Palmer JB, Skidmore IF, Lee TH. Corticosteroid pharmacokinetics in asthma. *Lancet* 1990; **336**: 1265.

Lewis-Tuffin LJ, Cidlowski JA. The physiology of human glucocorticoid receptor beta (hGRbeta) and glucocorticoid resistance. *Ann NY Acad Sci* 2006; **1069**: 1–9.

Lipworth BJ, Jackson CM. Safety of inhaled and intranasal corticosteroids: lessons for the new millennium. *Drug Saf* 2000; **23**: 11–33.

Lofdahl CG, Mellstrand T, Svedmyr N. Glucocorticoids and asthma. Studies of resistance and systemic effects of glucocorticoids. *Eur J Respir Dis Suppl* 1984; **136**: 69–79.

Mark PJ, Waddell BJ. P-glycoprotein restricts access of cortisol and dexamethasone to the glucocorticoid receptor in placental BeWo cells. *Endocrinology* 2006; **147**: 5147–5152.

Marzolini C, Paus E, Buclin T, Kim RB. Polymorphisms in human MDR1 (P-glycoprotein): recent advances and clinical relevance. *Clin Pharmacol Ther* 2004; **75**: 13–33.

McCormack PL, Plosker GL. Inhaled mometasone furoate: A review of its use in persistent asthma in adults and adolescents. *Drugs* 2006; **66**: 1151–1168.

Mortimer KJ, Harrison TW, Tang Y, Wu K et al. Plasma concentrations of inhaled corticosteroids in relation to airflow obstruction in asthma. *Br J Clin Pharmacol* 2006; **62**: 412–419.

Muller MB, Keck ME, Binder EB, Kresse AE et al. ABCB1 (MDR1)-type P-glycoproteins at the blood-brain barrier modulate the activity of the hypothalamic-pituitary-adrenocortical system: implications for affective disorder. *Neuropsychopharmacology* 2003; **28**: 1991–1999.

Naef R, Schmid C, Hofer M, Minder S, Speich R, Boehler A. Itraconazole comedication increases systemic levels of inhaled fluticasone in lung transplant recipients. *Respiration* 2007; **74**: 418–422.

Nayak AS, Banov C, Corren J, Feinstein BK et al. Once-daily mometasone furoate dry powder inhaler in the treatment of patients with persistent asthma. *Ann Allergy Asthma Immunol* 2000; **84**: 417–424.

Newman SP. Spacer devices for metered dose inhalers. *Clin Pharmacokinet* 2004; **43**: 349–360.

Newman SP, Weisz AW, Talaee N, Clarke SW. Improvement of drug delivery with a breath actuated pressurised aerosol for patients with poor inhaler technique. *Thorax* 1991; **46**: 712–716.

Okazaki K, Miyazaki M, Onishi S, Ito K. Effects of food intake and various extrinsic hormones on portal blood flow in patients with liver cirrhosis demonstrated by pulsed Doppler with the Octoson. *Scand J Gastroenterol* 1986; **21**: 1029–1038.

Pearce RE, Leeder JS, Kearns GL. Biotransformation of fluticasone: in vitro characterization. *Drug Metab Dispos* 2006; **34**: 1035–1040.

Pearlman DS, Berger WE, Kerwin E, Laforce C, Kundu S, Banerji D. Once-daily ciclesonide improves lung function and is well tolerated by patients with mild-to-moderate persistent asthma. *J Allergy Clin Immunol* 2005; **116**: 1206–1212.

Petrovsky N, Harrison LC. Diurnal rhythmicity of human cytokine production: a dynamic disequilibrium in T helper cell type 1/T helper cell type 2 balance? *J Immunol* 1997; **158**: 5163–5168.

Petrovsky N, McNair P, Harrison LC. Diurnal rhythms of pro-inflammatory cytokines: regulation by plasma cortisol and therapeutic implications. *Cytokine* 1998; **10**: 307–312.

Raaska K, Niemi M, Neuvonen M, Neuvonen PJ, Kivisto KT. Plasma concentrations of inhaled budesonide and its effects on plasma cortisol are increased by the cytochrome P4503A4 inhibitor itraconazole. *Clin Pharmacol Ther* 2002; **72**: 362–369.

Rohatagi S, Arya V, Zech K, Nave R, Hochhaus G, Jensen BK, Barrett JS. Population pharmacokinetics and pharmacodynamics of ciclesonide. *J Clin Pharmacol* 2003; **43**: 365–378.

Rohatagi S, Krishnaswami S, Pfister M, Sahasranaman S. Model-based covariate pharmacokinetic analysis and lack of cortisol suppression by the new inhaled corticosteroid ciclesonide using a novel cortisol release model. *Am J Ther* 2005a; **12**: 385–397.

Rohatagi S, Luo Y, Shen L, Guo Z et al. Protein binding and its potential for eliciting minimal systemic side effects with a novel inhaled corticosteroid, ciclesonide. *Am J Ther* 2005b; **12**: 201–209.

Rowland M, Tozer T. *Clinical Pharmacokinetics: Concepts and Applications* (3rd edn). New York: Lippincott Williams & Wilkins, 1995.

Russcher H, Smit P, van Rossum EF, van den Akker EL et al. Strategies for the characterization of disorders in cortisol sensitivity. *J Clin Endocrinol Metab* 2006; **91**: 694–701.

Saari SM, Vidgren MT, Koskinen MO, Turjanmaa VM, Waldrep JC, Nieminen MM. Regional lung deposition and clearance of 99mTc-labeled beclomethasone-DLPC liposomes in mild and severe asthma. *Chest* 1998; **113**: 1573–1579.

Sangsritavong S, Combs DK, Sartori R, Armentano LE, Wiltbank MC. High feed intake increases liver blood flow and metabolism of progesterone and estradiol-17beta in dairy cattle. *J Dairy Sci* 2002; **85**: 2831–2842.

Schäcke H, Rehwinkel H, Asadullah K. Dissociated glucocorticoid receptor ligands: compounds with an improved therapeutic index. *Curr Opin Invest Drugs* 2005; **6**: 503–507.

Scheer FA, Buijs RM. Light affects morning salivary cortisol in humans. *J Clin Endocrinol Metab* 1999; **84**: 3395–3398.

Schoemaker RC, Burggraaf J, Cohen AF. Assessment of hepatic blood flow using continuous infusion of high clearance drugs. *Br J Clin Pharmacol* 1998; **45**: 463–469.

Seckl JR, Yau J, Holmes M. 11Beta-hydroxysteroid dehydrogenases: a novel control of glucocorticoid action in the brain. *Endocr Res* 2002; **28**: 701–707.

Shitara Y, Horie T, Sugiyama Y. Transporters as a determinant of drug clearance and tissue distribution. *Eur J Pharm Sci* 2006; **27**: 425–446.

Smaldone GC. Advances in aerosols: adult respiratory disease. *J Aerosol Med* 2006; **19**: 36–46.

Stark JG, Werner S, Homrighausen S, Tang Y et al. Pharmacokinetic/pharmacodynamic modeling of total lymphocytes and selected subtypes after oral budesonide. *J Pharmacokinet Pharmacodyn* 2006; **33**: 441–459.

Stoilov I, Krueger W, Mankowski D, Guernsey L, Kaur A, Glynn J, Thrall RS. The cytochromes P450 (CYP) response to allergic inflammation of the lung. *Arch Biochem Biophys* 2006; **456**: 30–38.

Sutherland ER, Martin RJ. Targeting the distal lung in asthma: do inhaled corticosteroids treat all areas of inflammation? *Treat Respir Med* 2005; **4**: 223–229.

Tantisira KG, Weiss ST. The pharmacogenetics of asthma therapy. *Curr Drug Targets* 2006; **7**: 1697–1708.

Van der Deen M, de Vries EG, Timens W, Scheper RJ, Timmer-Bosscha H, Postma DS. ATP-binding cassette (ABC) transporters in normal and pathological lung. *Respir Res* 2005; **6**: 59.

Wiegand J, Schuler A, Kanzler S, Lohse A et al. Budesonide in previously untreated autoimmune hepatitis. *Liver Int* 2005; **25**: 927–934.

Wu K, Stark JL, Derendorf H, Hochhaus G. Effects of the Administration Time on the Cumulative Cortisol and Lymphocyte Suppression of Inhaled Corticosteroids. Nashville, TN: American Association of Pharmaceutical Scientists, 2005.

Yokogawa K, Shimada T, Higashi Y, Itoh Y et al. Modulation of mdr1a and CYP3A gene expression in the intestine and liver as possible cause of changes in the cyclosporin A disposition kinetics by dexamethasone. *Biochem Pharmacol* 2002; **63**: 777–783.

14

Improved Lung Deposition: New Inhaler Devices

Omar S. Usmani

14.1   Introduction

Inhalation has been successfully used as a convenient, effective and core mode of therapy to manage the majority of respiratory disorders and confers distinct therapeutic advantages by targeting drug directly to the lungs. Compared to systemic routes of delivery, a smaller dose of drug can be used, the onset of action is more rapid and the incidence of side effects is less. Recently, there has been increasing interest in the use of the respiratory tract as a portal for systemic drug delivery with a variety of aerosolized drugs, including insulin (Owens, 2002; Skyler et al., 2001), morphine (Dershwitz et al., 2000), peptides and hormones (Pattonet et al., 1994).

14.2   Historical Review of Inhaled Drug Therapy

Modern inhalation therapy celebrates its half-Centenary, however inhaling smokes and vapours for diseases of the lung has been utilized by many civilizations (Gandevia, 1975; Grossman, 1994; Sakula, 1988; Yernault, 1994). Classical Ayurvedic medicine in India, ca. 2000 BC, practiced the inhalation of fumes of the *Datura* plant species (an anticholinergic alkaloid) and, as described in Eber's papyrus, the ancient Egyptians treated respiratory ailments with inhaled vapours of the herb *Hyoscyamus* placed on heated bricks. Hippocrates and Galen advocated sea mists and hot vapours as inhaled remedies to ease airway obstruction and, in the 10th century, the Persian physician Ibn Sinna "Avicenna" described in his Cannon of Medicine the inhalation of essential oils from pine and eucalyptus

Overcoming Steroid Insensitivity in Respiratory Disease   Edited by Ian M. Adcock and Kian Fan Chung
© 2008 John Wiley & Sons, Ltd.

to alleviate respiratory symptoms, both compounds present in modern-day proprietary inhalation medicines.

In the early 1800s, pipe-smoking the leaves of *Datura* plant species became a standard remedy for asthma in England (Sims, 1812) and, as a result, proprietary brands of "asthma cigarettes" containing *Datura*–tobacco mixtures became very popular during the Industrial Revolution. The mid-19th century saw the development of an array of aerosol delivery devices particularly adapted for the delivery of liquids, the fore-runners of the modern-day nebulizer (Muers, 1997). By the early 1900s aerosolized adrenaline was in popular use (Barger and Dale, 1910; Camps, 1929), inhaled by hand-operated, squeeze-bulb compression nebulizer devices, and steadily replaced the anticholinergic burning powders. In the 1950s the benefit of nebulized cortisone inhaled by asthmatic patients was being realized (Gelfand, 1951).

Probably the most significant development in inhalation device technology was the advent of the pressurized metered dose inhaler (pMDI) developed by Riker Labs in 1956 (Freedman, 1956). Following a suggestion from the asthmatic daughter of Dr George Maison (then President of Riker Labs) to aerosolize her asthma medication "like hair spray" (Fink and Rau, 2000), within months the first pMDIs were manufactured with salts of isoprotenerol and adrenaline (Thiel, 1996). This era represented many of the technological advances in the chlorofluorocarbon (CFC)-propelled pMDIs, with further modifications leading to breath-actuated pMDIs in the early 1970s (Crompton, 1971) and the use of add-on spacers to complement inhaled drug therapy. The seminal publication that CFCs were contributing to depletion of the ozone layer (Molina and Rowland, 1974) led to the signing of the Montreal Protocol in 1987, with an agreed phase-out of all CFC products by 1996. In 1995, an exemption was granted for pMDIs (where worldwide CFC usage accounted for less than 1%) until such time as suitable alternatives could be found. This accelerated the development of the dry powder inhaler (DPI) and the quest for alternative propellants.

The first commercially available DPIs, which were propellant-free and relied on the patient's inspiratory flow to aerosolize the medication, were prompted by the safe and effective use of disodium cromoglycate, a synthetic analogue of khellin, delivered as a dry powder to atopic asthmatic subjects (Howell and Altounyan, 1967). Single-dose delivery devices (Bell et al., 1971; Hetzel and Clark, 1977) were quickly followed by multi-dose powder inhalers in the late 1980s (Brindley et al., 1995; Wetterlin, 1988). The first alternative propellant compounds to undergo industrial toxicity testing were tetrafluoroethanes, with physicochemical properties similar to the CFCs used in pMDIs, and these appeared to be a promising replacement (Dolovich, 1999).

The turn of this century has brought an increase in the scientific understanding of inhaled therapeutic aerosol delivery to the lungs and sophisticated technological advances in aerosol device development, with particular focus on a variety of new nebulizer devices.

14.3   Deposition of Aerosols within the Respiratory Tract

The human respiratory tract

Deposition is the process that determines the fraction of the inspired particles that will be caught in the respiratory tract and thus fail to exit with expired air. Deposition occurs when the inhaled particles do not follow but diverge from airflow streamlines and thereby come in contact with airway surfaces. The human respiratory tract has evolved to act as a series of filters that remove airborne particulate matter from the inspired air such that, in general, particles $> 100\,\mu m$ in size are usually trapped in the nasal cavity and oropharynx, whereas those particles $> 10\,\mu m$ tend not to penetrate the tracheobronchial tree.

Mechanisms of aerosol deposition

The three main mechanisms by which inhaled particles deposit in the human airways include inertial impaction, gravitational sedimentation and diffusional transport (Agnew, 1994; Yu and Chien, 1997);

Inertial impaction occurs when a particle's momentum prevents it from following the direction of the airstream in an area where there is a change in the direction of bulk airflow. Hence a drug particle, depending upon its momentum, may tend to continue in its original direction of flow, possibly impacting on an airway wall, particularly at branching junctions between larger airways where airflow velocities are high and rapid changes in airflow direction occur. The probability of impaction increases with increasing air velocity, breathing frequency and particle diameter.

Gravitational sedimentation describes particle deposition under the action of gravity. Sedimentation results when the gravitational force acting on a particle overcomes the total force of air resistance and, for a particle of given mass, is most efficient in the small airways where airflow velocities are low and there is increased time available for particles to settle within the airway (residence time). The probability of deposition by sedimentation increases with increasing particle diameter and particle density but decreases with increased breathing rate.

Diffusional transport refers to the random collision of gas molecules with very small particles that push these particles about in an irregular fashion, also called *Brownian motion*. Therefore, a particle in stationary air moves about in a random manner even in the absence of gravity and this can result in contact with airway surfaces. Consequently, the small airway dimensions of the lung periphery favour deposition by diffusion as airflow velocities are lowest, residence time is long and the distance a particle has to travel before it hits an airway wall is short.

The relative extent to which each of these three mechanisms contributes to the deposition of an inhaled drug particle within the respiratory tract depends upon the physical characteristics of the drug particle, airstream parameters, breathing patterns and the local airway geometry. All mechanisms act simultaneously, but inertial impaction and gravitational sedimentation are most important for the deposition of large particles of 1–10 μm, whereas diffusional transport is the main deposition determinant of smaller submicron (<1 μm) particles. As inspired aerosol flows through the upper respiratory tract at high velocity and remains in this region for a short period of time, particle deposition is primarily governed by inertial impaction, whereas the longer residence time of the aerosol in the lower respiratory tract is associated with low airflow velocity, so that particle deposition is governed by gravitational sedimentation and diffusional transport.

Secondary, less important, deposition mechanisms that occur within the human airways are electrostatic charge, interception and cloud settling, and other forces such as magnetic, thermal and radiational do not significantly contribute to the deposition of inhaled therapeutic medical aerosols within the human respiratory tract (Ariyananda et al., 1996).

Factors affecting aerosol deposition

The factors affecting the deposition of inhaled drug particles within the human airways can be divided into aerosol physical characteristics and patient variables (Table 14.1).

Particle size is the most important aerosol factor influencing the site and extent of inhaled drug deposition within the airways (Usmani et al., 2003, 2005) and this can have profound effects on the dose of drug required to achieve a given clinical response (Figure 14.1). Thus, 15 μg of salbutamol (particle size = 6 μm) is as effective as 200 μg

Table 14.1 Factors affecting the respiratory deposition of inhaled medical aerosols

Aerosol characteristics	Patient variables
Particle size	
Particle density	Inhalation manoeuvre
	• inspiratory flow
	• breathing frequency
	• inhaled aerosol volume
	• breath-hold pause
	• degree of lung inflation
Aerosol formulation	Airway diameter
• hygroscopicity	
• charge	
• surfactant	
Delivery device	Airway disease and severity
	Paediatric vs. adult airways

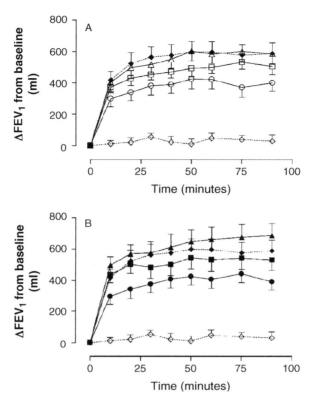

Figure 14.1   FEV$_1$ time–response profile curves. Placebo (dashed line, open diamonds) and salbutamol metered dose inhaler 200 µg (dotted line, closed diamonds) are shown on both graphs. Monodisperse salbutamol aerosols are shown as follows: 1.5 µm (circles), 3 µm (squares) and 6 µm (triangles) at (A) 15 µg (open symbols) and (B) 30 µg (closed symbols) doses. Data are presented as means (of 12 patients) of the maximal change in each patient's individual FEV1 response (from baseline value) at each time point ± SEM. (Reproduced with permission from Usmani et al., *Am J Resp Crit Care Med* [Official Journal of the American Thoracic Society] 2005; 172:1497–1504). © American Thoracic Society)

salbutamol delivered by conventional MDI (Usmani et al., 2005). As discussed, aerosol particle size affects the probabilities of both impaction and sedimentation and will determine in which particular lung region the drug particles will deposit. For a given particle size diameter (d), increasing the density (η) of the material from which the particle is made will result in an effectively bigger particle with an aerodynamic diameter (d_{ae}) for the particle of (Stuart, 1973):

$$d_{ae} = \eta^{\frac{1}{2}}d$$

Drug deposition in the lungs also may be enhanced using low-density gases such as helium (Corcoran and Gamard, 2004) and with large porous particles of low density (Edwards et al., 1998).

Water-soluble drug particles may enlarge as a result of their passage through the humid environment of the lungs and this phenomenon, described as hygroscopic growth, will cause particles to deposit more proximally than non-hygroscopic material. Hygroscopic growth, however, has only been demonstrated using non-therapeutic aerosols experimentally *in vitro* or in healthy subjects, but not with active pharmacological compounds (Phipps et al., 1994; Scherer et al., 1979).

In the clinical scenario, each component of the breathing manoeuvre is intrinsically related to the aerosol delivery device and can influence the efficacy and tolerability of the drug delivery system. Generally, a slow, deep inhalation coupled with a breath-hold pause is regarded as optimal for lung deposition from pMDIs, whereas rapid inhalation from pMDIs increases proximal airway deposition by impaction (Farr et al., 1995). In contrast, DPIs are dependent on the negative inspiratory pressure of the patient so that the powdered drug is disaggregated from its carrier molecule and aerosolized. Faster inspiratory flows, therefore, are needed for DPIs and will usually improve airway deposition compared to slow inhalation (Hindle and Byron, 1995; Tarsin et al., 2004). A greater inhaled aerosol volume allows more particles to be carried and deposited within the peripheral airways (Farr et al., 1998; Pavia et al., 1977), and actuation of aerosol from pMDIs at the beginning of inspiration results in enhanced total lung, conducting airway and alveolar deposition (Newman et al., 1981a, 1982). A breath-hold pause at the end of inhalation has also been shown to augment the peripheral regional lung deposition of inhaled drug by allowing the necessary airway residence time for particles to deposit by sedimentation or diffusion (Newman et al., 1981b).

The lung deposition of inhaled drug also depends upon airway calibre. Radiolabelling studies have shown greater total lung and peripheral airway deposition in healthy subjects compared to asthmatics (Melchor et al., 1993) and have demonstrated lower lung deposition following experimentally induced bronchoconstriction (Svartengren et al., 1986, 1989). Pharmacokinetic studies have concluded that smaller airway calibre leads to decreased total lung deposition of inhaled aerosol, as fenoterol plasma concentrations have been shown to be lower in asthmatic subjects compared to healthy subjects (Lipworth et al., 1995; Newnham et al., 1993), as have peak plasma salbutamol concentrations in severe asthmatics compared to mild-asthmatic subjects (Lipworth and Clark, 1997).

14.4 Assessing Drug Deposition in the Lungs

Predictive models of aerosol deposition

The general concepts regarding the deposition of inhaled particles within the human bronchial tree are primarily derived from indirect evidence, including theoretical mathematical calculations (Heyder, 1989; James and Stahlhofen, 1991) and experimental modelling (Gerrity et al., 1979; Heyder et al., 1986; Martonen et al., 2000b).

These models are based mainly upon the physics of fluid flowing through simple tubes and generally are in good agreement with each other. They have been applied to estimate therapeutic aerosol dosimetry and to predict the behaviour of inhaled medical aerosols within the human airways (Ferron, 1985). Measurements indicate that, in general, particles >8 μm in size deposit in the oropharyngeal region, those between 2–6 μm deposit in the conducting airways and particles < 1μm are directed to more distal alveolar regions in the peripheral lung. These models, however, are based upon idealized assumptions and conditions, such as morphology of the bronchial tree, physical aerosol characteristics, airway particle transport and breathing manoeuvre, to derive simple predictive equations of particle deposition in order to approximate the complexity of therapeutic aerosol deposition *in vivo*. These assumptions restrict the comprehensive application of current predictive deposition models to determine inhaled therapeutic aerosol behaviour within the human airways (Martonen et al., 2000a).

In vitro methods

In vitro test methods are mainly intended to analyse and monitor pharmaceutical quality control and performance output of aerosol delivery systems. These instruments fractionate the emitted aerosol cloud with respect to aerodynamic diameters in order to determine the particle size distributions and dose of the generated aerosol. The Andersen Cascade Impactor (Andersen, 1966), the Multi-Stage Liquid-Impinger and the Marple-Miler Impactor (Marple et al., 1998) are inertial multistage cascade impactors; optical light-scattering techniques are also used to analyse aerosol characteristics, and include laser diffraction analysers (Clark, 1995) and single-particle aerodynamic sizers (Mitchell and Nagel, 1999).

In vitro sizing measurements may enable a prediction of drug delivery to the lungs using pre-specified fractions of the aerosol distribution emitted from the inhaler device considered to be in an "acceptable" size range as indicating the potential for delivery of drug to the lower respiratory tract *in vivo*. However, *in vitro* characterization remains limited in reliably predicting aerosol deposition and there will remain a need for concurrent *in vivo* data (Borgstrom, 1999; Thiel, 1998).

Although a few drug-assay techniques have been used to quantify and estimate inhaled drug delivery to the lungs (Esmailpour et al., 1997; Ilowite et al., 1987), pharmacokinetic methods and radionuclide imaging techniques essentially remain the best approaches for the precise assessment of airway drug deposition *in vivo*.

Pharmacokinetic methods

Pharmacokinetic methods are an important means for investigating total lung deposition and for assessing the pulmonary and gastrointestinal contributions to

the systemic bioavailability of inhaled drug. Quantification of drug and its metabolites in plasma, or that excreted in the urine, may allow an indirect assessment
of deposition within the lungs. Drugs not absorbed from the gastrointestinal tract,
such as sodium cromoglycate (Auty et al., 1987; Richards et al., 1987) or those
that undergo complete first-pass hepatic metabolism such as fluticasone propionate
(Mollmann et al., 1998; Thorsson et al., 1997), have negligible oral bioavailability;
that is, it can be assumed that plasma and/or urine drug levels represent the inhaled
fraction or pulmonary bioavailability.

The pulmonary deposition of inhaled drug that is not metabolized in the lungs
may be evaluated by blocking the gastrointestinal absorption of the oropharyngeal
"swallowed" fraction (oral bioavailability) using a solution of activated charcoal.
Charcoal block has also been used to assess the absolute pulmonary bioavailability
for terbutaline (Borgstrom and Nilsson, 1990), salbutamol (Olsson et al., 1996) and
budesonide (Thorsson et al., 1994). Where accurate data on the oral bioavailability
of drug are known, such as budesonide, the unpleasant charcoal block technique
may be avoided and the lung dose calculated (Thorsson et al., 1994).

A urine-excretion pharmacokinetic method has been shown to indirectly evaluate the lung deposition of inhaled salbutamol (Hindle and Chrystyn, 1992). Urine
collected in the first 30 min post-dosing can estimate the lung deposition of inhaled
salbutamol, as the contribution of the swallowed fraction to systemic bioavailability
is negligible during this time. This method has also been used to investigate the
optimal inhaler technique (Hindle et al., 1993), to compare the lung bioavailability
of different inhaler devices (Hindle et al., 1995; Silkstone et al., 2002), to assess
the effect of inspiratory flow on lung deposition (Chege and Chrystyn, 2000) and
to determine the relative bioavailability for nedocromil (Aswania et al., 1998) and
sodium cromoglycate (Aswania et al., 1997). The same principle has been applied
to plasma salbutamol samples, although higher drug doses are required to assess
the pharmacodynamic response (Newnham et al., 1993). Pharmacokinetic methods, however, do not allow an assessment of regional deposition or distribution of
inhaled drug within the airways.

Radionuclide imaging of the lungs

Radionuclide imaging allows detailed visualization of the *in vivo* intrapulmonary
distribution of inhaled radiolabelled drug particles and a quantitative assessment
of their total and regional deposition patterns (Dolovich, 2001; Newman et al.,
2003). Scintigraphic scanning techniques are either two-dimensional planar or
three-dimensional single photon emission computed tomography (SPECT) and
positron emission tomography (PET).

Planar gamma scintigraphy has been the main technique employed in studies. The aerosolized drug formulation is radiolabelled with a gamma-emitting
isotope such as technetium-99m and, following inhalation, images encompassing

the oropharynx, lung fields and stomach are obtained (Newman et al., 1998). Lung ventilation images, obtained by tidally breathing radioactive gases such as krypton-81m (^{81m}Kr) or xenon-133 (^{133}Xe), are used to delineate the lung borders. Superimposition of the lung outline from the ventilation scan onto the images of radiolabelled drug deposition within the airways allows the lungs to be divided into a series of computer-generated zones or regions of interest for deposition analysis (Kim, 2000). Regions have been defined ranging from two-compartment (Melchor et al., 1993; Ruffin et al., 1981) and three-compartment areas (Agnew et al., 1984; Newman et al., 1998) to more complex six-compartment concentric lung sections (Pitcairn et al., 2002).

Three-dimensional imaging techniques such as SPECT and PET enable greater precision in the spatial resolution of the airways, where the lung is divided into a series of concentric shells so that it is easier to relate regional drug deposition patterns to lung anatomy (Chan, 1993; Fleming et al., 2003). SPECT detects gamma-ray intensities of radionuclides such as technetium-99m or iodine-123 using a 360° rotation of the gamma-camera and has been used to study the intrapulmonary deposition of terbutaline (Conway et al., 2000) and nedocromil sodium (Perring et al., 1994). PET utilizes radionuclides that emit positrons such as fluorine-18, oxygen-15, nitrogen-13 and carbon-11, which interact with tissue electrons to emit gamma-rays that are detected by the PET scanner (Jones, 1997). However, the requirement of large amounts of radionuclide coupled with the need for longer image acquisition times with SPECT, as well as the very short half-life of positron-emitting radionuclides and the greater hardware costs of both systems, have limited the use of these imaging modalities for assessing inhaled drug deposition.

14.5   Aerosol Generation Devices for Inhaled Drug Therapy

Several types of delivery system are used to generate inhaled therapeutic aerosols for use in clinical practice, including pMDIs, DPIs and nebulizers, and the major advantages and disadvantages of each type are listed in Table 14.2.

Pressurized metered dose inhaler

In a pMDI, the drug is suspended or dissolved with a liquid gaseous propellant under high pressure in a sealed canister. The canister contains a metering valve and chamber that releases an exact quantity of drug and propellant during each actuation. Upon actuation, the propellants undergo rapid vaporization, which provides the necessary force to aerosolize the liquid and propel the drug particles forward at high velocity through the actuator orifice. The velocity of the spray leaving the pMDI falls quickly and, as a result of propellant evaporation, aerosol particle size rapidly decreases (Dhand et al., 1988). Other formulation ingredients such as

Table 14.2 Advantages and disadvantages of various inhaler devices

Device	Advantages	Disadvantages
MDI	Compact and lightweight Cheap Precise and consistent doses Quick to use	Requires good coordination and technique (may not be suitable for elderly or young children) Cold freon effect Contains CFCs
MDI + spacer device (+/- face mask)	No need to coordinate inspiration with depression of canister Reduces drug deposition in the mouth Eliminates the cold freon effect Decreases the incidence of oral thrush	Attachments are cumbersome
Dry powder inhaler	Compact and lightweight Easy to use No breath coordination needed Does not need a spacer No CFCs	Require a high inspiratory flow to administer the drug Some patients dislike not being able to taste drugs
Nebulizer	Drug is inhaled with normal respiration	Noisy Not compact and travel friendly Expensive Requires regular maintenance

chemical preservatives and surfactant may be present, particularly in suspension aerosols, to prevent agglomeration of the solid drug particles. Chlorofluorocarbon (CFC) propellants are gradually being replaced by non-ozone-depleting propellants such as hydrofluorocarbons (HFCs) (Partridge et al., 1998).

Manually activated pMDIs are popular, compact, conveniently portable and generally inexpensive. Optimal results are obtained when the pMDI is actuated at the beginning of a deep-slow inhalation followed by a breath-hold pause of 10 s at the end of inspiration (Newman et al., 1982). The most frequently reported problem, however, is the difficulty many patients have in using the device efficiently (Hilton, 1990), which may be due to poor instruction in use (Guidry et al., 1992) or failure to understand the technique (De Blaquiere et al., 1989). Problems between coordination and inhalation are particularly present in elderly and physically impaired patients and to overcome these problems device- holding adaptors, add-on spacer attachments and breath-actuated pMDIs have been developed (Allen, 1997; Larsen et al., 1994). Breath-actuated inhalers rely on the patient's inhalation to trigger a spring mechanism that activates the inhaler (Hampson and Mueller, 1994). However, it has been shown that breath-actuated devices offer no added advantage over patients with good conventional pMDI inhaler technique (Newman et al., 1981b).

Recent advances in the design technology of pMDIs include the addition of a dose-counter.

Spacers

Spacer devices are used with pMDIs, designed to slow the emitted aerosol cloud and thereby reduce oropharyngeal deposition and promote ease of use (Newman, 2004; Terzano, 1999). Large drug particles are trapped on the plastic walls of the spacer, which decreases oropharyngeal impaction so that local unwanted side effects, particularly with corticosteroids, may be reduced and also a decrease in the amount of drug absorbed via the gastrointestinal tract is achieved, which could otherwise give rise to adverse systemic effects. In addition, increasing the distance the aerosolized drug has to travel before it is inhaled slows the emitted aerosol cloud and allows evaporation of the propellant, leading to relatively smaller particles that may enter the respiratory tract. Valved holding chambers provide a reservoir for the aerosolized drug from which the patient breathes tidally and they are particularly useful in patients with difficulty in inhaler actuation and breathing coordination (Allen, 1997), whereas extension devices are non-valved, add-on products that require a reasonable degree of coordination.

Dry powder inhalers

DPIs are propellant-free devices that contain finely-milled drug bound into loose aggregates or associated with carrier particles such as lactose and glucose (Frijlink and De Boer, 2004). They are breath-actuated and rely on the patient's inspiratory effort to de-aggregate the drug from its carrier particle and disperse the aerosol into drug particles of appropriate size to allow delivery to the lungs (Hindle and Byron, 1995). DPIs are highly dependent on a reliably generated inspiratory flow, with studies showing optimal drug deposition in the lungs with flows of 60 l/min or greater (Pedersen et al., 1990; Prime et al., 1999; Smith et al., 1998), particularly from devices with a high resistance (Assi and Chrystyn, 2000). Importantly, asthmatic patients and those with chronic obstructive pulmonary disease have been shown to inhale from DPIs using suboptimal inspiratory flows (Chodosh et al., 2001; Hawksworth et al., 2000). Single-dose delivery systems such as Spinhaler and Rotahaler (GlaxoSmithKline, UK), where individual drug doses are dispensed from punctured gelatine capsules, have mainly been replaced by multi-dose DPIs such as Turbuhaler (AstraZeneca, Sweden) and Clickhaler (Innovata, UK), where the drug powder is contained within a reservoir or where the drug is sealed in foil blisters individually as in Diskhaler (GlaxoSmithKline, UK), or on a strip as in Accuhaler (GlaxoSmithKline, UK). All these devices should be stored in a dry environment as deterioration of the drug may occur in damp and humid conditions.

A new generation of DPI devices have been developed that reduce the reliance of aerosol generation on the patient's inspiratory effort. The Spiros S2 System (Elan Pharmaceuticals, Ireland) and FlowCaps (Hovione, Portugal) require lower inspiratory flows of 15–30 l/min to adequately aerosolize the drug powder (Chan and Chew, 2003). The Nektar Pulmonary Inhaler (Nektar Therapeutics, USA) has been designed to deliver drug wholly independent of the patient's breathing manoeuvre, whereby a bolus of compressed air disperses powdered aerosol from a blister into a holding chamber, from which the patient inhales.

Conventional nebulizers

There are two main types of nebulizer widely used in clinical practice: jet nebulizers and ultrasonic nebulizers (Kendrick et al., 1997; Muers, 1997). Jet nebulizers use compressed gas, or an electrical compressor, to generate high air flows through a narrow opening and across the liquid drug solution/suspension to produce aerosolized particles. The liquid is drawn up by the high-velocity airstream and fragmented into droplets within the nebulizing chamber. Ultrasonic nebulizers produce aerosols by vibration of a piezoelectric crystal at a high frequency through the drug solution, which leads to the separation of liquid droplets to form an aerosol. Although smaller and less noisy, the ultrasonic nebulizers are usually more expensive, less robust and not as effective in nebulizing suspensions compared to jet nebulizers. There is great variation in the aerosol output and particle size distributions generated from these devices (Loffert et al., 1994) and, although nebulizers do not require patient coordination, the inhalation manoeuvre will affect drug deposition to the lungs, which is markedly reduced with shallow rapid inspirations or crying, as may occur with children.

New nebulizer technologies

A newer generation of nebulizers have been developed that offer a marked improvement in the efficiency and precision of pulmonary drug delivery over conventional nebulizer systems, and although the devices are more costly they may be cost-effective, particularly with expensive medication, by employing a reduced drug dose compared with that currently utilized (Geller, 2002; Smaldone, 2002).

Breath-enhanced "open vent" nebulisers such as Sidestream (Profile Therapeutics, UK) use the compressor airflow to entrain additional air through the nebulizer, whereas the Ventstream (Profile Therapeutics, UK), LC Plus and LCD (PARI GmbH, Germany) devices direct the patient's inspiratory flow through the nebulizer chamber. As with conventional systems, these nebulizers generate a continuous output of aerosol, but allow increased generation of drug aerosol during inspiration and reduced aerosol exhalation during expiration, leading to increased potential for drug deposition to the lungs (Coates and Ho, 1998).

The Circulaire nebulizer (Westmed, USA) relies on pre-existing jet nebulizer technology that has been adapted to provide a dosimetric system (Piper, 2000). A one-way exhalation valve in the mouthpiece directs the nebulizer output to a storage reservoir, which increases the drug available for inhalation during the next inspiration. Breath-actuated dosimetric nebulizers like AeroEclipse (Monaghan Medical, USA) have a valve that senses tidal breathing and triggers aerosol generation "on-demand" only during inspiration, eliminating the need for a storage reservoir bag (Leung et al., 2004).

Aerosol delivery systems that force pressurized liquid through nozzles include: the Respimat Soft-Mist Inhaler (Boehringer-Ingelheim, Germany), a multi-dose liquid device where a spring pushes drug solution through a nozzle, generating a slow-moving aerosol; and AERx (Aradigm, USA), where the drug solution supplied as unit-dose blister packs is forced through a number of small holes to produce a controlled spray and an aerosol dose that is timed with each breath and provides feedback to the patient to guide their inhalation technique.

New nebulizer technologies have utilized a vibration source from a piezoelectric crystal or ceramic element that leads to vibration of a mesh or plate with multiple apertures through which medication is extruded and liquid therapeutic aerosols are generated for inhalation. Devices include MicroAir (Omron Healthcare, USA), Aeroneb and Aerodose (Aerogen, USA), which are all portable and lightweight (Dhand, 2002). The e-flow nebulizer device (PARI GmbH, Germany) employs a similar principle using ultrasonic vibrating TouchSpray technology (TTP Technology Partnership, UK), where sonic pressure forces liquid aerosol through micron-sized holes perforated in a thin metal mesh membrane that vibrates due to a piezoelectric actuator, which leads to the controlled production of a low-velocity fine mist aerosol with consistent aerosol droplet particle size (Knoch and Keller, 2005). These devices achieve shorter nebulization times and are able to nebulize both drug solutions and suspensions. The main technical limitation is blockage of the small mesh holes, which can lead to altered characteristics of the generated aerosol rather than an inability to generate aerosol, which could have clinical implications, and hence these devices must be cleaned regularly.

The hand-held adaptive aerosol delivery system I-neb (Respironics, USA) is a battery-powered, computer-controlled "third-generation" device that adds further refinement to nebulized aerosol delivery (Denyer et al., 2004). Unlike its predecessors, this model incorporates vibrating mesh technology to generate aerosolized drug (rather than utilize compressed air) and has breathing mode features that can be adapted to the patient's preference. Aerosol delivery can occur during spontaneous tidal breathing or capable patients can be guided using vibratory feedback at the mouthpiece to perform slow and deep inhalation, which can increase lung deposition and shorten nebulization times. This nebulizer technology analyses the trend of the patient's preceding three spontaneous tidal breathing respiratory cycles by continually monitoring pressure changes and automatically adapts to deliver a controlled and precise drug dose constantly during the first half of the patient's inspiratory breath, thereby compensating for intrapatient variability in breathing patterns. The device is operated by a programmable microchip disc that records information on drug dosage, dosing frequency and patient compliance, and enables an accurate cumulative assessment of the volume of drug delivered per breath such that the total pre-programmed dose is correctly received by the patient, who also receives audible and visual feedback informing them that their treatment is complete (Nikander et al., 2003).

The AKITA system (Activaero GmbH, Germany) is also a computer-controlled device designed to maximize inhaled drug deposition to the lungs by controlling breathing patterns and tailoring drug delivery to each individual patient using personalized smart-card technology (Bennett, 2005). The device does not allow the patient to breathe tidally but takes control over inhalation, providing slow, deep and prolonged inhalation using an inspiratory resistance and, coupled with pulsing of the drug aerosol during any period in the inspiratory phase, the device promotes peripheral airway targeting of drug deposition and decreased dose exhalation (Brand et al., 2003). The smart-card stores the optimized pre-determined parameters of the patient's breathing pattern (inhalation flow, inhaled volume and breath-hold pause), displays feedback on the number of breaths remaining and, by recording the actual number of breaths and inhaled volumes, allows an integral assessment of patient compliance. Recently, this device technology has been combined with vibrating mesh technology to create a nebulizer combination that allows enhanced inhalation therapy by optimizing both patient breathing patterns and drug particle size distributions, to provide more selective and targeted regional drug deposition within the lungs. This requirement may be needed, as newer more expensive respiratory drugs with a narrow therapeutic index and significant tolerability profile may be safely delivered to the lungs only via the inhaled route.

References

Agnew JE. Physical properties and mechanisms of deposition of aerosols. In: Clarke SW, Pavia D (eds) *Aerosols and the Lung*. London: Butterworths 1999, pp. 49–70.

Agnew JE, Bateman JR, Pavia D, Clarke SW. A model for assessing bronchial mucus transport. *J Nucl Med* 1984; **25**: 170–176.

Allen SC. Competence thresholds for the use of inhalers in people with dementia. *Age Ageing* 1997; **26**: 83–86.

Andersen AA. A sampler for respiratory health hazard assessment. *Am Ind Hyg Assoc J* 1996; **27**: 160–165.

Ariyananda PL, Agnew JE, Clarke SW. Aerosol delivery systems for bronchial asthma. *Postgrad Med J* 1996; **72**: 151–156.

Assi K, Chrystyn H. The device resistance of recently introduced dry-powder inhalers. *J Pharm Pharmacol* 2000; **52**: 58.

Aswania OA, Corlett SA, Chrystyn H. Development and validation of an ion-pair liquid chromatographic method for the quantitation of sodium cromoglycate in urine following inhalation. *J Chromatogr B Biomed Sci Appl* 1997; **690**: 373–378.

Aswania OA, Corlett SA, Chrystyn H. Determination of the relative bioavailability of nedocromil sodium to the lung following inhalation using urinary excretion. *Eur J Clin Pharmacol* 1998; **54**: 475–478.

Auty RM, Brown K, Neale MG, Snashall PD. Respiratory tract deposition of sodium cromoglycate is highly dependent upon technique of inhalation using the Spinhaler. *Br J Dis Chest* 1987; **81**: 371–380.

Barger G, Dale HH. Chemical structure and sympathomimetic action of amines. *J Physiol* 1910; **41**: 19.

Bell JH, Hartley PS, Cox JS. Dry powder aerosols. I. A new powder inhalation device. *J Pharm Sci* 1971; **10**: 1559–1564.

Bennett WD. Controlled inhalation of aerosolised therapeutics. *Expert Opin Drug Deliv* 2005; **2**: 763–767.

Borgstrom L. In vitro, ex vivo, in vivo veritas. *Allergy* 1999; **54**: 88–92.

Borgstrom L, Nilsson M. A method for determination of the absolute pulmonary bioavailability of inhaled drugs: terbutaline. *Pharm Res* 1990; **7**: 1068–1070.

Brand P, Beckmann H, Maas Enriquez M, Meyer T et al. Peripheral deposition of alpha1-protease inhibitor using commercial inhalation devices. *Eur Respir J* 2003; **22**: 263–267.

Brindley A, Sumby B, Smith I, Prime D, Haywood P, Grant A. Design, manufacture and dose consistency of the Serevent Diskus. *Pharm Technol Eur* 1995; **7**: 16–17, 20–22.

Camps PWL. A note on the inhalation treatment of asthma. *Guy's Hosp Rep* 1929; **79**: 496–498.

Chan HK. Use of single photon emission computed tomography in aerosol studies. *J Aerosol Med* 1993; **6**: 23–36.

Chan HK, Chew NY. Novel alternative methods for the delivery of drugs for the treatment of asthma. *Adv Drug Deliv Rev* 2003; **55**: 793–805.

Chege JK, Chrystyn H. The relative bioavailability of salbutamol to the lung using urinary excretion following inhalation from a novel dry powder inhaler: the effect of inhalation rate and formulation. *Respir Med* 2000; **94**: 51–56.

Chodosh S, Flanders JS, Kesten S, Serby CW, Hochrainer D, Witek TJ Jr. Effective delivery of particles with the HandiHaler dry powder inhalation system over a range of chronic obstructive pulmonary disease severity. *J Aerosol Med* 2001; **14**: 309–315.

Clark AR. Spectral analysis of aerosols. *Int J Pharm* 1995; **115**: 69–78.

Coates AL, Ho SL. Drug administration by jet nebulization. *Pediatr Pulmonol* 1998; **26**: 412–423.

Conway JH, Walker P, Fleming JS, Bondesson E, Borgstrom L, Holgate ST. Three-dimensional description of the deposition of inhaled terbutaline sulphate administered via Turbuhaler. In: Dalby RN, Byron PR, Farr SJ, Peart J (eds) *Respiratory Drug Delivery*, Vol. VII. Raleigh: Serentec Press, 2000, pp. 607–609.

Corcoran TE, Gamard S. Development of aerosol drug delivery with helium oxygen gas mixtures. *J Aerosol Med* 2004; **17**: 299–309.

Crompton GK. Breath-activated aerosol. *Br Med J* 1971; **2**: 652–653.

De Blaquiere P, Christensen DB, Carter WB, Martin TR. Use and misuse of metered-dose inhalers by patients with chronic lung disease. A controlled, randomized trial of two instruction methods. *Am Rev Respir Dis* 1989; **140**: 910–916.

Denyer J, Nikander K, Smith NJ. Adaptive Aerosol Delivery (AAD) technology. *Expert Opin Drug Deliv* 2004; **1**: 165–176.

Dershwitz M, Walsh JL, Morishige RJ, Connors PM, Rubsamen RM, Shafer SL, Rosow CE. Pharmacokinetics and pharmacodynamics of inhaled versus intravenous morphine in healthy volunteers. *Anesthesiology* 2000; **93**: 619–628.

Dhand R. Nebulisers that use a vibrating mesh or plate with multiple apertures to generate aerosol. *Respir Care* 2002; **47**: 1406–1416.

Dhand R, Malik SK, Balakrishnan M, Verma SR. High speed photographic analysis of aerosols produced by metered dose inhalers. *J Pharm Pharmacol* 1988; **40**: 429–430.

Dolovich M. New delivery systems and propellants. *Can Respir J* 1999; **6**: 290–295.

Dolovich MB. Measuring total and regional lung deposition using inhaled radiotracers. *J Aerosol Med* 2001; **14**: S35–S44.

Edwards DA, Ben-Jebria A, Langer R. Recent advances in pulmonary drug delivery using large, porous inhaled particles. *J Appl Physiol* 1998; **85**: 379–385.

Esmailpour N, Hogger P, Rabe KF, Heitmann U, Nakashima M, Rohdewald P. Distribution of inhaled fluticasone propionate between human lung tissue and serum in vivo. *Eur Respir J* 1997; **10**: 1496–1499.

Farr SJ, Gonda I, Licko V. Physiochemical and physiological factors influencing the effectiveness of inhaled insulin. In: Dalby RN, Byron PR, Farr SJ (eds) *Respiratory Drug Delivery*, Vol. VI. Illinois: Interpharm Press, 1998, pp. 25–33.

Farr SJ, Rowe AM, Rubsamen R, Taylor G. Aerosol deposition in the human lung following administration from a microprocessor controlled pressurized metered dose inhaler. *Thorax* 1995; **50**: 639–644.

Ferron GA. Comparison of experimental and calculated data for total and regional lung deposition in the human lung. *J Aerosol Sci* 1985; **16**: 133–143.

Fink JB, Rau JL. New horizons in respiratory care. *Respir Care* 2000; **45**: 824–825.

Fleming JS, Conway JH, Bolt L, Holgate ST. A comparison of planar scintigraphy and SPECT measurement of total lung deposition of inhaled aerosol. *J Aerosol Med* 2003; **16**: 9–19.

Freedman T. Medihaler therapy for bronchial asthma. A new type of aerosol therapy. *Postgrad Med* 1956; **20**: 667–673.

Frijlink HW, De Boer AH. Dry powder inhalers for pulmonary drug delivery. *Expert Opin Drug Deliv* 2004; **1**: 67–86.

Gandevia B. Historical review of the use of parasympatholytic agents in the treatment of respiratory disorders. *Postgrad Med J* 1975; **51**: 13–20.

Gelfand ML. Administration of cortisone by the aerosol method in the treatment of bronchial asthma. *N Engl J Med* 1951; **245**: 293–294.

Geller DE. New liquid aerosol generation devices: systems that force pressurized liquids through nozzles. *Respir Care* 2002; **47**: 1392–1404.

Gerrity TR, Lee PS, Hass FJ, Marinelli A, Werner P, Lourenco RV. Calculated deposition of inhaled particles in the airway generations of normal subjects. *J Appl Physiol* 1979; **47**: 867–873.

Grossman J. The evolution of inhaler technology. *J Asthma* 1994; **31**: 55–64.

Guidry GG, Brown WD, Stogner SW, George RB. Incorrect use of metered dose inhalers by medical personnel. *Chest* 1992; **101**: 31–33.

Hampson NB, Mueller MP. Reduction in patient timing errors using a breath-activated metered dose inhaler. *Chest* 1994; **106**: 462–465.

Hawksworth GM, James L, Chrystyn H. Characterization of the inspiratory manoeuvre when asthmatics inhale through a Turbohaler pre- and post-counselling in a community pharmacy. *Respir Med* 2000; **94**: 501–504.

Hetzel MR, Clark TJ. Comparison of intravenous and aerosol salbutamol. *Br Med J* 1976; **2**: 919.

Heyder J. Assessment of airway geometry with inert aerosols. *J Aerosol Med* 1989; **2**: 89–97.

Heyder J, Gebhart J, Rudolf G, Schiller CF, Stahlhofen W. Deposition of particles in the human respiratory tract in the size range 0.005–15μm. *J. Aerosol Sci* 1986; **17**: 811–825.

Hilton S. An audit of inhaler technique among asthma patients of 34 general practitioners. *Br J Gen Pract* 1990; **40**: 505–506.

Hindle M, Byron PR. Dose emissions from marketed dry powder inhalers. *Int J Pharm* 1995; **116**: 169–177.

Hindle M, Chrystyn H. Determination of the relative bioavailability of salbutamol to the lung following inhalation. *Br J Clin Pharmacol* 1992; **34**: 311–315.

Hindle M, Newton DA, Chrystyn H. Investigations of an optimal inhaler technique with the use of urinary salbutamol excretion as a measure of relative bioavailability to the lung. *Thorax* 1993; **48**: 607–610.

Hindle M, Newton DA, Chrystyn H. Dry powder inhalers are bioequivalent to metered-dose inhalers. A study using a new urinary albuterol (salbutamol) assay technique. *Chest* 1995; **107**: 629–633.

Howell JB, Altounyan RE. A double-blind trial of disodium cromoglycate in the treatment of allergic bronchial asthma. *Lancet* 1967; **2**: 539–542.

Ilowite JS, Gorvoy JD, Smaldone GC. Quantitative deposition of aerosolized gentamicin in cystic fibrosis. *Am Rev Respir Dis* 1987; **136**: 1445–1449.

James AC, Stalhofen W. The respiratory tract deposition model proposed by the ICRP Task Group. *Rad Prot Dosim* 1991; **38**: 159–165.

Jones T. New opportunities in molecular imaging using PET. *Drug Inf J* 1997; **31**: 991–995.

Kendrick AH, Smith EC, Wilson RS. Selecting and using nebuliser equipment. *Thorax* 1997; **52**: S92–S101.

Kim CS. Methods of calculating lung delivery and deposition of aerosol particles. *Respir Care* 2000; **45**: 695–711.

Knoch M, Keller M. The customised electronic nebuliser: a new category of liquid aerosol drug delivery systems. *Expert Opin Drug Deliv* 2005; **2**: 377–390.

Larsen JS, Hahn M, Ekholm B, Wick KA. Evaluation of conventional press-and-breathe metered-dose inhaler technique in 501 patients. *J Asthma* 1994; **31**: 193–199.

Leung K, Louca E, Coates AL. Comparison of breath-enhanced to breath-actuated nebulizers for rate, consistency, and efficiency. *Chest* 2004; **126**: 1619–1627.

Lipworth BJ, Clark DJ. Effects of airway calibre on lung delivery of nebulised salbutamol. *Thorax* 1997; **52**: 1036–1039.

Lipworth BJ, Newnham DM, Clark RA, Dhillon DP, Winter JH, McDevitt DG. Comparison of the relative airways and systemic potencies of inhaled fenoterol and salbutamol in asthmatic patients. *Thorax* 1995; **50**: 54–61.

Loffert DT, Ikle D, Nelson HS. A comparison of commercial jet nebulizers. *Chest* 1994; **106**: 1788–1792.

Marple V, Olson BA, Miller NC. The role of inertial particle collectors in evaluating pharmaceutical aerosol delivery systems. *J Aerosol Med* 1998; **11**: S139–S153.

Martonen TB, Musante CJ, Segal RA, Schroeter JD et al. Lung models: strengths and limitations. *Respir Care* 2000a; **45**: 712–736.

Martonen TB, Schroeter JD, Hwang D, Fleming JS, Conway JH. Human lung morphology models for particle deposition studies. *Inhal Toxicol* 2000b; **12**: 109–121.

Melchor R, Biddiscombe MF, Mak VH, Short MD, Spiro SG. Lung deposition patterns of directly labelled salbutamol in normal subjects and in patients with reversible airflow obstruction. *Thorax* 1993; **48**: 506–511.

Mitchell JP, Nagel MW. Time-of-flight aerodynamic particle size analyzers: their use and limitations for the evaluation of medical aerosols. *J Aerosol Med* 1999; **12**: 217–240.

Molina MJ, Rowland FS. Stratospheric sink for chlorofluoromethanes: chlorine atom catalysed destruction of ozone. *Nature* 1974; **249**: 810–812.

Mollmann H, Wagner M, Meibohm B, Hochhaus G et al. Pharmacokinetic and pharmacodynamic evaluation of fluticasone propionate after inhaled administration. *Eur J Clin Pharmacol* 1998; **53**: 459–467.

Muers MF. Overview of nebuliser treatment. *Thorax* 1997; **52**: S25–S30.

Newman SP. Spacer devices for metered dose inhalers. *Clin Pharmacokin* 2004; **43**: 349–360.

Newman SP, Hirst PH, Pitcairn GR, Clark AR. Understanding regional lung deposition in gamma scintigraphy. In: Dalby RN, Byron PR, Farr SJ (eds) *Respiratory Drug Delivery*, Vol. VI. Illinois: Interpharm Press, 1998, pp. 9–15.

Newman SP, Pavia D, Clarke SW. How should a pressurized beta-adrenergic bronchodilator be inhaled? *Eur J Respir Dis* 1981a; **62**: 3–21.

Newman SP, Pavia D, Clarke SW. Improving the bronchial deposition of pressurized aerosols. *Chest* 1981b; **80**: 909–911.

Newman SP, Pavia D, Garland N, Clarke SW. Effects of various inhalation modes on the deposition of radioactive pressurized aerosols. *Eur J Respir Dis Suppl* 1982; **119**: 57–65.

Newman SP, Pitcairn GR, Hirst PH, Rankin L. Radionuclide imaging technologies and their use in evaluating asthma drug deposition in the lungs. *Adv Drug Deliv Rev* 2003; **55**: 851–867.

Newnham DM, McDevitt DG, Lipworth BJ. Comparison of the extrapulmonary beta2-adrenoceptor responses and pharmacokinetics of salbutamol given by standard metered dose-inhaler and modified actuator device. *Br J Clin Pharmacol* 1993; **36**: 445–450.

Nikander K, Arheden L, Denyer J, Cobos N. Parents' adherence with nebulizer treatment of their children when using an adaptive aerosol delivery (AAD) system. *J Aerosol Med* 2003; **16**: 273–281.

Olsson B, Asking L, Borgstrom L, Bondesson E. Effect of inlet throat on the correlation between the fine particle dose and lung deposition. In: Dalby RN, Byron PR, Farr SJ (eds) *Respiratory Drug Delivery*, Vol. V. Illinois: Interpharm Press, 1996, pp. 273–281.

Owens DR. New horizons–alternative routes for insulin therapy. *Nat Rev Drug Discov* 2002; **1**: 529–540.

Partridge MR, Woodcock AA, Sheffer AL, Wanner A, Rubinfeld A. Chlorofluorocarbon-free inhalers: are we ready for the change? *Eur Respir J* 1998; **11**: 1006–1008.

Patton JS, Tricnchera P, Paltz RM. Bioavailability of pulmonary delivery of peptides and proteins: alpha-interferon, calcitonins and parathyroid hormone. *J Cont Rel* 1994; **28**: 79–85.

Pavia D, Thomson M, Shannon HS. Aerosol inhalation and depth of deposition in the human lung. The effect of airway obstruction and tidal volume inhaled. *Arch Environ Health* 1977; **32**: 131–137.

Pedersen S, Hansen OR, Fuglsang G. Influence of inspiratory flow rate upon the effect of a Turbuhaler. *Arch Dis Child* 1990; **65**: 308–310.

Perring S, Summers Q, Fleming JS, Nassim MA, Holgate ST. A new method of quantification of the pulmonary regional distribution of aerosols using combined CT and SPECT and its application to nedocromil sodium administered by metered dose inhaler. *Br J Radiol* 1994; **67**: 46–53.

Phipps PR, Gonda I, Anderson SD, Bailey D, Bautovich G. Regional deposition of saline aerosols of different tonicities in normal and asthmatic subjects. *Eur Respir J* 1994; **7**: 1474–1482.

Piper SD. In vitro comparison of the circulaire and AeroTee to a traditional nebulizer T-piece with corrugated tubing. *Respir Care* 2000; **45**: 313–319.

Pitcairn GR, Joyson A, Hirst PH, Prior DV, Newman SP. Lung penetration profiles: a new method for analysing regional lung deposition data in scintigraphic studies. In: Dalby RN, Byron PR, Farr SJ, Peart J (eds) *Respiratory Drug Delivery*, Vol. VIII. Colorado: Davis Horwood, 2002, pp. 549–552.

Prime D, Grant AC, Slater AL, Woodhouse RN. A critical comparison of the dose delivery characteristics of four alternative inhalation devices delivering salbutamol: pressurized metered dose inhaler, Diskus inhaler, Diskhaler inhaler, and Turbuhaler inhaler. *J Aerosol Med* 1999; **12**: 75–84.

Richards R, Dickson CR, Renwick AG, Lewis RA, Holgate ST. Absorption and disposition kinetics of cromolyn sodium and the influence of inhalation technique. *J Pharmacol Exp Ther* 1987; **241**: 1028–1032.

Ruffin RE, Dolovich MB, Oldenburg FA Jr, Newhouse MT. The preferential deposition of inhaled isoproterenol and propranolol in asthmatic patients. *Chest* 1981; **80**: 904–907.

Sakula A. A history of asthma. The FitzPatrick Lecture (1987). *J R Coll Physicians Lond* 1988; **22**: 36–44.

Scherer PW, Haselton FR, Hanna LM, Stone DR. Growth of hygroscopic aerosols in a model of bronchial airways. *J Appl Physiol* 1979; **47**: 544–550.

Silkstone VL, Dennis JH, Pieron CA, Chrystyn H. An investigation of in vitro/in vivo correlations for salbutamol nebulised by 8 systems. *J Aerosol Med* 2002; **15**: 251–259.

Sims J. *Datura stramonium* or thorn apple as a cure or relief of asthma. *Edinburgh Med Surg J* 1812; **8**: 364–367.

Skyler JS, Cefalu WT, Kourides IA, Landschulz WH, Balagtas CC, Cheng SL, Gelfand RA. Efficacy of inhaled human insulin in type 1 diabetes mellitus: a randomised proof-of-concept study. *Lancet* 2001; **357**: 331–335.

Smaldone GC. Smart nebulizers. *Respir Care* 2002; **47**: 1434–1441.

Smith KJ, Chan HK, Brown KF. Influence of flow rate on aerosol particle size distributions from pressurized and breath-actuated inhalers. *J Aerosol Med* 1998; **11**: 231–245.

Stuart BO. Deposition of inhaled aerosols. *Arch Intern Med* 1973; **131**: 60–63.

Svartengren M, Philipson K, Linnman L, Camner P. Regional deposition of particles in human lung after induced bronchoconstriction. *Exp Lung Res* 1986; **10**: 223–233.

Svartengren M, Anderson M, Philipson K, Camner P. Individual differences in regional deposition of 6-micron particles in humans with induced bronchoconstriction. *Exp Lung Res* 1989; **15**: 139–149.

Tarsin W, Assi KH, Chrystyn H. In-vitro intra- and inter-inhaler flow rate-dependent dosage emission from a combination of budesonide and eformoterol in a dry powder inhaler. *J Aerosol Med* 2004; **17**: 25–32.

Terzano C. Metered dose inhalers and spacer devices. *Eur Rev Med Pharmacol Sci* 1999; **3**: 159–169.

Thiel CG. From Susie's question to CFC free: an inventor's perspective of 40 years of MDI development and regulation. In: Dalby RN, Byron PR, Farr SJ (eds) *Respirations Drug Delivery*, Vol. V. Illinois: Interpharm Press, 1996, pp. 115–123.

Thiel CG. Can in vitro particle size measurements be used to predict pulmonary deposition of aerosol from inhalers? *J Aerosol Med* 1998; **11**: S43–52.

Thorsson L, Dahlstrom K, Edsbacker S, Kallen A, Paulson J, Wiren JE. Pharmacokinetics and systemic effects of inhaled fluticasone propionate in healthy subjects. *Br J Clin Pharmacol* 1997; **43**: 155–161.

Thorsson L, Edsbacker S, Conradson TB. Lung deposition of budesonide from Turbuhaler is twice that from a pressurized metered-dose inhaler. *Eur Respir J* 1994; **7**: 1839–1844.

Usmani OS, Biddiscombe MF, Barnes PJ. Regional lung deposition and bronchodilator response as a function of β2-agonist particle size. *Am J Respir Crit Care Med* 2005; **172**: 1497–1504.

Usmani OS, Biddiscombe MF, Nightingale JA, Underwood SR, Barnes PJ. The effects of bronchodilator particle size in asthmatics using monodisperse aerosols. *J Appl Physiol* 2003; **95**: 2106–2112.

Wetterlin K. Turbuhaler.a new powder inhaler for administration of drugs to the airways. *Pharm Res* 1988; **5**: 506–508.

Yernault JC. Inhalation therapy: an historical perspective. *Eur Respir Rev* 1994; **4**: 65–67.

Yu J, Chien YW. Pulmonary drug delivery: physiologic and mechanistic aspects. *Crit Rev Ther Drug Carrier Syst* 1997; **14**: 395–453.

Index

Note: page numbers in *italics* refer to figures and tables

Overcoming Steroid Insensitivity in Respiratory Disease   Edited by Ian M. Adcock and Kian Fan Chung
© 2008 John Wiley & Sons, Ltd.